Nutritional Management of Gastrointestinal Disease

Editor

ANDREW UKLEJA

GASTROENTEROLOGY CLINICS OF NORTH AMERICA

www.gastro.theclinics.com

Consulting Editor
ALAN L. BUCHMAN

March 2018 • Volume 47 • Number 1

ELSEVIER

1600 John F. Kennedy Boulevard • Suite 1800 • Philadelphia, Pennsylvania, 19103-2899
http://www.theclinics.com

GASTROENTEROLOGY CLINICS OF NORTH AMERICA Volume 47, Number 1
March 2018 ISSN 0889-8553, ISBN-13: 978-0-323-58154-7

Editor: Kerry Holland
Developmental Editor: Sara Watkins

Gastroenterology Clinics of North America (ISSN 0889-8553) is published quarterly by Elsevier Inc., 360 Park Avenue South, New York, NY 10010-1710. Months of issue are March, June, September, and December. Business and Editorial Offices: 1600 John F. Kennedy Blvd., Suite 1800, Philadelphia, PA 19103-2899. Customer Service Office: 6277 Sea Harbor Drive, Orlando, FL 32887-4800. Periodicals postage paid at New York, NY and additional mailing offices. Subscription prices are $350.00 per year (US individuals), $100.00 per year (US students), $659.00 per year (US institutions), $383.00 per year (Canadian individuals), $220.00 per year (Canadian students), $809.00 per year (Canadian institutions), $458.00 per year (international individuals), $220.00 per year (international students), and $809.00 per year (international institutions). Foreign air speed delivery is included in all *Clinics* subscription prices. All prices are subject to change without notice. **POSTMASTER**: Send address changes to *Gastroenterology Clinics of North America*, Elsevier Health Sciences Division, Subscription Customer Service, 3251 Riverport Lane, Maryland Heights, MO 63043. **Telephone: 1-800-654-2452 (U.S. and Canada); 314-447-8871 (outside U.S. and Canada). Fax: 314-447-8029. E-mail: journalscustomerservice-usa@elsevier.com (for print support); journalsonlinesupport-usa@elsevier.com (for online support).**

Reprints. For copies of 100 or more, of articles in this publication, please contact the Commercial Reprints Department, Elsevier Inc., 360 Part Avenue South, New York, New York 10010-1710. Tel. 212-633-3874, Fax: 212-633-3820, E-mail: reprints@elsevier.com.

Gastroenterology Clinics of North America is also published in Italian by Il Pensiero Scientifico Editore, Rome, Italy; and in Portuguese by Interlivros Edicoes Ltda., Rua Commandante Coelho 1085, 21250 Cordovil, Rio de Janeiro, Brazil.

Gastroenterology Clinics of North America is covered in *MEDLINE/PubMed (Index Medicus), Excerpta Medica, Current Contents/Clinical Medicine, Science Citation Index, ISI/BIOMED*, and *BIOSIS*.

Contributors

CONSULTING EDITOR

ALAN L. BUCHMAN, MD, MSPH, FACP, FACN, FACG, AGAF
Medical Director, Health Care Services Corporation; and Visiting Clinical Professor of Surgery and Medical Director, Intestinal Rehabilitation and Transplant Center, University of Illinois at Chicago, Chicago, Illinois, USA

EDITOR

ANDREW UKLEJA, MD, CNSP, AGAF
Clinical Affiliate Assistant Professor of Clinical Biochemical Science, Florida Atlantic University, Boca Raton, Florida; Department of Gastroenterology, Digestive Diseases Institute, Cleveland Clinic Florida, Weston, Florida, USA

AUTHORS

DAWN WIESE ADAMS, MD, MS
Assistant Professor, Division of Gastroenterology, Hepatology, and Nutrition, Center for Nutrition, Vanderbilt University Medical Center, Nashville, Tennessee, USA

ABIMBOLA ADIKE, MD
Division of Gastroenterology and Hepatology, Mayo Clinic, Scottsdale, Arizona, USA

MANDY L. CORRIGAN, MPH, RD, LD, CNSC, FAND
Nutrition Manager, Home Nutrition Support and Center for Gut Rehabilitation and Transplant, Center for Human Nutrition, Cleveland Clinic, Cleveland, Ohio, USA

MARK H. DⓔLEGGE, MD
Professor of Medicine, The Medical University of South Carolina, Charleston, South Carolina, USA; Co-Founder, DeLegge Medical, Awendaw, South Carolina, USA

JOHN K. DⓘBAISE, MD
Professor of Medicine, Division of Gastroenterology and Hepatology, Mayo Clinic, Scottsdale, Arizona, USA

J. ENRIQUE DOMÍNGUEZ-MUÑOZ, MD, PhD
Director, Department of Gastroenterology and Hepatology, University Hospital of Santiago de Compostela, Santiago de Compostela, Spain

DONALD R. DUERKSEN, MD, FRCPC
Associate Professor of Medicine, University of Manitoba, Winnipeg, Manitoba, Canada

MARTIN H. FLOCH, MD, MACG, AGAF
Clinical Professor of Medicine, Section of Digestive Diseases, Yale School of Medicine, New Haven, Connecticut, USA

KRISTIAN ASP FUGLSANG, MD
Research Fellow, Department of Medical Gastroenterology, University Hospital of Copenhagen, Rigshospitalet, Copenhagen, Denmark

PRISCILA GARLA, MSc, RD
Department of Gastroenterology, School of Medicine, University of São Paulo, São Paulo, São Paulo, Brazil

KHURSHEED N. JEEJEEBHOY, MBBS, PhD, FRCPC
Emeritus, Professor of Medicine, University of Toronto, Department of Medicine, St. Michaels Hospital, Toronto, Ontario, Canada

PALLE BEKKER JEPPESEN, MD, PhD
Professor, Department of Medical Gastroenterology, University Hospital of Copenhagen, Rigshospitalet, Copenhagen, Denmark

DONALD F. KIRBY, MD, FACP, FACN, FACG, AGAF, FASPEN, CNSC, CPNS
Medical Director, Intestinal Transplant Program, Director, Center for Human Nutrition, Professor of Medicine, Cleveland Clinic, Cleveland, Ohio, USA

VANESSA KUMPF, PharmD, BCNSP
Clinical Specialist, Nutrition Support Center for Human Nutrition, Division of Gastroenterology, Hepatology, and Nutrition, Vanderbilt University Medical Center, Nashville, Tennessee, USA

BRIAN M. LAPPAS, MD, MPH
Department of Internal Medicine, Vanderbilt University Medical Center, Nashville, Tennessee, USA

LUIS F. LARA, MD
Division of Gastroenterology, Hepatology and Nutrition, Wexner Medical Center, The Ohio State University, Columbus, Ohio, USA

BERKELEY N. LIMKETKAI, MD, PhD
Clinical Assistant Professor, Division of Gastroenterology and Hepatology, Stanford School of Medicine, Stanford, California, USA

MIGUEL MALESPIN, MD
Division of Gastroenterology and Hepatology, University of Florida College of Medicine, Jacksonville, Florida, USA

GERARD E. MULLIN, MD
Division of Gastroenterology and Hepatology, The Johns Hopkins University School of Medicine, Baltimore, Maryland, USA

MARCIA NAHIKIAN-NELMS, PhD, RDN, LD, FAND
Academic Affairs, School of Health and Rehabilitation Sciences, College of Medicine, The Ohio State University, Columbus, Ohio, USA

RISHI D. NAIK, MD
Division of Gastroenterology, Hepatology, and Nutrition, Center for Nutrition, Vanderbilt University Medical Center, Nashville, Tennessee, USA

JULIE NANAVATI, MLS, MA
Clinical Informationist Welch Medical Library, The Johns Hopkins University School of Medicine, Baltimore, Maryland, USA

STEPHEN J.D. O'KEEFE, MBBS, MSc, MD, FRCP
Professor of Medicine, Division of Gastroenterology, University of Pittsburgh, Pittsburgh, Pennsylvania, USA

ALYSSA M. PARIAN, MD
Assistant Professor, Division of Gastroenterology and Hepatology, The Johns Hopkins University School of Medicine, Baltimore, Maryland, USA

DHYANESH PATEL, MD
Division of Gastroenterology, Hepatology, and Nutrition, Vanderbilt University Medical Center, Nashville, Tennessee, USA

MARY PHILLIPS, RD
Hepato-pancreatico-biliary Specialist Dietitian, Department of Nutrition and Dietetics, Royal Surrey County Hospital NHS Foundation Trust, Guildford, United Kingdom

SULIEMAN ABDAL RAHEEM, MD
Staff Gastroenterologist, Center for Human Nutrition, Cleveland Clinic, Cleveland, Ohio, USA

KRISTEN M. ROBERTS, PhD, RDN, LD
Medical Dietetics, Division of Gastroenterology, Hepatology and Nutrition, The Ohio State University School of Health and Rehabilitation Sciences, Columbus, Ohio, USA

AHMED SALEM, MD
Gastroenterology Department, University of Rochester Medical Center, Rochester, New York, USA

JAMES SCOLAPIO, MD
Division of Gastroenterology and Hepatology, University of Florida College of Medicine, Jacksonville, Florida, USA

DOUGLAS L. SEIDNER, MD, AGAF, FACG, FASPEN
Associate Professor of Medicine, Director of the Vanderbilt Center for Human Nutrition, Division of Gastroenterology, Hepatology, and Nutrition, Vanderbilt University Medical Center, Nashville, Tennessee, USA

ASIM SHUJA, MD
Division of Gastroenterology and Hepatology, University of Florida College of Medicine, Jacksonville, Florida, USA

RAJDEEP SINGH, MD
Department of Internal Medicine, Sinai Hospital, Baltimore, Maryland, USA

ALWEYD TESSER, RD
Department of Gastroenterology, School of Medicine, University of São Paulo, São Paulo, São Paulo, Brazil

ANDREW UKLEJA, MD, CNSP, AGAF
Clinical Affiliate Assistant Professor of Clinical Biochemical Science, Florida Atlantic University, Boca Raton, Florida, USA; Department of Gastroenterology, Digestive Diseases Institute, Cleveland Clinic Florida, Weston, Florida, USA

DAN LINETZKY WAITZBERG, PhD, MD
Department of Gastroenterology, School of Medicine, University of São Paulo, GANEP–Human Nutrition, São Paulo, São Paulo, Brazil

ANDREA WOLF, RD
Dietitian, Department of Clinical Nutrition, Stanford Health Care, Stanford, California, USA

Contents

Foreword: Nutrition and Disease xiii

Alan L. Buchman

Preface: Nutritional Management of Gastrointestinal Diseases xv

Andrew Ukleja

Malnutrition in Gastrointestinal Disorders: Detection and Nutritional Assessment 1

Khursheed N. Jeejeebhoy and Donald R. Duerksen

All patients with significant gastrointestinal disease should be clinically assessed for protein calorie malnutrition by using the subjective global assessment. Blood tests for anemia, electrolytes, calcium, phosphorus, magnesium, ferritin, vitamin B_{12}, and folate should be considered for the assessment of major micronutrients. Where malabsorption or inflammatory bowel disease is diagnosed, bone mineral density using dual beam x-ray absorptiometry, 25-OH vitamin D levels, and measurement of other vitamins and trace elements should be considered. In addition, in at-risk patients, vitamin and trace element clinical deficiency syndromes should be considered during patient assessment.

Enteral Access and Associated Complications 23

Mark H. DeLegge

Enteral access is the foundation for feeding in patients who are unable to meet their nutrition needs orally and have a functional gastrointestinal tract. Enteral feeding requires placement of a feeding tube. Tubes can be placed through an orifice or percutaneously into the stomach or proximal small intestine at the bedside or in specialized areas of the hospital. Bedside tubes can be placed by the nurse or the physician, such as in the intensive care unit. Percutaneous feeding tubes are placed by the gastroenterologist, surgeon, or radiologist. This article reviews the types of enteral access and the associated complications.

Parenteral Nutrition: Indications, Access, and Complications 39

Brian M. Lappas, Dhyanesh Patel, Vanessa Kumpf, Dawn Wiese Adams, and Douglas L. Seidner

Parenteral nutrition (PN) is a life-sustaining therapy in patients with intestinal failure who are unable to tolerate enteral feedings. Patient selection should be based on a thorough assessment to identify those at high nutrition risk based on both disease severity and nutritional status. This article reviews both the acute and chronic indications for PN as well as special formulation consideration in specific disease states, vascular access, and complications of both short-term and long-term PN.

Nutritional Therapy in Adult Short Bowel Syndrome Patients with Chronic
Intestinal Failure   61

Palle Bekker Jeppesen and Kristian Asp Fuglsang

Intestinal failure (IF) is the reduction of gut function below the minimum necessary for the absorption of macronutrients and/or water and electrolytes, such that parenteral support (PS) is required to maintain health and/or growth. This article critically revises the gaps in and evidence for providing general nutritional therapy recommendations in the population with short bowel syndrome-intestinal failure. It addresses the need for an individualized approach, aiming to reduce or even eliminate the need for PS, and emphasizes a need to focus on the effects of dietary interventions on the quality of life of these patients.

Nutritional Aspects of Acute Pancreatitis   77

Kristen M. Roberts, Marcia Nahikian-Nelms, Andrew Ukleja, and Luis F. Lara

The goal of nutritional support in acute pancreatitis is to reduce inflammation, prevent nutritional depletion, correct a negative nitrogen balance, and improve outcomes. Enteral nutrition (EN) in severe acute pancreatitis (SAP) should be preferred to parenteral nutrition. It maintains the integrity of the gut barrier, decreases intestinal permeability, downregulates the systemic inflammatory response, maintains intestinal microbiota equilibrium, and reduces the complications of the early phase of SAP, improving morbidity and possibly improving mortality, and it is less expensive. Further studies to understand the optimal timing of nutrition, the route of delivery of EN, and the type of nutrition and nutrients are necessary.

Nutritional Therapy in Chronic Pancreatitis   95

J. Enrique Domínguez-Muñoz and Mary Phillips

Malnutrition is a frequent complication in patients with chronic pancreatitis. Maldigestion as a consequence of pancreatic exocrine insufficiency is the major cause of malnutrition in these patients. Together with that, toxic habits and alterations of the gastroduodenal transit may play a relevant role. Malnutrition in chronic pancreatitis is associated with osteoporosis, sarcopenia, poor quality of life, and increased mortality. An adequate nutritional evaluation including anthropometric, biochemical, and morphologic parameters is recommended in these patients. Nutritional advice and support together with an adequate pancreatic enzyme replacement therapy are indicated.

The Role of Diet in the Treatment of Irritable Bowel Syndrome: A Systematic
Review   107

Rajdeep Singh, Ahmed Salem, Julie Nanavati, and Gerard E. Mullin

Irritable bowel syndrome (IBS) is a multifaceted illness involving maladaptive shifts in the gut microbiota that affect the enteric nervous and immune systems, mucosal barrier function, the balance of neurotransmitters and hormones, and emotional well-being. There is abundant evidence indicating that certain foods elicit symptoms in IBS. Numerous elimination-type diets have been shown to alleviate symptoms. However, among these, the most controversial is a group of foods called fructo, oligo-, di-, and monosaccharides and polyols (FODMAPs). This article reviews the role of diet and systematically analyzes the literature for the role of FODMAPs in IBS.

Nutritional Consideration in Celiac Disease and Nonceliac Gluten Sensitivity   139

Rishi D. Naik, Douglas L. Seidner, and Dawn Wiese Adams

Celiac disease is an autoimmune disorder due to the inflammatory response to gluten in genetically predisposed individuals. It causes an enteropathy associated with several nutritional complications. Strict compliance to a gluten-free diet (GFD) is the current primary therapy. Nonceliac gluten sensitivity (NCGS) is a condition in which gluten ingestion leads to systemic symptoms but is not associated with small bowel atrophy or abnormal celiac serologies. A GFD heals celiac disease enteropathy and improves symptoms in NCGS. However, a long-term GFD can be associated with nutritional deficiencies and requires monitoring and guidance.

Nutritional Interventions in the Patient with Inflammatory Bowel Disease   155

Berkeley N. Limketkai, Andrea Wolf, and Alyssa M. Parian

Nutritional strategies have been explored as primary or adjunct therapies for inflammatory bowel disease (IBD). Exclusive enteral nutrition is effective for the induction of remission in Crohn disease and is recommended as a first-line therapy for children. Dietary strategies focus on adjusting the ratio of consumed nutrients that are proinflammatory or antiinflammatory. Treatments with dietary supplements focus on the antiinflammatory effects of the individual supplements (eg, curcumin, omega-3 fatty acids, vitamin D) or their positive effects on the intestinal microbiome (eg, prebiotics, probiotics). This article discusses the role of diets and dietary supplements in the treatment of IBD.

The Role of Prebiotics and Probiotics in Gastrointestinal Disease   179

Martin H. Floch

With the advent of the scientific realization that the microbiota of the gastrointestinal tract was more than the cells that exist in the body, the full importance of prebiotics and probiotics has come forth. The importance has been stressed and is available in the new textbook entitled, "The Microbiota in Gastrointestinal Pathophysiology: Implication for Human Health, Prebiotics, Probiotics and Dysbiosis." There is enough evidence published in the literature so that the scientific world now believes that prebiotics and probiotics are important in gastrointestinal disease.

Small Intestinal Bacterial Overgrowth: Nutritional Implications, Diagnosis, and Management   193

Abimbola Adike and John K. DiBaise

Small intestinal bacterial overgrowth (SIBO), characterized by the presence of excessive bacteria in the small intestine, is typically described as a malabsorptive syndrome occurring in the context of gut stasis syndromes. SIBO is now considered to be a disorder associated with diverse clinical conditions without classic risk factors for SIBO and a cause of several nonspecific gastrointestinal and nongastrointestinal symptoms. Because there is currently no gold standard for diagnosing SIBO, its prevalence and role in the pathogenesis of other diseases remain uncertain as does optimal treatment of patients with relapsing symptoms.

Nutritional Interventions in Chronic Intestinal Pseudoobstruction   209

Donald F. Kirby, Sulieman Abdal Raheem, and Mandy L. Corrigan

Although chronic intestinal pseudoobstruction (CIPO) is a rare disorder, it presents a wide spectrum of severity that ranges from abdominal bloating to severe gastrointestinal dysfunction. In the worst cases, patients may become dependent on artificial nutrition via parenteral nutrition or choose to have an intestinal transplant. However, whatever the severity, a patient's quality of life can be seriously compromised. This article defines the disorder and discusses the spectrum of disease and challenges to providing adequate nutrition to help improve a patient's quality of life.

The Need to Reassess Dietary Fiber Requirements in Healthy and Critically Ill Patients   219

Stephen J.D. O'Keefe

This article provides evidence that current dietary fiber intake levels may be insufficient to maintain colonic mucosal health and defense and reduce inflammation and cancer risk in otherwise healthy people. Current commercial tube feeds generally overlook the metabolic needs of the colon and may predispose patients to dysbiosis, bacterial overgrowth with pathogens such as *Clostridium difficile*, and acute colitis. These results raise concern about the wide-scale use of prophylactic antibiotics in the intensive care unit and the use of elemental, fiber-depleted tube feeds. Nutrition support is not complete without the addition of sufficient fiber to meet colonic nutritional needs.

Nutritional Therapy in Gastrointestinal Cancers   231

Priscila Garla, Dan Linetzky Waitzberg, and Alweyd Tesser

Malnutrition is the most frequent nutritional disorder in patients with gastrointestinal cancer and is associated with cachexia syndrome, worsening of prognosis, and shortened survival rate. Early nutrition screening, assessment, and intervention are able to favorably modify the clinical evolution of affected patients. The adequate provision of nutritional requirements has been associated with improvement of immunologic status and avoidance of further complications related to poor nutritional status, surgical treatment, and anticancer therapy. In malnourished patients, the supplementation of perioperative immunonutrition might contribute to fewer infectious and noninfectious complications, shorter length of hospitalization, and improved wound healing.

Nutritional Considerations in Liver Disease   **243**

Asim Shuja, Miguel Malespin, and James Scolapio

Malnutrition occurs in most patients with advanced liver diseases and is associated with higher rates of morbidity and mortality. In this article, the authors discuss the pathophysiology of malnutrition and methods to optimize nutrition status in liver disease and include a brief section on perioperative and postoperative nutrition.

GASTROENTEROLOGY
CLINICS OF NORTH AMERICA

FORTHCOMING ISSUES

June 2018
Gastrointestinal Transplantation
Enrico Benedetti and Ivo G. Tzvetanov,
Editors

September 2018
Gastrointestinal Imaging
Perry J. Pickhardt, *Editor*

December 2018
Pediatric Gastroenterology
Robert J. Shulman, *Editor*

RECENT ISSUES

December 2017
**Complementary and Alternative Medicine
in Inflammatory Bowel Disease**
Ali Keshavarzian and Ece A. Mutlu, *Editors*

September 2017
Crohn's Disease
Edward V. Loftus, *Editor*

June 2017
Liver Pathology
Jay H. Lefkowitch, *Editor*

Foreword
Nutrition and Disease

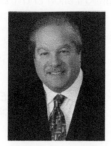

Alan L. Buchman, MD, MSPH, FACP, FACN, FACG, AGAF
Consulting Editor

Nutrition starts and ends in the gastrointestinal tract. Although "nutrition" itself is only directly responsible for "undernutition" (eg, malnutrition) or overnutrition (eg, obesity), it contributes via metabolism to virtually every bodily function and disease process. There are many things in nutrition that are "so obvious," yet on closer inspection are not actually true, while at the same time there are things that make little sense, but that's the way it is. "Nutrition" is the culmination of complex interactions between the host, oral nutrient and fluid intake, the genome, and the intestinal microbiome. Genetics plays a role in metabolism and possibly in food choices. Those choices and that metabolism affect the microbiome, which then in turn has effects on metabolism and disease. Disease may regulate the microbiome, and the microbiome may in turn regulate disease. This ain't the four food groups we're talking about any more.

In this issue of *Gastroenterology Clinics of North America*, Dr Ukleja has attempted to address these areas by engaging noted authors and investigators to discuss the assessment of nutritional status and how it is affected by disease, the provision of specialized nutrition made necessary due to disease, and the prevention and treatment of disease using nutritional interventions.

Knowledge of the relationship of nutrition and disease as well as therapeutic nutrition to prevent and to treat disease is perhaps some of the most important medical information that can be disseminated, yet as Dr Ukleja has pointed out, also the least valued and understood. If I could, I'd order that all clinicians read this issue cover to cover, but

Gastroenterol Clin N Am 47 (2018) xiii–xiv
https://doi.org/10.1016/j.gtc.2017.12.002
0889-8553/18/© 2017 Published by Elsevier Inc.

gastro.theclinics.com

I can't. Hopefully though, it will serve to interest and teach those who are willing to recognize the true importance of nutrition and where it fits within the modern treatment armamentarium.

Alan L. Buchman, MD, MSPH, FACP, FACN, FACG, AGAF
Intestinal Rehabilitation and Transplant Center
Department of Surgery
University of Illinois at Chicago
Health Care Services Corporation
300 E. Randolph Street
Chicago, IL 60601, USA

E-mail address:
buchman@uic.edu

Preface

Nutritional Management of Gastrointestinal Diseases

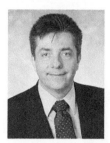

Andrew Ukleja, MD, CNSP, AGAF
Editor

It is my great pleasure to introduce you to an issue of *Gastroenterology Clinics of North America* focused on nutrition.

Food (nutrition) is one of the greatest pleasures of our life. While food is a main source of energy, vitamins and trace minerals, vital components of our diet, are involved in many critical steps of cellular functions. Dietary deficiencies play a role as a potential pathogenic factor in the development of a disease state. Poor nutrition has a major impact on the development of most chronic conditions. For example, malnutrition, very common in hospitalized patients, has been associated with prolonged hospitalization, longer intensive care unit (ICU) stay, and higher hospital costs. Malnutrition has also been linked to worse outcomes of outpatient surgical procedures. Therefore, identifying patients at risk by nutritional assessment and early initiation of nutrition interventions have been associated with improved clinical outcomes.

In general, only a few areas of the medical field are completely free from nutritional issues. Without any doubt, nutrition has been an integral part of the management of digestive disorders. There is also a great interest in nutritional supplements, diets, and nutritional interventions among practicing physicians, researchers, and patients, as well as the general public. Because of broad access to medical and nonmedical information via the Internet, patients and the general public are often facing misinformation about scientific evidence regarding nutrition and nutritional therapies.

Basic scientific research has shed a new light on the role of nutritional factors in disease states. Those positive results led to clinical studies with documented positive outcomes and subsequently to changes in clinical practice. Several new developments took place over the last decade that altered our approach to nutritional interventions in our daily clinical practice (**Table 1**).

In this editorial, I will highlight only a few topics reviewed in this issue of *Gastroenterology Clinics of North America*. Gluten-free diet (GFD) gained popularity particularly

Gastroenterol Clin N Am 47 (2018) xv–xx
https://doi.org/10.1016/j.gtc.2017.12.001
0889-8553/18/© 2017 Published by Elsevier Inc.

gastro.theclinics.com

Table 1
Examples of major advancements in the field of nutrition in relation to gastrointestinal diseases over the last decade

GI Disease or Nutrition Interventions	Major Advancements	Outcomes
Acute pancreatitis[5]	Enteral feeding as a primary therapy in SAP	No need for bowel rest and parenteral nutrition in most cases of SAP Early oral feeding in mild pancreatitis
Short bowel syndrome–intestinal failure[7]	Teduglutide (Gattex, Shire) approved for short bowel syndrome adult patients dependent on parenteral nutrition/IV hydration (2012) First drug targeted for intestinal adaptation	In research protocols with Teduglutide: >10% of patients were able to wean off parenteral support (PS) >60% patients were able to reduce weekly PS volume by ≥20% by 24 wk >50% patients were able to get ≥1 d off PS per week
Celiac disease[8]	New drugs in development for control of celiac disease (phase 2 studies) 1. Immusan T: peptide-based celiac disease vaccine designed to reprogram gluten-specific T cells 2. ALV003: recombinant gluten-specific proteases (cysteine protease [EP-B2]) and a prolyl endopeptidase shown in vitro to degrade gluten 3. Larazotide acetate: tight junction regulator	Possibly no need for strict celiac diet in the future

	Established criteria for diagnosis and testing	Avoidance of gluten is not required in healthy individuals
NCGS[1]		
IBS[9]	FODMAP diet proven to alter IBS-related symptoms	Improvement in GI symptoms with dietary measures (FODMAP)
GI surgical nutrition[10]	Immunonutrition (IEN) is beneficial in perioperative setting in GI cancer surgery	Reduced infections and length of hospital stay found with IEN
Parenteral nutrition[11]	Approval of SMOFlipid for treatment of surgical ICU patients and those with liver enzyme elevation First lipid with anti-inflammatory properties approved in United States (2016)	SMOF-based lipid emulsions (LE) may have nutritional advantages over soybean oil–based LEs and are similarly safe SMOFlipid may modify inflammatory and immune processes in ways to influence patient outcome SMOFlipid should be considered in surgical ICU patients and those with elevated liver enzymes
Enteral nutrition[12]	New improved guided nasoenteric (NE) tube placement at the bedside Passage of nasogastric or nasojejunal tubes at the bedside without the use of fluoroscopic visualization can be achieved with use of either an electromagnetic placement device or an optical imaging device for visualization during placement	Rapid NE tube placement allows for initiation of early EN in ICU setting Potential benefits include reduced ICU stay, days of mechanical ventilation, and infectious complications

Abbreviations: NE, nasoenteric tube; SMOF, soy oil, medium chain triglycerides, olive oil, fish oil.

because of support by celebrities, athletes, the food industry, and nonmedical professionals. However, the scientific evidence does not support the use of GFD in healthy individuals. It is now recognized that gluten-free products, highly advertised and broadly available, are more expensive and higher in total calories. Nonceliac gluten sensitivity (NCGS) has been better characterized, and the consensus has been developed on diagnosis, testing, and management, while additional research is still needed for better understanding of the pathogenesis of this condition.[1] NCGS pathogenesis is complex with many contributing factors, including low-grade intestinal inflammation, increased intestinal barrier function, and alterations in the gut microbiota, while innate immunity may play a pivotal role with suspected inducer to be amylase-trypsin inhibitor, a protein present in wheat endosperm.

Another area of tremendous research involves human gut macrobiome. A growing body of evidence indicates that microbiota plays a crucial role in our body because of an ability to manipulate intestinal barrier function, modulation of the immune system, influence on the host antigen production, and bile acid metabolism, and has a pivotal role in host energy homeostasis.[2] The importance of intestinal microbiota composition has been recently shown in disease states such as severe acute malnutrition, obesity, anorexia nervosa, and sepsis. It is now widely acknowledged that the gut bacterial flora significantly contributes to the immunopathogenesis of inflammatory bowel disease.[3] Diet and its components can modulate the gut microbiome and several metabolic pathways. Nutraceuticals, products derived from food sources, are involved in several biological processes, such as antioxidant defenses, gene expression, and cell proliferation, which could account for the maintenance of the mucosal barrier integrity, control of the inflammatory pathways, and the modulation of immune responses. Nutraceuticals are often accepted as a safe alternative or supplement to standard therapy. Special interest has been given to probiotics and prebiotics, safe and effective dietary supplements, with the therapeutic potential to alter the gut microbiota of the host. While we have a much better understanding of the basics of probiotic effects in many digestive disorders, the true benefits of probiotics in clinical practice must be clarified in large prospective studies. The unanswered questions regarding probiotics include the duration of supplementation, dosage, and type of probiotics used to achieve maximum health benefit.

Increased interest in the interactions between the diet and the functional gastrointestinal (GI) symptoms has been observed, including irritable bowel disease (IBS). Dietary restrictions of short-chain fermentable carbohydrates, the low fermentable oligosaccharide, disaccharide, monosaccharide, and polyol (FODMAP) are now increasingly used in clinical practice.[4] Recent advances have been made in the understanding of the mechanisms by which the low FODMAP diets impact the symptoms in IBS.[5] For example, polyols can provoke dose-dependent symptoms of flatulence, abdominal discomfort, and laxative effects when consumed by healthy volunteers and patients with IBS. Studies demonstrated that short-chain fermentable carbohydrates increase small bowel water volumes and colonic gas production in individuals with visceral hypersensitivity and induce GI symptoms. While well-designed clinical trials have demonstrated benefits of the low FODMAP diet in IBS patients, more recent trials have also shown that the FODMAP diet was linked to profound changes in the gut microbiota. At present, the impact of the FODMAP diet on the human microbiome and its clinical relevance is unknown. There is also the risk of compromising nutritional status with a restrictive diet since undernutrition is common in patients with IBS.

Finally, I would like to address the importance of nutritional therapy in acute pancreatitis (AP). AP is associated with significant morbidity, and if severe, with significant mortality. Management of severe acute pancreatitis (SAP) creates especially unique nutritional challenges. Of all the interventions that treat severe pancreatitis, none is more important than nutrition. High-quality evidence supports the use of enteral nutrition (EN) as the optimal nutritional intervention in SAP.[5] EN has been demonstrated to reduce mortality and infectious complications as compared to parenteral nutrition in SAP. The optimal route of EN remains unclear, but nasogastric tube feeding in SAP seems to be safe if tolerated. Most studies have utilized nasojejunal tubes for enteral feeding in SAP. Without any doubt, optimal nutritional support in SAP often requires an individualized approach with close monitoring of its effectiveness and safety. The optimal timing of initiating EN should be within 48 hours of the onset of SAP. Clinicians must be aware of the pivotal role of nutritional interventions in SAP to prevent pancreatitis-related complications.

Some of the major challenges of nutrition trials include limitations to retrospective studies, small number of participants, and the use of combined nutrients, making it difficult to detect the real effect of a single component. Therefore, it is often hard to extrapolate data to clearly prove the effects of nutritional interventions in the disease states. In addition, most of the nutrition studies involve a heterogeneous patient population, making a final conclusion quite difficult for interpretation. We need to understand that many of the recommendations for nutritional interventions are based on expert opinions and available meta-analyses rather than large randomized placebo controlled studies. In addition, some of the results found in animal studies cannot be achieved in humans.

We covered in this issue nutritional screening and nutritional interventions, including enteral and parenteral support. I believe that this is an important part of our practice: to recognize a nutritional risk and act on it. There is a need for solid nutrition knowledge and clinical skills to provide the optimal outcomes.

I would like to take a stand to remind you that currently, nutritional education in the US medical schools is quite limited. A recent publication showed that many US medical schools failed to provide sufficient nutrition education.[6] Physicians should be able to recognize the importance of nutritional issues and take the initiative to make nutrition a key part of their practice, including nutrition assessment. Since patients often ask for nutritional guidance, we should be able to recognize the need for a nutritional evaluation, explain the importance of nutritional interventions, and refer the patient if appropriate to the nutrition professionals.

I am very glad that we have nutrition experts who will clarify for us those difficult questions that we are facing in our daily practice in this issue of *Gastroenterology Clinics of North America*. I would like to express my gratitude to all the outstanding contributors who dedicated their time and shared their expertise in writing for this issue devoted entirely to nutrition.

This issue includes multidisciplinary and international distinguished authors to create a highly valuable resource. I believe that the content of this issue will be very helpful in your practice and will serve as a clinically useful tool. The challenges and future tasks within the nutrition field are well addressed. I also found this issue to be a great stimulus for further nutrition research.

Andrew Ukleja, MD, CNSP, AGAF
Department of Gastroenterology and Hepatology
Beth Israel Deaconess Medical Center
Harvard Medical School
330 Brookline Avenue
Boston, MA 02215, USA

E-mail address:
aukleja@bidco.org

REFERENCES

1. Catassi C, Elli L, Bonaz B, et al. Diagnosis of non-celiac gluten sensitivity (NCGS): the Salerno Experts' Criteria. Nutrients 2015;7:4966–77.
2. Plaza-Díaz J, Ruiz-Ojeda FJ, Vilchez-Padial LM, et al. Evidence of the anti-inflammatory effects of probiotics and synbiotics in intestinal chronic diseases. Nutrients 2017;9(6) [pii:555].
3. König J, Wells J, Cani PD, et al. Human intestinal barrier function in health and disease. Clin Transl Gastroenterol 2016;7:e196.
4. Lenhart A, Chey WD. A systematic review of the effects of polyols on gastrointestinal health and irritable bowel syndrome. Adv Nutr 2017;8:587–96.
5. McClave SA, Taylor BE, Martindale RG, et al, Society of Critical Care Medicine, American Society for Parenteral and Enteral Nutrition. Guidelines for the provision and assessment of nutrition support therapy in the adult critically ill patient: Society of Critical Care Medicine (SCCM) and American Society for Parenteral and Enteral Nutrition (A.S.P.E.N.). JPEN J Parenter Enteral Nutr 2016;4:159–211.
6. Adams KM, Butsch WS, Kohlmeier M. The state of nutrition education at US medical schools. J Biomed Educ 2015. https://doi.org/10.1155/2015/357627.
7. Jeppesen PB. New approaches to the treatments of short bowel syndrome-associated intestinal failure. Curr Opin Gastroenterol 2014;30:182–8.
8. Gottlieb K, Dawson J, Hussain F, et al. Development of drugs for celiac disease: review of endpoints for phase 2 and 3 trials. Gastroenterol Rep (Oxf) 2015;3:91–102.
9. Varjú P, Farkas N, Hegyi P, et al. Low fermentable oligosaccharides, disaccharides, monosaccharides and polyols (FODMAP) diet improves symptoms in adults suffering from irritable bowel syndrome (IBS) compared to standard IBS diet: a meta-analysis of clinical studies. PLoS One 2017;12:e0182942.
10. Osland E, Hossain MB, Khan S, et al. Effect of timing of pharmaconutrition (immunonutrition) administration on outcomes of elective surgery for gastrointestinal malignancies: a systematic review and meta-analysis. JPEN J Parenter Enteral Nutr 2014;38:53–69.
11. Dai YJ, Sun LL, Li MY, et al. Comparison of formulas based on lipid emulsions of olive oil, soybean oil, or several oils for parenteral nutrition: a systematic review and meta-analysis. Adv Nutr 2016;7:279–86.
12. Powers J, Luebbenhusen M, Spitzer T, et al. Verification of an electromagnetic placement device compared with abdominal radiograph to predict accuracy of feeding tube placement. JPEN J Parenter Enteral Nutr 2011;35:535–9.

Malnutrition in Gastrointestinal Disorders
Detection and Nutritional Assessment

Khursheed N. Jeejeebhoy, MBBS, PhD[a],*, Donald R. Duerksen, MD[b]

KEYWORDS

- Malnutrition • Gastrointestinal disorders • Subjective Global Assessment
- Macronutrient malnutrition • Nutritional assessment

KEY POINTS

- The detection and management of malnutrition in patients with gastrointestinal disease are important, and influence patient outcome and costs.
- Malnutrition occurs when net nutrient intakes does not meet the body's requirements.
- All patients with significant gastrointestinal disease should be clinically assessed for protein calorie malnutrition by using the Subjective Global Assessment.
- All patients should be have blood tests for anemia, electrolyte and micronutrient deficiency.
- Pateints with inflammatory bowel disease and malabsorption should have measurement of bone mineral deficiency an 25-OH vitamin D levels.

INTRODUCTION

In a recent study of 18 Canadian hospitals encompassing 1015 patients, of whom 30.4% had gastrointestinal disease, 45% were malnourished.[1] Malnutrition was related independently to a prolonged duration of hospital stay and the cost of hospital stay was 31% to 34% more than that of well-nourished patients.[2] Hence, the detection and management of malnutrition in patients with gastrointestinal disease are important and influence the outcome and costs.

Nutritional health requires the intake and absorption of protein, lipids, and carbohydrate that, together, maintain the structure and meet the energy requirements of tissues. They are referred to as macronutrients. In addition, relatively small to minute amounts of other substances are required for the function of tissues and protection

Disclosure: The authors have nothing to disclose.
[a] Department of Medicine, University of Toronto, 784 Alexander Road, Hamilton, Ontario L9G 3E9, Canada; [b] University of Manitoba, C 5120 409 Tache Avenue, Winnipeg, Manitoba R2H 2A6, Canada
* Corresponding author.
E-mail address: khushjeejeebhoy@hotmail.com

Gastroenterol Clin N Am 47 (2018) 1–22
https://doi.org/10.1016/j.gtc.2017.09.002
0889-8553/18/© 2017 Elsevier Inc. All rights reserved.

from infection. They are collectively referred to as micronutrients and are composed of electrolytes, vitamins, and trace elements.

MACRONUTRIENT MALNUTRITION

Malnutrition occurs when net nutrient intake (nutrient intake corrected for absorption and for abnormally large fecal or urinary losses) is less than requirements. Recently, the following definition has been given: "Malnutrition includes both the deficiency or excess (or imbalance) of energy, protein and other nutrients. In practice, undernutrition or inadequate intake of energy, protein and nutrients is the focus."[3] The phenotype of progressive macronutrient malnutrition is loss of body mass and weakness. In patients with gastrointestinal disease, malnutrition owing to lack of nutrients interacts with 2 other factors that also cause the same phenotype, namely, body wasting and weakness. These factors are concurrent disease (usually inflammatory or cancer) and the effects of aging.

Protein–Energy Deficit

Malnutrition owing to lack of macronutrients, namely, protein, carbohydrates, and fats, leads to a depletion of liver glycogen, followed by the use of body fat to meet energy requirements in an effort to preserve muscle and essential organs (**Fig. 1**A). With pure protein–energy malnutrition, blood count, electrolytes, and plasma protein levels are maintained at normal levels. Once body fat is depleted, muscle is catabolized for energy and, ultimately, extreme weakness and death occurs.

Disease-Induced Body Wasting: Cachexia

Disease-induced wasting and fatigue, which is called cachexia, can be a feature of infection, sepsis, cancer, heart failure, systemic inflammatory disorders, and chronic pulmonary disease (**Fig. 1**B). A consensus document on cachexia has pointed out that the term malnutrition has often been used to describe cachexia and should be avoided because cachexia "cannot be successfully treated with nutrition alone." A major difference between an imbalance of protein–energy status and cachexia is the early and profound loss of muscle mass seen with cachexia.[4] In contrast, muscle loss is a late manifestation of protein–energy imbalance. Cachexia with profound muscle loss may be associated with increased body fat called cachectic obesity. In a recent systematic literature review, the authors pointed out that the analysis was clouded by the variety of definitions used to include patients defined as being cachectic. This review pointed out that cachexia does not respond to nutritional support and there is a negative protein energy balance owing to both reduced intake and abnormal metabolism, leading to progressive functional impairment.[5] The recognition of cachexia is based on weight loss of at least 5% body weight or body mass index (BMI) of less than 20 kg/m² in the absence of simple starvation and the presence of 3 of the following 5 criteria.[4]

1. Decreased muscle strength.
2. Fatigue.
3. Anorexia.
4. Low fat-free mass index (<7.26 kg/m² in men and <5.45 kg/m² in women).
5. Abnormal biochemistry including increased C-reactive protein, reduced albumin, and anemia.

In addition, reduced muscle function disproportionate to loss of muscle mass occurs and causes profound weakness. In contrast, pure imbalance of protein–energy does not cause early fatigue. For example, anorexic patients are hyperactive and rarely fatigued.

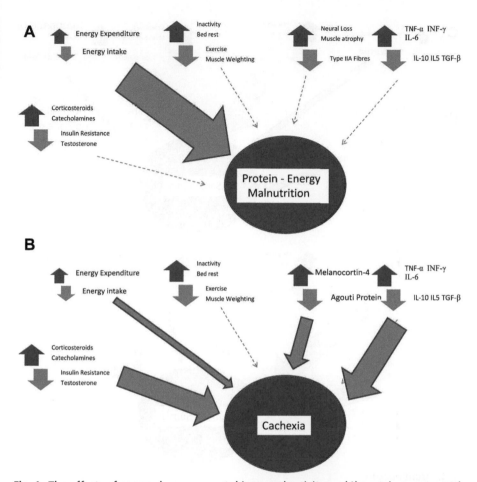

Fig. 1. The effects of energy, hormones, cytokines, and activity on (*A*) protein energy nutrition status, (*B*) the development of cachexia, (*C*) sarcopenia, and (*D*) acute illness. Factors that increase the condition are shown as *up arrows* and those that decrease as *down arrows*. Thickness of the *arrows* shows the extent the parameter influences the change of the condition. IL, interleukin; TGF, transforming growth factor; TNF, tumor necrosis factor. (*From Jeejeebhoy KN. Malnutrition, fatigue, frailty, vulnerability, sarcopenia and cachexia: overlap of clinical features. Curr Opin Clin Nutr Metab Care 2012;15:215; with permission.*)

Acute illness causing cachexia

Acute illness results in rapidly developing cachexia (**Fig. 1**D). Acute trauma is associated with uncontrolled hypercatabolism the so-called ebb phase, followed by a phase during which anabolism increases and there is restoration of lost body components, called the flow phase. A prolonged hypercatabolic phase can lead to profound muscle wasting and cachexia. Sepsis causes marked tissue wasting owing to hypercatabolism and reduced muscle anabolism owing to a combination of increased cytokine activity and hypothalamic activation, causing AN increased output of corticosteroids.[6] These changes are augmented by an imbalance of reduced intake with increased requirements. However, wasting is not entirely owing to a relative or absolute reduction in nutrient intake, because increased protein energy feeding maintains or even increases body fat, but lean body loss continues.[7] A combination of increased

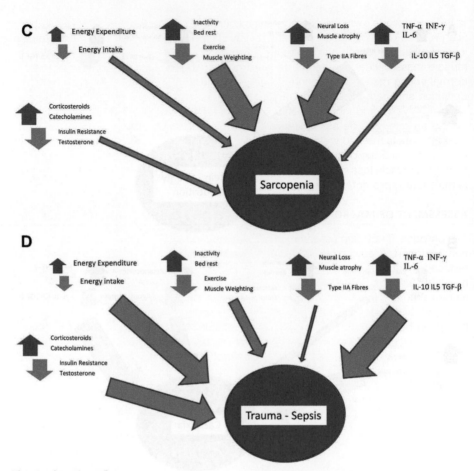

Fig. 1. (*continued*)

corticosteroid output, cytokine expression such as tumor necrosis factor alpha and interleukin 6 contribute to muscle loss owing to mechanisms similar to those seen with cachexia.

Mechanisms of illness-related wasting

Direct effect of cytokines Two proinflammatory cytokines tumor necrosis factor-alpha and interferon-gamma activate nuclear factor-kappa B, resulting in the subsequent activation of the ubiquitin–proteasome pathway, which promotes myofibrillar proteolysis and muscle loss.[8,9]

Hypothalamic effects Inflammation and cancer in the peripheral tissues increase levels of cytokines in the hypothalamus resulting in increased metabolic rate, anorexia and lethargy. Increased secretion of adrenocorticotrophic hormone and glucocorticoids also occur and together increase muscle catabolism.[10]

Age-Related Wasting (Sarcopenia and Frailty)

The term sarcopenia was coined by Irwin Rosenberg to describe age-related muscle loss (**Fig. 1**C).[11] After the age of 30 years, the basal metabolic rate falls at a rate of 3%

to 8% per decade owing to decreases in muscle mass. After the age of 50 years, there is a 1% to 2% loss of muscle per year, mainly of type IIa fibers.[12] This change results in loss of muscle strength and endurance. Sarcopenia can be defined by appendicular muscle mass divided by height squared greater than 2 standard deviations below normal young men and women (<7.23 kg/m^2 and in women at <5.67 kg/m^2).[13] This definition shows the prevalence of sarcopenia is 14% in those between the ages of 65 and 70 years and increases to 53% in those greater than 80 years of age.[14] The loss in muscle may be associated with increased body fat so that, despite normal weight, there is marked weakness, a condition called sarcopenic obesity.[15] A sedentary lifestyle and the presence of inflammatory arthritis-activating cytokines secretion promotes muscle loss in the elderly. Deficiency of hormones, particularly testosterone in males, also promotes muscle loss.

ASSESSMENT OF MACRONUTRIENT MALNUTRITION

The purpose of nutrition assessment is to identify patients who will benefit from nutritional support. Traditionally, malnutrition has been recognized by the phenotype of reduced weight, muscle wasting, loss of body fat, reduced plasma proteins, and immune dysfunction.[16] The recognition of malnutrition based entirely on these features alone, although intuitively obvious, has several pitfalls. First, there is a range of body habitus in otherwise normal individuals, making the recognition of malnutrition based on body composition alone very unreliable. Second, if we use the presence of body wasting to start nutritional care, then we fail to prevent malnutrition or identify the early stages of malnutrition. Third, the phenotype of a wasted body owing to lack of nutrient intake cannot be distinguished from the same features owing to cachexia and aging, which may not respond to nutritional support.

Hence, any method of assessing nutritional status needs to ideally fulfill the following criteria.

1. Does the method specifically show that it can predict the development of complications resulting from malnutrition?
2. Can the method identify the risk of developing malnutrition or malnutrition in early stages so that prophylactic nutritional therapy can be instituted?
3. Can the assessment technique distinguish between protein–energy malnutrition on the one hand and cachexia and age-related changes on the other?

CRITICAL ANALYSIS OF NUTRITIONAL ASSESSMENT TECHNIQUES
Traditionally Used Methods of Nutritional Status

The assessment of nutritional status has previously been focused on the fact that the obvious effect of protein–energy deficiency was weight loss, loss of body fat and muscle mass, circulating proteins, and immune competence. Unfortunately, as discussed, this phenotype of the thin muscle and fat wasted person can be owing to factors other than a simple deficiency of nutrients.

Body weight and weight loss
Body weight is a simple measure of the total mass of body components and is compared with an ideal or desirable weight. This comparison can be made by using formulas such as the Hamwi formula or to normalized tables. However, a simple approach that gives as much information as tables is the calculation of the body mass or Quetelet index (BMI). BMI is calculated as weight in kilograms divided by height in meters squared. A BMI of less than 15 kg/m^2 is associated with significant mortality. However, measurements of body weight in patients in hospital and

intensive care units, as well as those with liver disease, cancer, and renal failure are confounded by changes in body water owing to underhydration, edema, ascites, and dialysate in the abdomen. Two studies, one conducted in a Germany and the other in India, concluded that BMI did not predict the development of complications and increased duration of hospital stay.[17,18] In contrast, a simple history of unintentional and progressive weight loss is a good prognosticator of clinical outcome.[19,20]

Anthropometry

Triceps and subscapular skinfold thicknesses provide an index of body fat and midarm muscle circumference provides a measure of muscle mass. Although these measurements seem to be useful in population studies, their reliability in individual patients is less clear.[21] The most commonly used standards for triceps skinfold thickness and midarm muscle circumference are based on their measurements of white males and females participating in the National Health and Nutrition Examination Survey data. The use of these standards to identify malnutrition in many patients is problematic[22] because of the absence of correction factors for ethnicity, age, hydration status, and physical activity on anthropometric parameters. Several studies have demonstrated that 20% to 30% of healthy control subjects would be considered malnourished based on these standards.[22,23]

Measurement of Body Composition

A more sophisticated way of determining the loss of body weight, fat, and muscle is by a formal evaluation of body components using techniques discussed elsewhere in this article. However, although objective, they cannot be easily applied at the bedside and therefore are usually used as research tools.

Isotope dilution

Total body water maintains a relatively stable relationship to fat-free body mass and thus measured water isotope dilution volumes allow prediction of fat-free body mass and fat (ie, body weight minus fat-free body mass). The relationship of this measurement to outcome has not been studied.

Bioimpedance analysis

Bioimpedance analysis is a method of estimating body fluid volumes by measuring the resistance to a high-frequency, low-amplitude, alternating electric current (50 kHz at 500–800 mÅ).[24] The amount of resistance measured is inversely proportional to the volume of electrolytic fluid in the body. In healthy adults, it is possible to predict total body water within 2 to 3 L. From body water and body weight, the lean and fat masses can be calculated[25] easily at the bedside. A recent article by Pichard and colleagues[26] showed that patients who had a low fat-free mass defined as being less than 17.4 and less than 15.0 kg/m^2 in men and women, respectively, were more likely to have a longer duration of stay in hospital.

Dual-energy x-ray absorptiometry

Dual-energy x-ray absorptiometry was developed originally for the measurement of bone density and bone mass. Systems today also quantify soft tissue composition, and it is possible to measure total and regional fat, bone mineral, and bone mineral free lean components with dual-energy x-ray absorptiometry. Again, there are no data indicating whether dual-energy x-ray absorptiometry can predict outcome in hospital patients unrelated to treatment.

Whole body counting

Total body potassium can be estimated by whole body counters measuring the gamma-ray decay of naturally occurring ^{40}K. The method is safe and can be used in children and pregnant women. The ^{40}K counts can be used to estimate total body potassium, which in turn can be used to calculate body cell mass because all cells have a fixed amount of potassium. Loss of total body potassium is a good predictor of poor outcome in a variety of conditions associated with malnutrition.[27–30]

Computed tomography and MRI

These methods measure components at the tissue-system level of body composition, including skeletal muscle, adipose tissue, visceral organs, and brain. Computed tomography systems measure x-ray attenuation as the source and detector rotate in a perpendicular plane around the subject. MRI systems measure nuclear relaxation times from the nuclei of atoms with a magnetic moment that are aligned within a powerful magnetic field. Clinical systems are based on hydrogen, although it is possible to create images and spectrographs from phosphorus, sodium, and carbon. The collected data are transformed into high-resolution images, and this allows the quantification of whole or regional body composition. A large number of phantoms, cadavers, and in vivo studies validate these methods. There are no studies of imaging methods in relation to outcome.

Body composition and outcomes

Although these methods of measuring body composition can accurately assess different components, they are difficult to apply in the clinical setting, except in specialized units. The only method that can be available for wide clinical application in nutritional assessment is bioimpedance analysis. As discussed elsewhere in this article, reduced fat-free mass as measured by bioimpedance analysis is associated with increased duration of stay in hospital patients but, unlike composite clinical evaluation described in the section on Subjective Global Assessment (SGA), this method has not been shown to predict complications, except in cancer patients.[31] Body composition measurements are also limited by a single measurement at a specific moment in time and unless repeated, do not provide information about the trajectory of body composition. For example, an individual with dysphagia owing to a tight esophageal stricture may have a BMI that has decreased by 5 from 27 to 22 kg/m^2. Although this value is within the normal range, this person is likely malnourished when assessed by other criteria such as the SGA (as described elsewhere in this article).

Serologic Measurements

Albumin

Several studies have demonstrated that a low serum albumin concentration correlates with an increased incidence of medical complications.[32–34] In practice, it is an not an index of malnutrition as exemplified by the fact that prolonged protein calorie restriction induced experimentally in human volunteers [35] or observed clinically in patients with anorexia nervosa,[36] causes marked reductions in body weight but little change in plasma albumin concentration. A protein-deficient diet with adequate calories in elderly persons causes a decrease in lean body mass and muscle function without a change in plasma albumin concentration.[37] In states of acute inflammation, albumin levels decrease largely owing to increased vascular permeability and shift toward the production of inflammatory proteins in the liver.

Prealbumin

Prealbumin is a transport protein for thyroid hormones and exists in the circulation as a retinol-binding–prealbumin complex. The turnover rate of this protein is rapid with a half-life of 2 to 3 days. It is synthesized by the liver and is partially catabolized in the kidneys. Protein–energy malnutrition reduces the levels of prealbumin and refeeding restores levels. Prealbumin levels are influenced by a number of factors other than malnutrition, including infections, renal failure,[38] and liver failure. Although, prealbumin is responsive to nutritional changes, it is influenced by several disease-related factors making it unreliable as an index of nutritional[39,40] status in patients. Similar to albumin, acute inflammation causes a decrease in prealbumin levels.

CLINICAL ASSESSMENT OF NUTRITIONAL STATUS
Subjective Global Assessment

It is clear that use of the traditional nutrition assessment techniques, estimation of body composition, and serologic measurements do not identify the risk of nutritional associated complications, cannot be used in a busy clinical practice, have a wide range of normal values, and are influenced by disease. In a critical assessment of various techniques traditionally used to measure nutritional status, it was clear that these techniques were inadequate,[41] and an alternative method would have to be used to identify the interacting clinical factors that resulted in malnutrition. These factors are shown in **Fig. 2**. In

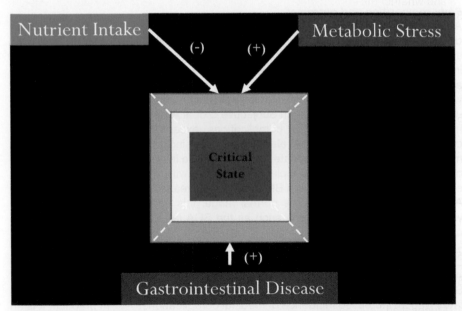

Fig. 2. Interaction of factors affecting nutritional status. The *central square* represents body components essential for normal function. As these components diminish, this a critical state influencing survival is reached. Factors that promote this progression are marked with a + sign and those preventing progression a – sign. The nutritional status of the individual is represented by the square box in the center of the slide. This box contracts or expands depending on the nutrient intake, metabolic stress, and state of the gastrointestinal tract, which determines the ability to feed orally and digest and absorb nutrients. Based on the interaction of these 3 factors, the clinical course of the individual is determined. (*From* Jeejeebhoy KN. Nutritional assessment. In: Buchman AL, editor. Care of pat with gastro dis. Boca Raton (FL): CRC Press; 2015. p. 1–14; with permission.)

this figure, the initial nutritional and functional status is shown as a purple square, which is positively (+, increases size of square) or negatively (-, decreases size of square) influenced by nutrient intake, gastrointestinal disease (which impedes intake and/or prevents absorption) and inflammatory disease or cancer (which increases energy and nutrient requirements).

We hypothesized that a composite evaluation of these parameters together with their effect on the direction and rapidity of change in body mass and function evaluated at the bedside would identify outcome without the need to exactly determine weight, BMI, arm muscle circumference, fat in skin fold thickness, and albumin levels.

A clinical method referred to these parameters for evaluating nutritional status, was termed SGA, encompassing historical, symptomatic, and physical parameters. The history used in the SGA focuses on 5 areas.

1. An important factor is the loss of body weight in the previous 6 months and continuing in last 2 weeks. The direction of change rather than absolute weight is important to note. The pattern of loss is also important, and it is possible for a patient to have significant weight loss but still be considered well-nourished if body weight (without edema or ascites) recently increased. For example, a patient who has had a 10% body weight loss but regained 3% of that weight over the past month could be considered well-nourished.
2. Dietary intake is classified as normal or abnormal as judged by a change in intake and whether the current diet is nutritionally adequate to meet dietary requirements.
3. The presence of persistent gastrointestinal symptoms, such as anorexia, nausea, vomiting, diarrhea, and abdominal pain, which have occurred almost daily for at least 2 weeks, is noted. All of these factors may influence the ability to meet nutritional requirements and place the patient at risk for malnutrition.
4. The patient's functional capacity is defined as bedridden, suboptimally active, or full capacity.
5. The last feature of the history concerns the metabolic demands of the patient's underlying disease state. Examples of high-stress illnesses are inflammation, such as acute colitis. Moderate -stress diseases might be a mild infection or a limited malignant tumor.

The features of the physical examination are noted as normal, mild or moderate, or severe alterations. They include the following:

1. Loss of subcutaneous fat measured in the triceps region and the midaxillary line at the level of the lower ribs.
2. Muscle wasting, particularly in the temporal areas, shoulder areas, deltoids, and quadriceps, as determined by loss of bulk and tone detectable by palpation.
3. The presence of edema in the ankle and sacral regions and the presence of ascites are noted.
4. Mucosal and cutaneous lesions are noted, as are the color and appearance of the patient's hair.

The findings on the history and physical examination are used as a global composite to categorize patients as being well-nourished (category A) having no abnormal features, moderate or suspected malnutrition (category B), or having severe malnutrition (category C). The rank is assigned on the basis of subjective weighting. We have shown that clinical evaluation accurately predicted nutrition associated complications.[42] Detsky and associates[43] found that the use of the SGA in evaluating hospitalized patients gives reproducible results and there was more than 80% agreement when 2 blinded observers assessed the same patient. Detsky and colleagues[44] subsequently showed it had better sensitivity and specificity than individual traditional parameters in predicting outcome.

Since the publication of the SGA in 1982,[42] a number of similar techniques have been published to identify hospital malnutrition. In 1995, Lennard-Jones and colleagues[45] recommended that all patients at admission answer 4 questions: (1) Did they experience unintentional weight loss? (2) Did they experience unintentional reduced food intake? (3) What is their height? (4) What is their weight? A screening tool was later developed based on these questions.[46] In 1994, a Mini Nutritional Assessment (MNA) for geriatric patients was described.[47] This lengthy assessment was later shortened to a short form (MNA-SF) and validated as compared with the full MNA.[48]

Kondrup and colleagues[49] described the Nutritional Risk Screening finalized in the year 2002 (NRS 2002). This method used parameters from controlled clinical trials to select those that were associated with response to nutritional support. The NRS 2002 assessed the risk for malnutrition by assigning a score to each of the following:

1. Degree of weight loss,
2. BMI,
3. Food intake,
4. Severity of disease, and
5. Age.

The Malnutrition Universal Screening Tool,[50] which was developed by the British Association for Parenteral and Enteral Nutrition, used the following parameters:

1. BMI graded as obese, normal, or reduced,
2. Weight loss less than 5%, 5% to 10%, or greater than 10%, and
3. Disease-related decrease in food intake.

Recently, a Canadian Nutrition Screening tool[51] was developed and shown to predict the occurrence of nutrition-associated complications. It is based on 2 questions: Have you lost weight in the past 6 months without trying to lose this weight? Have you been eating less than usual for more than a week?

Examination of these different methods show that they all use the same parameters first described for the SGA, namely, progressive weight loss, reduced food intake, loss of function (mobility in the MNA-SF), and stress of disease. Unlike the SGA, the other measures all include an anthropometric parameter such as BMI or limb muscle circumference, but do not include aspects of physical examination.

Comparison of Different Methods in Predicting Outcome

A comparison of medical inpatients showed excellent agreement between the Malnutrition Universal Screening Tool and the SGA,[22] although the SGA did not use BMI. In another study[52] in elderly patients in the intensive care unit, it was shown that the MNA-SF, MNA (full), SGA, and NRS (using only the nutrition score and eliminating the points for age and disease) were in excellent agreement with each other (kappa of 0.91–0.96). The NRS, however, if used in its complete form, falsely increased the incidence of malnutrition in the elderly and sick owing to scores given for age and acute illness, resulting in the loss of specificity.[52] They all showed that duration of hospital stay was increased in patients identified as malnourished. In addition, all methods showed that malnutrition resulted in a significantly reduced proportion of patients discharged home and an increased proportion discharged to a hospice or those who died.

That the predictability of outcome by SGA, which does not include evaluation of BMI or limb circumference, is comparable with other techniques that include these measurements indicates that it is unnecessary to use any anthropometrics to complement the SGA. Thus, the SGA remains a simpler and effective tool to assess malnutrition clinically.

Implementation of the Subjective Global Assessment in the assessment of nutritional status

The SGA can be implemented at the bedside by completing the SGA form (**Fig. 3**) according to directions given in **Fig. 4**. On the basis of the criteria given in **Fig. 4**, a nutrition assessment classifying individuals into well-nourished, mild or moderately malnourished, or severely malnourished can be made.

Mechanisms of Protein–Calorie Malnutrition

The mechanisms contributing to protein calorie malnutrition can be divided into 3 major categories: decreased oral intake, malabsorption of nutrients, and increased energy expenditure (**Box 1**). In many cases, the cause of protein–calorie malnutrition in individuals with gastrointestinal disorders is multifactorial and includes decreased oral intake.

MICRONUTRIENT MALNUTRITION

Only clinically important micronutrients related to gastrointestinal disorders are considered in this section on micronutrients.

ELECTROLYTES

Water with dissolved sodium, potassium, magnesium, and phosphorus constitutes about 73% of lean body mass; therefore, in addition to macronutrients, attention to the fluid and electrolyte status is critical to good nutrition.

Sodium and Chloride

Sodium with chloride are the main extracellular ions responsible for maintaining the tonicity and volume of extracellular fluid. Diarrhea and vomiting associated with gastrointestinal disease results in sodium and chloride depletion. Although any gastrointestinal disorder with significant diarrhea can be associated with electrolyte abnormalities, the gastrointestinal condition associated with major losses of sodium and chloride is short bowel syndrome.

Assessment

Clinically absent jugular filling on lying flat and a postural drop in systolic blood pressure of 20 mm Hg are signs of severe salt and water deficiency. Because losses of intestinal contents in short bowel syndrome may be isotonic, the blood level of sodium is not a good index of depletion. Depletion is monitored by urine sodium output which in deficiency falls below 50 mmol/24 hours.

Potassium, Magnesium, and Phosphorus

With protein–caloric malnutrition there is loss of the intracellular ions potassium (K^+)[30,53] and magnesium (Mg^{2+}),[54] together with a gain in sodium (Na^+)[55] and water.[56] On refeeding, it is necessary to give potassium,[57] magnesium,[58] phosphorus (as monovalent or divalent phosphate),[55] and zinc (Zn^{2+})[59] to ensure optimum nitrogen

Patient name: _____   Date: _____/ _____/ _____

DIETARY INTAKE
1. ☐ No change; adequate
2. Inadequate; duration of inadequate intake _____
   ☐ Suboptimal solid diet   ☐ Full fluids or only oral nutrition supplements   ☐ Minimal intake, clear fluids or starvation
3. Dietary Intake in past 2 weeks*
   ☐ Adequate _____   ☐ Improved but not adequate _____   ☐ No improvement or inadequate _____

WEIGHT   Usual weight _____   Current weight _____
1. **Non fluid weight change past 6 months**   Weight loss (kg) _____
   ☐ <5% loss or weight stability   ☐ 5-10% loss without stabilization or increase   ☐ >10% loss and ongoing
   If above not known, has there been a subjective loss of weight during the past six months?
   ☐ None or mild   ☐ Moderate   ☐ Severe
2. **Weight change past 2 weeks***   Amount (if known) _____
   ☐ Increased   ☐ No change   ☐ Decreased

SYMPTOMS (Experiencing symptoms affecting oral intake)
1. ☐ Pain on eating   ☐ Anorexia   ☐ Vomiting   ☐ Nausea   ☐ Dysphagia   ☐ Diarrhea
   ☐ Dental problems   ☐ Feels full quickly   ☐ Constipation
2. ☐ None   ☐ Intermittent/mild/few   ☐ Constant/severe/multiple
3. **Symptoms in the past 2 weeks***
   ☐ Resolution of symptoms   ☐ Improving   ☐ No change or worsened

FUNCTIONAL CAPACITY (Fatigue and progressive loss of function)
1. **No dysfunction**
2. Reduced capacity; duration of change _____
   ☐ Difficulty with ambulation/normal activities   ☐ Bed/chair-ridden
3. **Functional Capacity in the past 2 weeks***
   ☐ Improved   ☐ No change   ☐ Decrease

METABOLIC REQUIREMENT
High metabolic requirement   ☐ No   ☐ Yes

PHYSICAL EXAMINATION

Loss of body fat   ☐ No   ☐ Mild/Moderate   ☐ Severe
Loss of muscle mass   ☐ No   ☐ Mild/Moderate   ☐ Severe
Presence of edema/ascites   ☐ No   ☐ Mild/Moderate   ☐ Severe

SGA RATING
☐ A Well-nourished   ☐ B Mildly/moderately malnourished   ☐ C Severely malnourished
Normal   Some progressive nutritional loss   Evidence of wasting and progressive symptoms
or
☐ **CACHEXIA** (wasting due to disease and inflammation)
☐ **SARCOPENIA** (reduced muscle mass and strength)
*See page 2 SGA Rating for more description.

Fig. 3. Subjective Global Assessment (SGA) form. (*From* Jeejeebhoy KN. Malnutrition, fatigue, frailty, vulnerability, sarcopenia and cachexia: overlap of clinical features. Curr Opin Clin Nutr Metab Care 2012;15:213–9; with permission.)

retention. Therefore, it is essential that the level of these elements be monitored to avoid malnutrition and protein depletion in particular.

Assessment
The plasma levels of these elements should be monitored and repleted, but because the major body content of these elements are in tissues it is possible to have depleted body stores with normal plasma levels.

SUBCUTANEOUS FAT

Physical examination	Normal	Mild/Moderate	Severe
Under the eyes	Slightly bulging area	Somewhat hollow look, Slightly dark circles	Hollowed look, depression, dark circles
Triceps	Large space between fingers	Some depth to fat tissue, but not ample. Loose fitting skin.	Very little space between fingers or fingers touch
Ribs, lower back, sides of trunk	Chest is full; ribs do not show. Slight to no protrusion of the iliac crest	Ribs obvious, but indentations are not marked. Iliac Crest somewhat prominent	Indentation between ribs very obvious. Iliac crest very prominent

MUSCLE WASTING

Physical examination	Normal	Mild/Moderate	Severe
Temple	Well-defined muscle	Slight depression	Hollowing, depression
Clavicle	Not visible in males; may be visible but not prominent in females	Some protrusion; may not be all the way along	Protruding/prominent bone
Shoulder	Rounded	No square look; acromion process may protrude slightly	Square look; bones prominent
Scapula/ribs	Bones not prominent; no significant depressions	Mild depressions or bone may show slightly; not all areas	Bones prominent; significant depressions
Quadriceps	Well defined	Depression/atrophy medially	Prominent knee, Severe depression medially
Interosseous muscle between thumb and forefinger (back of hand)**	Muscles protrudes; could be flat in females	Slightly depressed	Flat or depressed area

FLUID RETENTION

Physical examination	Normal	Mild/Moderate	Severe
Edema	None	Pitting edema of extrimities / pitting to knees, possible sacral edema if bedridden	Pitting beyond knees, sacral edema if bedridden, may also have generalized edema
Ascites	Absent	Present (may only be present on imaging)	

A - Well-nourished no decrease in food intake; <5% weight loss; no/minimal symptoms affecting food intake; no deficit in function; no deficit in fat or muscle mass or an individual with some criteria for SGA B or C but with recent adequate food intake; non-fluid weight gain; significant recent improvement in symptoms allowing adequate oral intake; significant recent improvement in function.

B - Mildly/moderately malnourished definite decrease in food intake; 5%—10% weight loss without stabilization or gain; mild/some symptoms affecting food intake; moderate functional deficit or recent deterioration; mild/moderate loss of fat and/or muscle mass or an individual meeting some criteria for SGA C but with improvement (but not adequate) of oral intake, recent stabilization of weight, decrease in symptoms affecting oral intake, and stabilization of functional status.

C - Severely malnourished severe deficit in food intake; >10% weight loss which is ongoing; significant symptoms affecting food intake; severe functional deficit; recent significant deterioration obvious signs of fat and/or muscle loss.

Cachexia - If there is an underlying predisposing disorder (eg, malignancy) and there is evidence of reduced muscle and fat and no or limited improvement with optimal nutrient intake, this is consistent with cachexia. **Sarcopenia** – If there is an underlying disorder (eg, aging) and there is evidence of reduced muscle and strength and no or limited improvement with optimal nutrient intake.
**In the elderly prominent tendons and hollowing is the result of aging and may not reflect malnutrition.

Fig. 4. Subjective Global Assessment (SGA) guidance for body composition. (*From* Jeejeebhoy KN. Malnutrition, fatigue, frailty, vulnerability, sarcopenia and cachexia: overlap of clinical features. Curr Opin Clin Nutr Metab Care 2012;15:213–9; with permission.)

Calcium

Calcium in the plasma is tightly regulated by parathormone and 1,25-dihydroxy vitamin D levels, and is not influenced by nutrition. However, cumulative dietary calcium intake does influence bone mass where the bulk of body calcium is present, and dietary calcium is not the only factor influencing bone. Total body calcium can be estimated by measuring bone mass using DEXA and compared with normals.

TRACE ELEMENTS

Cotzias[60] defined an essential trace element as one that has the following characteristics: (1) present in the healthy tissues of all living things, (2) constant tissue concentration from one animal to the next, (3) withdrawal leads to a reproducible functional

---

Box 1
Mechanisms of protein calorie malnutrition in patients with gastrointestinal disorders

Decreased oral intake
- Anorexia from underlying disease
- Chronic nausea and/or vomiting
- Gastrointestinal tract obstruction
- Oropharyngeal ulceration
- Medication side effects
- Dysphagia
- NPO for diagnostic workup

Malabsorption
- Underlying disease, for example, celiac disease
- Extensive surgical resection of small bowel, for example, short bowel syndrome
- Small intestinal bacterial overgrowth
- Fistulizing disease

Increased energy expenditure
- Underlying inflammatory gastrointestinal disorder, for example, Crohn's disease
- Sepsis

---

and/or structural abnormality, (4) addition of the element prevents the abnormality, (5) the abnormality is associated with a specific biochemical change, and (6) the biochemical change is prevented and/or cured along with the observed clinical abnormality by giving the nutrient.

In animal studies, 15 elements have been found to be essential for health. They are iron, zinc, copper, chromium, selenium, iodine, cobalt, manganese, nickel, molybdenum, fluorine, tin, silicon, vanadium, and arsenic. However, using the strict criteria suggested by Cotzias,[58] only the first 7 elements have been shown to be necessary for health in humans. Of these, cobalt is essential only insofar as it is part of the corrin ring in vitamin B_{12}.

Trace elements are absorbed as inorganic substances and as organic compounds. In natural foods, the latter often predominate. Because the absorption of the 2 forms may differ, results of studies with inorganic test substances cannot be equated with the availability of the same elements in organic form in food. For example, heme iron is absorbed very efficiently,[61] and the availability of this form of iron cannot be judged from studies with element iron.

Absorbed trace elements circulate as protein-bound complexes that are not always in free equilibrium with tissue stores. For example, the exchangeable plasma copper is present in very small amounts bound to albumin.[62] In contrast, the major form of circulating copper, ceruloplasmin, is not freely exchangeable.[63] For this and other reasons, total circulating levels may not reflect the availability of an element for nutritional needs.

Tissue stores of a trace element may not be available to meet needs during a period of deficient supply because of 2 factors. First, they may be incorporated in enzyme proteins that do not exchange with the free pool. Second, during anabolism there is net flow of trace elements into cells, so that cellular stores cannot be mobilized. The converse applies as well in catabolism. For example, in hypercatabolic states, even though zinc is being lost and the patient is in negative zinc balance, deficiency does not occur and plasma zinc is normal because of net outflow from tissue stores. When nutritional support is given, resulting in protein synthesis, a positive zinc balance occurs, but plasma levels decrease and deficiency will result unless exogenous zinc is given. Because the action of trace elements depends on other factors such as age, metabolic and nutritional states (anabolic or catabolic), and the availability of agonists and antagonists, clinical deficiency cannot be predicted by simple demonstration of a low blood level of the element. As an example of this complexity, it has been found that at least some degree of selenium deficiency can be overcome by giving vitamin E. Also, children with selenium-responsive Keshan disease have levels of plasma selenium no lower than those in children with phenylketonuria receiving artificial diets, and yet the latter do not show a clinical deficiency.[64]

These findings make it imperative to look for subclinical functional changes to enable us to define needs. For example, even in patients who do not have overt clinical deficiency of zinc, Wolman and colleagues (65) have shown that a negative zinc balance was associated with reduced nitrogen retention and carbohydrate tolerance, thus justifying the need for maintaining balance. Finally, the route of excretion of most trace elements, excepting chromium, is mainly through the gastrointestinal tract. This raises the possibility that abnormal gastrointestinal losses may increase requirements in patients with disease of the gastrointestinal tract. Another consequence of the gastrointestinal route of excretion is that renal disease does not reduce the need for giving these elements.

Specific Trace Elements

Iron
Gastrointestinal disorders (iron malabsorption in celiac disease and increased losses owing to gastrointestinal disease) are frequently associated with iron deficiency and iron deficiency anemia.

Assessment Plasma ferritin levels are a good index of iron stores. For ferritin, 1 µg/L indicates 10 mg of body iron stores. However, ferritin is an acute phase reactant and inflammation increases levels, potentially masking deficiency.

Zinc
Zinc is an important constituent of enzymes, DNA polymerase, and structures called zinc fingers. Functionally, zinc is important for the expression of immunity. These experimental findings about zinc and nucleic acids are interesting in view of the clinical observation that a number of functions dependent on protein synthesis are suppressed by zinc deficiency. These include growth, cellular immunity, fertility, hair growth, wound healing, and plasma protein levels. Thus, it is obvious that zinc deficiency leads to profound disturbances of protein synthesis. In addition, in volunteer studies, experimental mild zinc deficiency reduced thymulin levels and the CD4/CD8 ratio.[65]

Assessment Although circulating zinc levels decrease in the deficient state, there are other causes of low circulating zinc levels that make this measurement unreliable. Hair zinc levels are low when there is low-grade chronic deficiency, but in acute deficiency hair does not grow, and with profound deficiency hair loss occurs, although the remaining hair may have normal zinc concentrations.[66] Currently, the best way of assessing zinc status and requirements is through multiple clinical parameters. Abnormal gastrointestinal losses, hypercatabolism, or amino acid infusions increase the need for zinc supplementation. The clinical syndrome of acrodermatitis enteropathica confirms the need for zinc supplementation. This syndrome consists of scaly, red, desquamating lesions involving the nasolabial folds and hands. In severe cases, it extends to the trunk, resulting in extensive exfoliation and secondary skin infection. There is often associated loss of hair.

Copper
The major effects of copper deficiency are expressed through the consequences of ceruloplasmin and lysyl oxidase deficiencies. Ceruloplasmin is an iron oxidase.

Ceruloplasmin oxidizes ferrous iron and aids in the transfer of iron from stores to trans-ferrin.[67] Therefore, copper deficiency results in conditioned iron deficiency. Mature collagen and elastin are characterized by the presence of crosslinks formed from pre-cursor peptides. This process depends on the copper-containing enzyme lysyl oxi-dase. In addition to the effects on iron and collagen, another result of copper deficiency leukopenia.[68]

Assessment Plasma copper is reduced in copper deficiency and is also affected by a variety of factors that alter the serum concentration of ceruloplasmin. These include reduced synthesis caused by protein–calorie malnutrition and increased loss in pa-tients with nephrosis, both being situations in which reduced levels of copper are found. Infections, inflammatory conditions, leukemia, and Hodgkin's disease all in-crease the levels of serum copper. Oral contraceptive agents likewise increase plasma copper levels to 300 ± 7 µg/dL from a mean normal of 118 ± 2 µg/dL.[69]

Selenium

Selenium is incorporated into tissue proteins as selenocysteine.[70] Glutathione perox-idase is an enzyme made up of 4 subunits, each containing selenocysteine as an in-tegral part of the molecule.[71] In association with superoxide dismutase, it controls the levels of superoxide and peroxide and protects cells from peroxidation.

Assessment Plasma selenium and glutathione peroxidase levels are sensitive to sele-nium intake and can be used to assess the need for this element.

FAT-SOLUBLE VITAMINS
Vitamin A

Vitamin A exists in 3 forms. All-trans-retinol or A_1 and 3-dehydroretinol or A_2 and the precursor beta-carotene. Vitamin A has 2 important functions. First, it facilitates the transfer of carbohydrate for glycoprotein synthesis. In the retina, in the form of 11-cis-retinal, it is associated with a protein, opsin, to form the light-sensitive pigment rhodopsin.

Assessment

Clinical deficiency presents as night blindness and xerophthamia. The ocular findings include shiny gray foamy triangular areas on the conjunctiva called Bitot's spots. Bio-chemically, circulating retinol levels decrease to less than 10 µg/mL (**Table 1**).

Vitamin E

Natural alpha tocopherol is biologically the most potent and is composed of only one isomer. It is called RRR-alpha-tocopherol. The synthetic compound has 8 isomers and is only 74% as potent is the natural compound. It is called all-rac-alpha-tocopherol. Dietary tocopherol is expressed as RRR-alpha-tocopherol equivalents (alpha-TE). One alpha-TE is equal to the activity of 1 mg of RRR-alpha-tocopherol. Vitamin E con-trols the formation of hydroperoxides in the fatty acid residues of phospholipids, a pro-cess that depends on the antioxidant role of the vitamin and also involves its entering into a structural relation with membrane phospholipids.

Assessment

In patients with severe steatorrhea (as in abetalipoproteinemia and biliary atresia), vitamin E deficiency has been shown to be responsible for neurologic syndromes associated with spinocerebellar degeneration and neuropathy. The diagnosis of defi-ciency can be made from blood levels (see **Table 1**).

Table 1
Normal values and deficient levels of serum and blood vitamins

Vitamin	Units	Normal	Deficient
Retinol	µg/dL	10–100	<10
25-Hydroxy D	µg/dL	0.8–5.5	<0.7
1,25-Dihydroxy D	ng/dL	2.6–6.5	
alpha-Tocopherol	µg/dL	7.0–20.0	<5
Blood thiamin	µg/dL	2.5–7.5	<1.7
Urine thiamin	µg/g creatinine	>66	<27
Blood riboflavin	µg/dL	10–50	<10
Urine riboflavin	µg/g creatinine	>79	<27
Plasma vitamin B_6	µg/dL	>5.0	<2.5
Urine vitamin B_6	µg/g creatinine	>20	<20
Serum niacin	µg/dL	300–600	<300
Urinary N1-methylnicotinamide	mg/d	2.2–9.4	<0.5
Ascorbic acid	mg/d	0.4–1.5	<0.3
Plasma biotin	ng/d	30–74	
Urinary biotin	mg/dL	6–50	<6
Carotenoids	µg/dL	80–400	
Vitamin B_{12}	pg/mL	205–867	<140
Folic acid	ng/mL	3.3–20	<2.5

Vitamin D

Vitamin D is a critically essential nutrient irrespective of the presence of inflammatory bowel disease and is necessary in every person. Vitamin D is produced by action of sunlight on the skin which converts 7-dehydrocholesterol to cholecalciferol or vitamin D_3.

In northern climates, the cold temperature reduces exposure to sunlight during late fall, winter, and early spring, resulting in widespread vitamin D deficiency or insufficiency. This condition is especially prevalent in ethnic groups with pigmented skin. In food, it is present as vitamin D_3 or as ergocalciferol (vitamin D_2). Vitamin D_3 and D_2 are hydroxylated in the liver to 25-OH vitamin D. This is the form of vitamin D that is measured to determine deficiency. The 25-OH vitamin D is converted into the active 1,25-dihydroxyvitamin D by the kidney regulated by plasma parathyroid hormone levels.[72]

Assessment

The levels of 25-OH vitamin D needed to provide a nadir plateau of parathyroid hormone levels and maximal intestinal transport of calcium is considered to be the level of vitamin D sufficiency. Based on those considerations, deficiency is defined as a level less than 50 nmol/L, insufficiency 52 to 72 nmol/L, and sufficiency greater than 75 nmol/L.[73]

WATER-SOLUBLE VITAMINS

These vitamins are distinguished by the fact that most contain nitrogen (unlike fat-soluble vitamins) and are components of coenzymes catalyzing biochemical reactions. Five of these vitamins are especially concerned with energy metabolism: thiamin, riboflavin, niacin, biotin, and pantothenate.

Assessment

Deficiency can be monitored from blood and urinary levels. The normal and deficient levels are given in **Table 1**.

Thiamin

This vitamin catalyzes the decarboxylation of alpha-keto acids, in which thiamin pyrophosphate converts pyruvate to acetyl coenzyme A and CO_2, and alpha-ketoglutarate to succinyl coenzyme A and CO_2.

Assessment Clinically, deficiency presents as 3 different syndromes commonly seen in alcoholics. They are Wernicke-Korsakoff syndrome, and wet and dry beriberi. Wernicke syndrome is an acute disease presenting as ophthalmoplegia, nystagmus, ataxia, and confusion. Korsakoff syndrome is a chronic condition of impaired short-term memory and confabulation with a normal cognitive state. Wet beriberi presents as a high-output cardiac failure and dry beriberi as a peripheral neuropathy. Deficiency results in high blood lactate levels detected at the bedside and confirmed by blood and urine tests (see **Table 1**).

Vitamin B₁₂ and folic acid

These vitamins are intimately connected. Both are critical for DNA and RNA synthesis. Folate supplies methyl groups for DNA synthesis and vitamin B_{12} is a cofactor in recycling 5-methyl tetrahydrpfolate to tetrahydrofolate, which can donate 1-carbon compounds required for synthesis of DNA.

Assessment Clinically, deficiency of both vitamins result in megaloblastic anemia and delayed maturation of neutrophils. In addition, there is atrophy of buccal mucosa causing glossitis and stomatitis. Vitamin B_{12} deficiency causes paresthesias, gait disturbance, and degeneration of the dorsal columns of the spinal cord, resulting in a loss of position sense and ataxia, as well as cognitive changes. The blood levels of vitamin B_{12} and folate are good indices of deficiency (see **Table 1**). In some elderly patients deficiency, may present as low normal levels of B_{12}, but they may have increased urine output of methylmalonate as an index of deficiency. This functional test of vitamin B_{12} deficiency is clinically available.

Riboflavin, niacin, pyridoxine, biotin, and pantothenate

Riboflavin is phosphorylated to the coenzyme flavin adenine mononucleotide, which is then converted to flavin adenine dinucleotide. These coenzymes participate in numerous oxidation-reduction reactions and through the respiratory chain in energy production. Niacin is a component of nicotine adenine dinucleotide and its phosphate, which are coenzymes of dehydrogenases used in redox reactions and for the generation of adenosine triphosphate. Pyridoxine functions as a coenzyme, which is involved in the metabolism of amino acids, 1-carbon chain, and lipids, and the biosynthesis of neurotransmitters. Biotin is a component of 5 carboxylases that are critical for energy production and synthetic reactions. Pantothenate is a component of coenzyme A that is critical for transferring acyl groups, beta-oxidation of fatty acids and oxidative degradation of amino acids. Hence, these vitamins are very important in energy production from substrates, biosynthetic functions and redox reactions. Deficiency of other B vitamins can be detected by blood levels (see **Table 1**).

Vitamin C

The main action of vitamin C in collagen synthesis is hydroxylation at lysine and proline residues, making it possible for collagen to form a triple helix, giving the tissue strength and stability.

Assessment The syndrome of deficiency is called scurvy and first presents as perifollicular hyperkeratosis. Advanced deficiency results in perifollicular hemorrhages, followed by hemorrhages into skin, joints, and nails, and swelling, friability, and bleeding of the gums. There may be terminal seizures, fever, and edema. Plasma levels of ascorbic acid can be used to detect and confirm deficiency (see **Table 1**).

SUMMARY

All patients with significant gastrointestinal disease should be clinically assessed for protein calorie malnutrition by using the SGA. Blood tests for anemia, electrolytes, calcium, phosphorus, magnesium, ferritin, vitamin B_{12}, and folate should be considered for assessment of major micronutrients. Where malabsorption or inflammatory bowel disease is diagnosed, bone mineral density using DEXA, 25- OH vitamin D levels, and measurement of other vitamins and trace elements should be considered. In addition, in at-risk patients, vitamin and trace element clinical deficiency syndromes should be considered during patient assessment.

REFERENCES

1. Allard JP, Keller H, Jeejeebhoy KN, et al. Malnutrition at hospital admission—contributors and effect on length of stay: a prospective cohort study from the Canadian Malnutrition Task Force. JPEN J Parenter Enteral Nutr 2016;40: 487–97.
2. Curtis LJ, Bernier P, Jeejeebhoy K, et al. Costs of hospital malnutrition. Clin Nutr 2017;36(5):1391–6.
3. McKinlay AW. Malnutrition: the spectre at the feast. J R Coll Physicians Edinb 2008;38:317–21.
4. Fearon K, Strasser F, Anker SD, et al. Definition and classification of cancer cachexia: an international consensus. Lancet Oncol 2011;12:489–95.
5. Blum D, Omlin A, Baracos VE, et al. Cancer cachexia: a systematic literature review of items and domains associated with involuntary weight loss in cancer. Crit Rev Oncol Hematol 2011;80:114–44.
6. Chiolero R, Revelly JP, Tappy L. Energy metabolism in sepsis and injury. Nutrition 1997;13(9 Suppl):45S–51S.
7. Hart DW, Wolf SE, Herndon DN, et al. Energy expenditure and calorie balance after burns: increased feeding leads to fat rather than lean mass accretion. Ann Surg 2002;235:152–61.
8. Mitch WE, Price SR. Transcription factors and muscle cachexia: is there a therapeutic target? Lancet 2001;337:734–5.
9. Zoico E, Roubenoff R. The role of cytokines in regulating protein metabolism and muscle function. Nutr Rev 2002;60:39–51.
10. Grossberg AJ, Scarlett JM, Marks DL. Hypothalamic mechanisms in cachexia. Physiol Behav 2010;100:478–89.
11. Rosenberg IH. Sarcopenia: origins and clinical relevance. Clin Geriatr Med 2011; 27:337–9.
12. Hughes VA, Frontera WR, Roubenoff R, et al. Longitudinal changes in body composition in older men and women: role of body weight change and physical activity. Am J Clin Nutr 2002;76:473–81.
13. Fielding RA, Vellas B, Evans WJ, et al. Sarcopenia: an undiagnosed condition in older adults. current consensus definition: prevalence, etiology, and consequences. International Working Group on Sarcopenia. J Am Med Dir Assoc 2011;12:249–56.

14. Baumgartner RN, Waters DL, Gallagher D, et al. Predictors of skeletal muscle mass in elderly men and women. Mech Ageing Dev 1999;107:123–36.
15. Alfonso JC-J, Baeyens JP, Baeuer JM, et al. Sarcopenia: European consensus on definition and diagnosis. Age Ageing 2010;39:412–23.
16. Blackburn GL, Bistrian BR, Maini BS, et al. Nutritional and metabolic assessment of the hospitalized patient. JPEN J Parenter Enteral Nutr 1977;1:11.
17. Pirlich M, Schutz T, Norman K, et al. The German hospital malnutrition study. Clin Nutr 2006;25:563–72.
18. Shirodkar M, Mohandas KM. Subjective global assessment: a simple and reliable screening tool for malnutrition among Indians. Indian J Gastroenterol 2005;24: 246–50.
19. Stanley KE. Prognostic factors for survival in patients with inoperable lung cancer. J Natl Cancer Inst 1980;65:25.
20. DeWys WD, Begg C, Lavin PT, et al. Prognostic effect of weight loss prior to chemotherapy in cancer patients. Am J Med 1980;69:491.
21. Morgan DB, Hill GL, Burkinshaw L. The assessment of weight loss from a single measurement of body weight: the problems and limitations. Am J Clin Nutr 1980; 33:2101.
22. Thuluvath PJ, Triger DR. How valid are our reference standards of nutrition? Nutrition 1995;11:731.
23. Harries AD, Jones LA, Heatley RV, et al. Malnutrition in inflammatory bowel disease: an anthropometric study. Hum Nutr Clin Nutr 1982;36C:307.
24. Lukaski HC, Johnson PE, Bolonchuk WW, et al. Assessment of fat-free mass using bioelectrical impedance measurements of the human body. Am J Clin Nutr 1985;41:810–7.
25. Kyle UG, Genton LC, Slosman DO, et al. Fat-free and fat-mass percentiles in 5225 healthy subjects aged 15 to 98 years. Nutrition 2001;17:534–41.
26. Pichard C, Kyle UG, Morabia A, et al. Nutritional assessment: lean body mass depletion at hospital admission is associated with an increased length of stay. Am J Clin Nutr 2004;79:613–8.
27. Kotler DP, Tierney AR, Wang J, et al. Magnitude of body-cell-mass depletion and the timing of death from wasting in AIDS. Am J Clin Nutr 1989;50:444–7.
28. Halliday AW, Benjamin IS, Blumgart LH. Nutritional risk factors in major hepatobiliary surgery. JPEN J Parenter Enteral Nutr 1988;12:43–8.
29. Lehr K, Schober O, Hundeshagen H, et al. Total body potassium depletion and the need for preoperative nutritional support in Crohn's disease. Ann Surg 1982;196:709–14.
30. Mann MD, Bowie MD, Hansen JD. Total body potassium and serum electrolyte concentrations in protein energy malnutrition. S Afr Med J 1975;49:76–8.
31. Fritz T, Hollwarth I, Romaschow M, et al. The predictive role of bioelectrical impedance analysis (BIA) in postoperative complications of cancer patients. Eur J Surg Oncol 1990;16:326–31.
32. Anderson CF, Wochos DN. The utility of serum albumin values in the nutritional assessment of hospitalized patients. Mayo Clin Proc 1982;57:181.
33. Reinhardt GF, Myscofski JW, Wilkens DB, et al. Incidence and mortality of hypoalbuminemic patients in hospitalized veterans. JPEN J Parenter Enteral Nutr 1980;4:357.
34. Apelgren KN, Rombeau JL, Twomey PL, et al. Comparison of nutritional indices and outcome in critically ill patients. Crit Care Med 1982;10:305.
35. Keys A, Brozek J, Henschel A, et al. The biology of human starvation. Minneapolis University of Minnesota Press; Minneapolis MS, 1950.

36. Russell DMcR, Prendergast PJ, Darby PL, et al. A comparison between muscle function and body composition in anorexia nervosa: the effect of refeeding. Am J Clin Nutr 1983;38:229–37.
37. Castenada C, Charnley JM, Evans WJ, et al. Elderly women accommodate to a low-protein diet with losses of body cell mass, muscle function, and immune response. Am J Clin Nutr 1995;62:30.
38. Cano N, Costanzo-Dufetel J, Calaf R, et al. Pre-albumin retinol binding protein-retinol complex in hemodialysis patients. Am J Clin Nutr 1988;47:664–7.
39. Hedlund JU, Hansson LO, Ortqvist AB. Hypoalbuminemia in hospitalized patients with community-acquired pneumonia. Arch Intern Med 1995;155:1438.
40. Feitelson M, Winkler MS, Gerrior SA, et al. Use of retinol-binding protein and pre-albumin as indicators of response to nutrition therapy. J Am Dent Assoc 1989;89: 684–7.
41. Jeejeebhoy KN, Baker JP, Wolman SL, et al. Critical evaluation of the role of clinical assessment and body composition studies in patients with malnutrition and after total parenteral nutrition. Am J Clin Nutr 1982;35(5 Suppl.):1117–27.
42. Baker J, Detsky AS, Wesson DE, et al. Nutritional assessment: a comparison of clinical judgment and objective measurements. N Engl J Med 1982;306:969–72.
43. Detsky AS, McLaughlin JR, Baker JP, et al. What is subjective global assessment of nutritional status? JPEN J Parenter Enteral Nutr 1987;11:8.
44. Detsky AS, Baker JP, Mendelson RA, et al. Evaluating the accuracy of nutritional assessment techniques applied to hospitalized patients: methodology and comparisons. JPEN J Parenter Enteral Nutr 1984;8:153.
45. Lennard-Jones JE, Arrowsmith H, Davison C, et al. Screening by nurses and junior doctors to detect malnutrition when patients are first assessed in hospital. Clin Nutr 1995;14:336–40.
46. Weekesa CE, Elia M, Emery PW. The development, validation and reliability of a nutrition screening tool based on the recommendations of the British Association for Parenteral and Enteral Nutrition (BAPEN) clinical nutrition. Clin Nutr 2004;23: 1104–12.
47. Guigos Y, Vallas BJ, Garry PJ. Mini nutritional assessment. In: BJ Vellas, Y Guigoz, Garry PJ, and Albarede JL, editors. a practical tool for grading the nutritional state of elderly patients. New York: Sprager; Facts Res Gerontol 1994;4(suppl2):15–59.
48. Kaiser MJ, Bauer JM, Ramsch C, et al, MNA-International Group. Validation of the Mini Nutritional Assessment Short-Form (MNA®-SF): a practical tool for identification of nutritional status. J Nutr Health Aging 2009;13:782–8.
49. Kondrup J, Rasmussen HH, Hamberg O, et al, Ad Hoc ESPEN Working Group. Nutritional Risk Screening (NRS 2002): a new method based on an analysis of controlled clinical trials. Clin Nutr 2003;22(3):321–36.
50. Stratton RJ, Hackston A, Longmore D, et al. Malnutrition in hospital outpatients and inpatients: prevalence, concurrent validity and ease of use of the 'Malnutrition Universal Screening Tool' ('MUST') for adults. Br J Nutr 2004;92:799–808.
51. Laporte M, Keller HH, Payette H, et al. Validity and reliability of the new Canadian Nutrition Screening Tool in the 'real-world' hospital setting. Eur J Clin Nutr 2015; 69:558–64.
52. Sheean PM, Peterson SJ, Chen Y, et al. Utilizing multiple methods to classify malnutrition among elderly patients admitted to medical and surgical intensive care units. Clin Nutr 2013;32(5):752–7.
53. Garrow JS. Total body potassium in kwashiorkor and marasmus. Lancet 1965;2: 455–8.

54. Montgomery RD. Magnesium metabolism in infantile protein malnutrition. Lancet 1960;2:74–6.
55. Garrow JS, Smith R, Ward EE. Electrolyte metabolism in severe infantile malnutrition. Oxford (United Kingdom): Pergamon Press; 1968. p. 56.
56. Brinkman GL, Bowie MD, Frus-Hansen B, et al. Body water composition in kwashiorkor before and after loss of edema. Pediatrics 1965;36:94–103.
57. Rudman D, Millikan WJ, Richardson TJ, et al. Elemental balances during intravenous hyperalimentation of underweight adult subjects. J Clin Invest 1975;33: 94–104.
58. Freeman JB. Magnesium requirements are increased during total parenteral nutrition. Surg Forum 1977;28:61–2.
59. Wolman SL, Anderson GH, Marliss EB, et al. Zinc in total parenteral nutrition. Requirements and metabolic effects. Gastroenterology 1979;76:458–67.
60. Cotzias GC. Role and importance of trace substances in environmental health. In: Hemphill DD, editor. Proceedings of the First Annual Conference on Trace Substances and Environmental Health, 1. Columbia (MO): University of Missouri; 1967. p. 5–19.
61. Finch CA, Hubers H. Perspectives in iron metabolism. N Engl J Med 1982;306: 1320–8.
62. Bush JA, Mahoney JP, Gubler CJ, et al. Studies on copper metabolism; transfer of radio-copper between erythrocytes and plasma. J Lab Clin Med 1936;47: 898–906.
63. Sternlieb I, Morell AG, Tucker WD, et al. The incorporation of copper into ceruloplasmin in vivo: studies with copper-64 and copper-67. J Clin Invest 1961;40: 1834–40.
64. Diplock AT. Metabolic and functional defects in selenium deficiency. Philos Trans R Soc Lond B Biol Sci 1981;294:105–17.
65. Prasad AS, Meftah S, Abdallah J, et al. Serum thymulin in human zinc deficiency. J Clin Invest 1988;82:1202–10.
66. Hambidge KM. Zinc deficiency in man: its origins and effects. Phil Trans R Soc Lond B Biol Sci 1981;294:129–44.
67. Osaki S, Johnson DA, Freiden E. The possible significance of the ferrous oxidase activity of ceruloplasmin in normal human serum. J Biol Chem 1966;241:2746–51.
68. Cordano A, Baertl JM, Graham GG. Copper deficiency in infancy. Pediatrics 1964;34:324–36.
69. Halsted JA, Hackley BM, Smith JC. Plasma zinc and copper in pregnancy and after oral contraceptives. Lancet 1968;2:278–9.
70. Burk RF. Molecular biology of selenium with implications for its metabolism. FASEB J 1991;5:2274–9.
71. Rotruck JT, Pope AL, Ganther HE, et al. Selenium: biochemical role as a component of glutathione peroxidase. Science 1973;179:588–90.
72. Horlick M. Vitamin D. In: Shike M, Ross C, Cabalerro B, et al, editors. Modern nutrition in health and disease. 10th edition. New York: Lippincott Williams & Wilkins; 2006. p. 376–95.
73. Horlick MF. Vitamin D deficiency. N Engl J Med 2007;357:266–81.

Enteral Access and Associated Complications

Mark H. DeLegge, MD[a,b],*

KEYWORDS

- Enteral access • Nutrition • Complications • Nasoenteric tubes • Gastrostomy tube
- Jejunostomy tube • Gastrojejunostomy

KEY POINTS

- Enteral access is the foundation for feeding in patients who are unable to meet their nutrition needs orally and have a functional gastrointestinal tract.
- Tubes can be placed through an orifice such as the mouth or the nose, or percutaneously into the stomach or proximal small intestine.
- Although there are a number of commonalities between the techniques used for placing tubes, there are also a number of considerable differences.

INTRODUCTION

Enteral access is the foundation for feeding in those patients who are unable to meet their nutrition needs orally and have a functional gastrointestinal tract. Enteral feeding (tube feeding) requires placement of a feeding tube. The tubes can be placed through an orifice such as the mouth or the nose, or percutaneously into the stomach or proximal small intestine. These tubes can be placed at the bedside or in specialized areas of the hospital, such as the endoscopy suite, operating room, or radiology department. Bedside tubes can be placed by the nurse or the physician, such as in the intensive care unit. Percutaneous feeding tubes are placed by the gastroenterologist, surgeon, or radiologist (**Table 1**). This article reviews the types of enteral access and the associated complications.

NASOENTERIC TUBES

Bedside nasoenteric tube placement is the most common enteral access technique used in the hospital setting. Either a nasogastric (NG) or nasojejunal (NJ) tube may be placed.

Disclosure: The author has nothing to disclose.
[a] Department of Medicine, Medical University of South Carolina, 25 Courtenay Street, Charleston, SC 29425, USA; [b] DeLegge Medical, 4057 Longmarsh Road, Awendaw, SC 29429, USA
* Department of Medicine, Medical University of South Carolina, 25 Courtenay Street, Charleston, SC 29425, USA
E-mail address: DrMark@deleggemedical.com

Gastroenterol Clin N Am 47 (2018) 23–37
https://doi.org/10.1016/j.gtc.2017.09.003
0889-8553/18/© 2017 Elsevier Inc. All rights reserved.

gastro.theclinics.com

Table 1
Enteral access procedures

Location	Oral	Nasal	Percutaneous
Gastric	Oral gastric tube	Nasal gastric tube	• Percutaneous endoscopic gastrostomy • Radiologic gastrostomy • Surgical gastrostomy
Gastrojejunal	Oral gastrojejunal tube	Nasal gastrojejunal tube	• Percutaneous endoscopic gastrojejunostomy • Radiologic gastrojejunostomy • Surgical gastrojejunostomy
Jejunal	Oral jejunal tube	Nasal jejunal tube	• Direct percutaneous endoscopic jejunostomy • Radiologic jejunostomy • Surgical jejunostomy

These tubes can also be placed orally if desired. There are many techniques available for passing bedside NG tubes. Typically, an 8 to 12-Fr NG tube is passed into the stomach after the tube has been lubricated, the head is flexed, and the patient ingests sips of water to assist in passing the tube into the stomach.[1] Many centers promote bedside auscultation of the abdomen or aspiration of gastric contents for confirmation of an adequate position of the NG tube before use. However, this process can be misleading, because inappropriate tube locations, such as in the lung, in the pleural cavity after perforation, or coiled in the esophagus may be misinterpreted as being in proper position by bedside auscultatory techniques. For this reason, every patient should have a radiograph to confirm proper position of a blindly placed bedside NG tube before initiating feedings.[2]

It is not unusual to be faced with a patient who is comatose and therefore unable to assist with the passage of an NG tube. In these instances, the tube can again be passed at the bedside after tube lubrication and head flexion. Auscultation of the abdominal cavity and a radiograph can confirm proper tube location. Patients with nasal or facial fractures may be more appropriate for orogastric tubes.

In general, placement of an NG tube is technically "easier" than placement of an NJ tube for the simple reason that the NG tube has to pass the esophagus and arrive in a gastric location, whereas an NJ tube must pass the esophagus and stomach, make its way through the pylorus, and end its journey in the jejunum. A number of techniques have been promoted for blind, bedside placement of an NJ tube. **Table 2** details some of these techniques that have been reported in the literature.

Table 2
Bedside nasal jejunal tube placement

Author	Technique
Thurlow,[3] 1986	Stiffen nasal jejunal tube with internal stylet and use corkscrew motion with advancement
Zaloga,[4] 1991	Thurlow technique with 90% success rate
Ugo et al,[5] 1992	Patient in right lateral decubitus position and tube position tracked with auscultation during advancement
Lord et al,[6] 1993	Use of unweighted nasal jejunal tubes associated with greater successful placement than weighted nasal jejunal tubes
Roubenoff & Ravich,[7] 1981	Advance tube to esophagus, get radiograph to ensure esophageal location before advancing into stomach or small bowel

There have been many attempts to position a tube beyond the pylorus with the use of pharmacologic agents. The results have been mixed. Selfert and colleagues[8] and Kittinger and colleagues[9] reported no benefit of the use of metoclopramide in assisting NJ tube placement.

In contrast, Whatley and colleagues[10] and Kalafarentzos and colleagues[11] noted a benefit of the use of metoclopramide for NJ tube placements with a reported success rate of up to 90%. There cannot be a definitive statement either for or against the use of pharmacologic agents to promote NJ tube passage.

More recently, technology has developed to allow passage of NG or NJ tubes at the bedside without the use of fluoroscopic visualization. These technologies vary, but include either an electromagnetic placement device (EMPD) or an optical imaging device that uses a very narrow caliber optic fiber placed through the NJ tube for visualization during placement. Some of these fiberoptic systems also allow minor mechanical directional movement of the tip of the feeding tube.

The EMPD device has the greatest body of literature. An electromagnetic signal from the distal tip creates an image on a receiver that allows interpretation by the technician to detect the direction of passage of the NJ tube through the esophagus and stomach, and into the small intestine.[12] This technology has reported good success rates with both physicians and nurses passing the NJ tube into a jejunal position. The technique has been approved by the US Food and Drug Administration for confirmation of the final tip position without the need for radiographic confirmation.[12] However, a recent review of the adverse medical device reports in the United States (MAUDE) with regard to EMPD has noted 54 adverse events between January 1, 2006, and February 29, 2016. Most events (98%) involved feeding tube placement into the lungs. Some of these misplacements resulted in death. When EMPD bedside tracings were reviewed, it was discovered that in 89% of the insertion image tracings, clinicians had failed to recognize lung placement.[13]

Failure to blindly pass an NJ tube at the bedside requires the use of fluoroscopic or endoscopic methods of passage. The preference of either technique depends on local health center care expertise. In those centers with available C-arm fluoroscopy and modified fluoroscopy beds, fluoroscopic passage of NJ tubes can be done at the patient's bedside. Success of fluoroscopic guidance of NJ tube passage can approach 100%.[14] However, in those institutions without bedside fluoroscopic capabilities, transport of patients to the radiology suite may be required. Hospital transport of patients—especially critically ill patients—can be time consuming, expensive, and hazardous.[15]

NG and NJ tube placement and use are associated with complications (**Box 1**).[16] In general, the longer these tubes remain in place the greater the risk of developing complications. These tubes can be uncomfortable after prolonged use and are cosmetically unappealing for the patient who is awake and alert. In general, nasoenteric tubes are believed to be recommended for enteral feeding that is going be required for 4 weeks or less.[17]

Endoscopic placement of NJ feeding tubes can be done at the bedside with conscious sedation. **Table 3** lists the techniques for bedside, endoscopic nasoenteric tube passage. These techniques are focused on directing the nasoenteric tube into a proximal jejunal position. These techniques require practice and familiarity with the techniques to ensure success. In general, any looping of the NJ tube remaining within the stomach after placement will result in ultimate migration of the NJ tube tip from the small bowel into the stomach.

The decision to use a jejunostomy tube also should warrant some very specific instructions regarding its care. The lumen of these tubes is much smaller than a gastric

---

Box 1
Complications associated with nasoenteric tube placement and use

Pharyngitis

Otitis media

Nasal mucosal ulceration

Sinusitis

Pneumothorax

Aspiration

Tracheoesophageal ulceration

Gastrointestinal ulceration

Data from Prabhakaran S, Doraiswamy VA, Nagaraja V, et al. Nasoenteric tube complications. Scan J Surg 2012;101:147–55.

---

tube and, therefore, is prone to clogging. Jejunal feeding tubes should never be checked for residual content because they are a poor indicator of residual content of the small bowel. In addition, checking residuals through these small bore tubes increases their probability of clogging. These tubes should be flushed after every tube feeding and medication instillation. Only liquid medications, or completely dissolved medications, should be placed through a jejunostomy tube to reduce the chances of tube occlusion.

PERCUTANEOUS GASTROSTOMY TUBE PLACEMENT

Gastrostomy tubes may be placed endoscopically, surgically, or radiologically. The choice of procedure depends on local resources and expertise, anatomic considerations that may affect the ability to place the tube endoscopically or radiologically (eg, inability to endoscopically identify an appropriate placement site because of prior surgery or obesity), and whether the patient is undergoing surgery for another reason

---

Table 3
Endoscopic techniques for nasoenteric tube placement

Author	Technique
Stark et al,[18] 1991	Suture on tip of the endoscope grabbed with forceps and nasal jejunal tube pulled into position
Patrick et al,[19] 1997	Guidewire placed through endoscope orally, exchanged to nasal position and nasal jejunal tube pushed over the guidewire with fluoroscopic or endoscopic visualization
Fang et al,[20] 2005	Guidewire passed through the nose with nasal endoscope and nasal jejunal tube placed over the guidewire under fluoroscopic guidance
Wiggins & DeLegge,[21] 2006	Nasal jejunal tube stiffened with guidewires and passed through the nose into small bowel under endoscopic visualization
Brandt & Mittendorf,[22] 1999	Small nasal jejunal tube passed through the working channel of the endoscope into the small bowel with subsequent nasal exchange

and operative gastrostomy can be performed in the operating room in combination with the primary surgical procedure.

Percutaneous Endoscopic Gastrostomy

Percutaneous endoscopic gastrostomy (PEG) was developed by Ponsky-Gauderer in the early 1980s. The procedure involves the placement of a percutaneous gastrostomy tube after endoscopic transillumination of the stomach for appropriate PEG access position. The use of prophylactic antibiotics before the procedure is important in the prevention of postprocedure infections.[23] Placement of a PEG tube may be by either the Sachs-Vine (push), Ponsky (pull) techniques, or by external dilation (Russell) technique[24] (**Table 4**). A decision to use either technique is simply a matter of physician preference and is usually based on how they were trained.[26]

Prospective evaluations of PEG tube placement have found this procedure to be associated with few major procedure-related complications. However, the most common intraprocedure complications are orotracheal aspiration during the endoscopic procedure and bowel perforation from inadvertent trocar access through the colon as the stomach is being accessed. Prevention of orotracheal aspiration includes attention to mouth and tracheal secretion suctioning during the procedure, head of the bed elevation, and avoidance of oversedation of the patient.[28] Inadvertent bowel perforation can be minimized by avoiding trocar access of the gastric cavity unless adequate endoscope light transillumination and finger palpation are present. Postprocedure complications are described in **Table 5**.[29]

Proper placement of the external bolster after PEG tube placement is critical. The bolster should be placed such that it allows 1 to 2 cm of "in-and-out" movement of the PEG tube into the stoma (**Fig. 1**). Looser apposition of the bolster to the abdominal wall does not result in peritoneal leakage, because an early gastrostomy tract forms as a result of tissue edema and associated tissue secretions.[30] If the tissue between the internal and external bolsters is compressed by placement of the external bolster too tightly against the abdominal wall, it may lead to tissue pressure necrosis, buried bumper syndrome, or breakdown of the gastrostomy tract (**Fig. 2**). **Table 6** lists brief treatment approaches to PEG postprocedure complications.

Surgical Gastrostomy

Surgical gastrostomy, or placement of a gastrostomy tube into the stomach using an operative procedure, was first developed by Stamm in the 1800s.[31] A standard feeding tube, such as a red rubber catheter, is placed during an open surgical procedure directly into the stomach. Alternatively, balloon gastrostomy replacement tubes may be used as the surgical gastrostomy tube (**Fig. 3**). Studies comparing surgical

Table 4 Methods of PEG placement	
PEG Procedure	**Description**
Ponsky pull[25]	After endoscopy, a PEG tube is pulled through the abdominal wall by an attached guidewire.
Sachs-Vine push[26]	After endoscopy, a PEG tube is pushed over a guidewire into position.
Russell external dilator[27]	After endoscopy, an external tract is dilated in the abdominal wall and a PEG tube is placed into the stomach.

Abbreviation: PEG, percutaneous endoscopic gastrostomy.

Table 5
PEG postprocedure complications

Complication	Description
Wound infection	Generally from skin and/or oral bacteria
Stomal leakage	Gastric and wound secretions around the tube
Peritonitis	Typically from gastric/abdominal wall stoma tract breakdown and leakage of enteral contents into the peritoneal cavity
Necrotizing fasciitis	Necrosis of the abdominal wall
Inadvertent tube removal	Usually from external traction on the tube
Tube occlusion	Medication or tube feeding
Tumor seeding	Generally oral or pharyngeal tumors seeding the abdominal wall
Buried bumper syndrome	Burrowing of the internal bolster into the gastric wall
Colocutaneous fistula	Inadvertent puncture of the colon with initial PEG tube placement (through and through injury of the colon)

Abbreviation: PEG, percutaneous endoscopic gastrostomy.
Modified from Rhanemai-Azar AA, Rhanemaiazar AA, Naghshizadian R, et al. Percutaneous endoscopic gastrostomy: Indications, technique, complications and management. World J Gastroenterol 2014;20:7743; with permission.

gastrostomy with PEG tubes have shown no difference in morbidity or mortality.[32] However, PEG is less expensive than surgical gastrostomy and has a reduced procedure time. Thus, surgical gastrostomy is typically reserved for patients who are already going to the operating room for another surgical procedure. In the 1990s, with the advent of laparoscopy, the surgical approach was modified to use laparoscopic techniques. In general, subsequent trials have not demonstrated an improvement in postoperative mortality or procedure time between an open and laparoscopic surgical gastrostomy. Postoperative morbidity has been reported as greater with laparoscopic gastrostomy as compared with open gastrostomy in one small series.[33]

Radiologic Gastrostomy

Placement of a gastrostomy tube under radiologic guidance was first described in 1983.[34] Radiology-inserted gastrostomy (RIG) tubes are placed using fluoroscopic

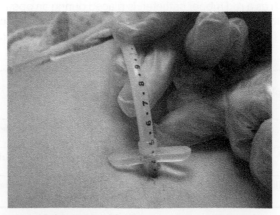

Fig. 1. Loose placement of the external bumper.

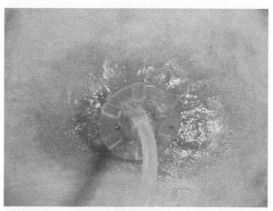

Fig. 2. Tissue damage from a tight external bolster.

or other imaging guidance. Radiologic insertion of a gastrostomy tube requires that the stomach first be distended with air, often with use of an NG tube. Once the stomach is insufflated, T-fasteners are placed into the stomach to secure the abdomen to the anterior gastric wall. This is known as gastropexy.[35] Gastropexy involves the use of between 2 and 4 T-fasteners. T-fasteners are delivered through a small trocar device into the stomach. Once in the stomach, the T-portion of the T-fastener rests against the gastric mucosa. Gentle traction is applied to the T-fastener sutures at the abdominal wall skin surface to approximate the stomach to the abdominal wall. Gastropexy reduces the risk of initial peritoneal catheterization and gastric leakage into the peritoneal cavity.[36] A trocar and guidewire are subsequently placed into the stomach between the T-fasteners. The trocar is removed and the guidewire is left in place. Dilators are placed over the guidewire to create a stomal tract. A feeding tube, sometimes with an inflatable internal bolster, is passed over the guidewire into position in

Table 6	
PEG postprocedure complication management	
Complication	**Description**
Wound infection	Antibiotic or antifungal
Stomal leakage	Skin protectant barrier cream. Severe leakage requires PEG tube removal and placement at a new site.
Peritonitis	Antibiotics and abdominal surgery.
Necrotizing fasciitis	Antibiotics and emergent surgery.
Inadvertent tube removal	Replacement of a new PEG tube and confirmation of location of internal PEG tube tip position. Often can use original PG tube placement site.
Tube occlusion	Warm water syringe injection or mechanical device tube cleaning.
Tumor seeding	Surgical and oncology consult.
Buried bumper syndrome	Remove PEG tube and place new PEG tube. Often can use original PEG tube placement site.
Colocutaneous fistula	Allow stomal tract to completely heal (at least 1 mo) and remove PEG tube or surgery.

Abbreviation: PEG, percutaneous endoscopic gastrostomy.

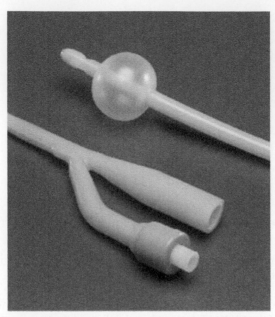

Fig. 3. Balloon gastrostomy tube.

the stomach. The guidewire is removed. Contrast material is injected to confirm correct tube placement. An alternative to this procedure is the placement of a guidewire through a trocar passed into an insufflated stomach, which is guided retrograde up the esophagus to the pharynx, where it is captured and pulled out of the mouth. The gastrostomy tube is attached to the guidewire at the mouth. The guidewire at the abdominal skin surface is pulled moving the gastrostomy tube into position in a technique similar to the 'pull" PEG endoscopic procedure. A standard "PEG" gastrostomy tube with a distensible internal bolster can be used. These gastrostomy tubes are not susceptible to internal bolster balloon deflation and inadvertent dislodgement as seen with balloon internal bolster gastrostomy tubes.

Whether there is a difference in morbidity and between endoscopic and radiologic gastrostomy tube placement is not clear. A metaanalysis comparing surgical with PEG and RIG tubes noted worse outcomes with surgical gastrostomy and a higher success rate and lower complication rate of RIG tubes compared with PEG tubes.[37] However, the radiology group in this metaanalysis was younger and had less neurologic disease. A 2010 prospective study comparing RIG tubes with PEG tubes noted similar 30-day and 1-year mortality rates.[38]

Gastrostomy tube dislodgement is the most common associated complication seen with RIG tubes. Tube dislodgment is one of the leading causes for repeat intervention. One report found that 46 of 83 repeat procedures (55%) were for tube dislodgment.[39] Catheter occlusion requiring tube replacement is also a common complication as often RIG tubes are of smaller diameter than PEG tubes.

PERCUTANEOUS JEJUNOSTOMY TUBE PLACEMENT
Direct Percutaneous Endoscopic Jejunostomy

Direct percutaneous jejunostomy (DPEJ) is the placement of a commercially available PEG tube into the small bowel (jejunum) for jejunal feeding. Compared with PEG jejunal tube (PEG/J), the DPEJ tube is larger (18–24 Fr) and less likely to clog and become displaced as compared with the smaller jejunostomy tube used commonly in PEG/J (9–12 Fr).[40] This procedure can be done in the endoscopy suite under moderate or deep sedation. The original DPEJ technique was first described by Shike and colleagues[41] more than 20 years ago. It is considerably more technically challenging than PEG insertion. The key to DPEJ placement is successful endoscopic intubation of a suitable superficial loop of the jejunum. The chosen jejunal loop should allow adequate transillumination and digital indentation, because this condition minimizes the risk of inadvertently puncturing other loops of bowel that may be interspersed between the chosen jejunal loop and the abdominal wall.[42]

The technique commonly used in DPEJ includes the use of a "seeker needle." A 19 or 20-G needle is passed into the small bowel lumen after an appropriate insertion site is identified on the abdominal wall with the use of transillumination and finger palpation.[43] An antiperistaltic agent is given to reduce small bowel motility. Often a pediatric colonoscope is used to reach the appropriate jejunal position. Once the seeker needle is in the small bowel, it is snared. This maneuver traps the small bowel from being pushed aside when trocar access is initiated. Once the trocar is in the small bowel, the snare is removed from the seeker needle and placed around the trocar (**Fig. 4**). From this point a standard pull PEG (now DPEJ) procedure is used to place the feeding tube directly into the small bowel.[44] The use of a double balloon enteroscope has been reported successful in DPEJ placement with reported improved endoscope and small bowel control as compared with the use of a standard endoscope or colonoscope.[45]

The complications of DPEJ are similar to PEG with one exception of a reported small bowel volvulus occurring after DPEJ placement.[46]

Surgical Jejunostomy

Surgical jejunostomy is an operative procedure in which a tube is placed into the lumen of the proximal jejunum. The first person to accomplish this procedure was Bush in 1858 in a patient with a nonoperable cancer.[47] In 1891, Witzel first described the most well known technique for jejunostomy, which has subsequently undergone a number of modifications.[48]

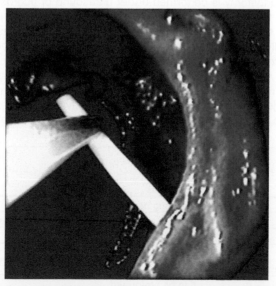

Fig. 4. Trocar placed into the small bowel for direct percutaneous endoscopic jejunostomy.

The decision to place an operative jejunostomy follows the same decision analysis as the decision to place any jejunal feeding tube. Typically, patients who are intolerant to gastric feedings or patients in whom the stomach is either diseased or surgically absent will receive a surgical jejunostomy. Surgical jejunostomy is also a common procedure in trauma patients. In a review by Meyers and colleagues,[49] patients received surgical jejunostomies as an additional technique during major abdominal surgery in 95% of cases and as the sole surgical technique in 5% of cases. Approximately 20% of the major abdominal surgical cases were trauma related.

In the standard operative jejunostomy, a transverse celiotomy is performed and a jejunal loop is identified. A purse string suture is placed in the jejunal loop and a small enterostomy is made. This enterostomy–purse string suture is subsequently attached to the abdominal wall and an 8 to 12-Fr silicone or rubber catheter is inserted through the abdominal wall and into the jejunum. A modification of this procedure is a needle catheter jejunostomy. This procedure involves the placement of a 5 or 7-Fr catheter into the jejunum via a submucosal tunnel. It was hypothesized that this technique would have fewer complications compared with standard jejunostomy because the entrance to the jejunum was much smaller in comparison. However, the small size of the tube was subsequently found to result in frequent tube occlusion and dislodgement.[50]

Holmes and colleagues[51] reported a complication rate of 10% and a mortality rate of 1.4% in trauma patients receiving a surgical jejunostomy directly related to the procedure. Complications of surgical jejunostomy are noted in **Table 7**.

Radiologic Jejunostomy

Radiology-inserted jejunal access under image guidance can be obtained by direct puncture of the jejunum or by access of the jejunum through a gastrostomy site. Jejunal access through a gastrostomy site involves the same gastric access procedure to perform RIG tube insertion. However, the tube passed into the stomach is guided down into the small bowel resulting in a jejunal feeding tube tip location. Direct radiologic percutaneous jejunostomy is more difficult than gastrostomy (RIG tube) techniques. Direct jejunostomy is performed under ultrasound or fluoroscopic guidance, using an NJ tube to distend the jejunum. The jejunal loop is punctured using a Cope suture anchor for small bowel stabilization. Water-soluble contrast material is injected through the needle to document an intraluminal position, and an anchor is inserted. With the guidewire in place, the track is dilated and a 10-Fr pigtail catheter is inserted into the jejunum. Antiperistaltic agents can also be used to assist safe jejunal puncture.[52] The most important complication of percutaneous jejunostomy is inadvertent placement of the jejunostomy tube into the peritoneal cavity or intraperitoneal leakage, which can cause peritonitis and death. Intraperitoneal leakage may be caused by

Table 7 Complications of surgical jejunostomy	
Complications	**Comments**
Wound infection	Including necrotizing fasciitis
Bleeding	Intraperitoneal, intraabdominal wall or at the skin surface
Intraperitoneal leakage	Often with peritonitis
Volvulus	Small bowel torsion
Tube dislodgement	Tube falls out of jejunal stoma site
Ileus	Can be prolonged

catheter malposition or early dislodgment, but may also be caused by pericatheter leakage if the small bowel does not adhere to the abdominal wall after placement. Reports of intraperitoneal leakage have ranged from 2% to 13%.[53]

PERCUTANEOUS ENDOSCOPIC GASTROJEJUNOSTOMY AND JEJUNOSTOMY PLACEMENT
Percutaneous Endoscopic Gastrojejunostomy and Jejunostomy

The first use of a jejunal extension tube placed through a PEG was reported by Ponsky and Aszodi in 1984.[54] In this procedure, a jejunal feeding tube is placed through an existing PEG tube. The literature has a number of names for this tube system, but the most common used are PEG/J or jejunal extension tube through a PEG. In general, these are 2-piece systems consisting of a PEG tube with a separate jejunostomy tube threaded through the PEG tube down into the small intestine. The jejunal tube is of smaller diameter than the PEG tube. This allows feeding through the jejunostomy tube through 1 port and suction through the PEG tube using a second port (**Fig. 5**). A modification of this design is that some PEG/J tubes are of a single tube construction (the G portion and J portion are molded together). The feeding tube is placed through the gastrostomy site on the abdominal wall with the feeding end of the tube in the small bowel. These tubes system generally do not allow suctioning of the stomach, but do allow feeding into the small intestine. There are a number of endoscopic placement techniques for PEG/J that have been described in the literature (**Table 8**).

A retrospective analysis compared feeding tube outcomes in patients receiving PEG/J or DPEJ.[40] The DPEJ patient population has significantly fewer reinterventions (endoscopic, surgical, bedside) than the PEG/J group. More recently, another retrospective analysis compared DPEJ and PEG/J with regard to procedure success rate and clinical outcomes.[59] PEG/J had a higher success rate of completion. Short- and long-term complications noted only a difference in dislocation of the jejunostomy tube, which was higher in the PEG/J patient group. The average duration of the jejunostomy tube was 272 ± 414 days in the DPEJ.

Surgical Gastrojejunostomy

In general, G/J feeding tubes are infrequently placed in the operating room unless the patient is in the operating room for another surgical procedure. The gastrostomy tube is placed as described in the surgical gastrostomy section. Subsequently, a jejunal

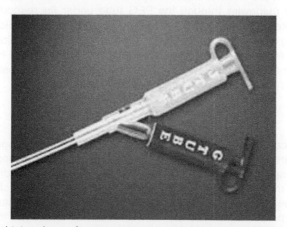

Fig. 5. Gastric and jejunal port for percutaneous endoscopic gastrojejunostomy.

Table 8
Methods of percutaneous endoscopic gastrojejunostomy placement

Technique	Description
Pediatric colonoscope guidewire method[55]	A guidewire passed through the PEG is grasped and pulled into the small bowel. The J tube passed over the guidewire.
Ultrathin endoscope guidewire method[56]	Ultrathin endoscopy of a PEG tube into the small bowel. The guidewire is passed through the endoscope. The endoscope is removed and the jejunal tube is passed over guidewire.
Through the gastrostomy guidewire method[57]	PEG tube removed 4 weeks after placement. A guidewire is passed through the gastrostomy site into the small bowel. One piece of the percutaneous endoscopic gastrojejunostomy is threaded over the guidewire into the small bowel.
PEG tube guidance method[58]	Peg tube internal bolster placed over the pylorus. The J tube is pushed through the PEG into the small bowel and locked into the PEG tube. The PEG tube is pulled back so the internal bolster is resting against the gastric mucosa.

Abbreviations: J, jejunostomy; PEG, percutaneous endoscopic gastrostomy.

tube is handfed down into the small bowel through the gastrostomy tube during an open abdominal procedure. Alternatively, after the gastrostomy tube is placed operatively, a jejunal tube can be threaded through the gastrostomy tube into the small bowel using fluoroscopy. Commercially, a 1-piece gastrojejunal tube is sold. This 1-piece G/J tube can be placed through a surgical gastrostomy site into the small bowel by either direct hand manipulation during an open procedure or by using fluoroscopy.

Radiologic Gastrojejunostomy

Fluoroscopy can be used to place a G/J feeding tube.[60] To place a G/J feeding tube, a puncture of the stomach by an access needle is first performed with attempts to direct the needle, and ultimately the feeding tube, to face toward the pylorus as opposed to antrum of the stomach. This makes passage of a jejunal tube through the gastrostomy easier. Subsequently, a gastropexy is performed and a gastrostomy tube is placed. A stiff catheter or metal cannula is advanced through the gastrostomy tube into the small bowel. A guidewire is placed through the catheter or cannula. The jejunostomy tube is placed over the guidewire through the PEG tube under fluoroscopic guidance. A recent report noted good longevity of G/J feeding tubes placed radiologically with a mean functioning time of 28 ± 10 months.[61] This series did note 2 major complications in the 5 patients reported; a colocutaneous fistula and a migration of the gastrostomy tube internal bumper through the pylorus resulting in gastric outlet obstruction, bezoar formation and a requirement for a surgical intervention.

SUMMARY

Enteral access can be provided by either the endoscopist, radiologist, or surgeon. Although there are a number of commonalities between the techniques used by these various medical specialties, there are also a number of considerable differences. Even within the same medical specialty, there are considerable technical choices of how a procedure can be performed; for example, with a PEG/J. The physician performing an enteral access procedure should be familiar with the technique they know well, including the potential complications and their resolution.

REFERENCES

1. Fan L, Liu Q, Gui L. Efficacy of non-swallow nasogastric tube intubation: a randomized controlled trial. J Clin Nurs 2016;21–22:3326–32.
2. Bennetzen LV, Hakonsen SJ, Svenningsen H, et al. Diagnostic accuracy of methods to verify nasogastric tube position in mechanically ventilated adult patients: a systematic review. JBI Database System Rev Implement Rep 2015;13:188–223.
3. Thurlow PM. Bedside enteral feeding tube placement into duodenum and jejunum. JPEN J Parenter Enteral Nutr 1986;10(1):104–5.
4. Zaloga GP. Bedside method for placing small bowel feeding tubes in critically ill patients. Chest 1991;100:1643–6.
5. Ugo PJ, Mohler PA, Wilson GL. Bedside post-pyloric placement of weighted feeding tubes. Nutr Clin Pract 1992;7:284–7.
6. Lord LM, Weiser-Mamone A, Pulhamus M, et al. Comparison of weighted vs unweighted enteral feeding tubes for efficacy or transpyloric passage. JPEN 1993;17:271–3.
7. Roubenoff R, Ravich WJ. The technique of avoiding feeding tube misplacement. J Crit Illness 1989;4:75–9.
8. Selfert CS, Cuddy PG, Pemberton B, et al. A randomized trial of metoclopramide's effect on the transpyloric intubation of weighted feeding tubes. Nutr Supp Serv 1987;11:11–3.
9. Kittinger JM, Sandler RS, Heizer W. Efficacy of metoclopramide as an adjunct to duodenal placement of small-bore feeding tubes: a randomized, placebo controlled, double-blind study. JPEN 1987;11:33–7.
10. Whatley K, Turner WW Jr, Dey M, et al. When does metoclopramide facilitate transpyloric intubation? JPEN 1984;8:679–81.
11. Kalafarentzos F, Alivizatos V, Panagopoulos K, et al. Nasoduodenal intubation with the use of metoclopramide. Nutr Supp Sev 1987;7:33–4.
12. Powers J, Luebbenhusen M, Spitzer T, et al. Verification of an electromagnetic placement device compared with abdominal radiograph to predict accuracy of feeding tube placement. J Parent Enteral Nut 2011;35:535–9.
13. Bourgalt AM, Aguirre L, Ibrahim J. Comprehensive review of adverse events in the Maude database. Am J Crit Care 2017;26:149–56.
14. Baskin WN, Johansen JF. An improved approach to the delivery of enteral nutrition in the intensive care unit. Gastrointest Endosc 1995;42:161–5.
15. Beckmann U, Gillies DM, Berenholtz SM, et al. Incidents related to intra-hospital transfer of critically ill patients. Intensive Care Med 2005;30:1579–85.
16. Prabhakaran S, Doraiswamy VA, Nagaraja V, et al. Nasoenteric tube complications. Scan J Surg 2012;101:147–55.
17. Delegge MH. Enteral access – the foundation of feeding. J Parenter Enteral Nutr 2001;25(suppl 2):S8–14.
18. Stark SP, Sharpe JN, Larson JM. Endoscopically placed nasoenteral feeding tubes: indications and techniques. Am Surg 1991;57:203–5.
19. Patrick PG, Marulenmdra S, Kirby DF, et al. Endoscopic naso-gastric-jejunal feeding tube placement in critically ill patients. Gastrointest Endosc 1997;45:72–6.
20. Fang JC, Hilden K, Holubkov R, et al. Transnasal endoscopy vs fluoroscopy for the placement of nasoenteric feeding tubes in critically ill patients. Gastrointest Endosc 2005;62:661–6.

21. Wiggins TF, DeLegge MH. Evaluation of a new technique for endoscopic nasoenteric feeding-tube placement. Gastrointest Endosc 2006;63:590–5.
22. Brandt CP, Mittendorf EA. Endoscopic placement of nasojejunal feeding tubes in ICU patients. Surg Endosc 1999;12:1211–4.
23. Jafri NS, Mahid SS, Minor KS, et al. Meta-analysis: antibiotic prophylaxis to prevent peristomal infection following percutaneous endoscopic gastrostomy. Aliment Pharmacol Therap 2006;25:647–56.
24. Gauderer MW. Percutaneous endoscopic gastrostomy – 20 years later: a historical perspective. J Pediatr Surg 2001;36:217–9.
25. Gauderer MW, Ponsky JL, Izant RJ. Gastrostomy without laparotomy: a percutaneous endoscopic technique. J Pediatr Surg 1980;15:872–5.
26. Hogan RB, DeMarco DC, Hamilton JK, et al. Percutaneous endoscopic gastrostomy-to push or to pull: a prospective, randomized trial. Gastrointest Endosc 1986;32:253–8.
27. Russell TR, Brotman M, Norris F. Percutaneous gastrostomy. A new simplified and cost-effective technique. Am J Surg 1984;148:132–7.
28. Johnston SD, Tham TCK, Mason M. Death after PEG: results of the national confidential enquiry int0 patient outcome and death. Gastrointest Endosc 2008;68: 223–7.
29. Rhanemai-Azar AA, Rhanemaiazar AA, Naghshizadian R, et al. Percutaneous endoscopic gastrostomy: indications, technique, complications and management. World J Gastroenterol 2014;20:7739–51.
30. McClave SA, Neff RL. Care and long-term maintenance of percutaneous endoscopic gastrostomy tubes. JPEN J Parenter Enteral Nutr 2006;30(1 Suppl): S27–38.
31. Meyers JG, Page CP, Stewart RM. Atlas of nutrition support techniques. Boston: Little Brown; 1989. p. 167–74.
32. Steigman GV, Goff JS, Silas D, et al. Endoscopic versus operative gastrostomy: final results of a prospective, randomized trial. Gastrointest Endosc 1990;36:1–5.
33. Bankhead RG, Fisher CA, Rolandelli RH. Gastrostomy tube placement outcomes. Comparison of surgical, endoscopic and laparoscopic methods. Nutr Clin Pract 2005;20:2005–12.
34. Sacks BA, Vine HS, Palestrant AM, et al. A non-operative technique for establishment of a gastrostomy in the dog. Invest Radiol 1983;18:485–7.
35. Saini S, Mueller PR, Gaa J, et al. Percutaneous gastrostomy with gastropexy: experience in 125 patients. Am J Roentgenol 1990;154:1003–6.
36. Thornton FJ, Fotheringham T, Haslam PJ, et al. Percutaneous radiological gastrostomy with and without T-fastener gastropexy: a randomised comparison study. Cardiovasc Intervent Radiol 2002;25:467–71.
37. Wollman BD'Agosino HB, Walus –Wigle JR, Easter DW, et al. Radiologic, endoscopic and surgical gastrostomy: an institutional evaluation and meta-analysis of the literature. Radiology 1995;197:699–704.
38. Leeds JS, McAlindon ME, Grant J, et al. Survival analysis after gastrostomy: a single-centre observational study comparing radiological and endoscopic insertion. Eur J Gastroenterol Hepatol 2010;22:591–6.
39. Dewald CL, Hiette PO, Sewall LE, et al. Percutaneous gastrostomy and gastrojejunostomy with gastropexy; experience in 701 procedures. Radiology 1999;211: 651–6.
40. Fan AC, Baron TH, Rumalla A, et al. Comparison of direct percutaneous endoscopic jejunostomy and PEG with jejunal extension. Gastrointest Endosc 2002; 56:890–4.

41. Shike M, Schroy P, Ritchie MA, et al. Percutaneous endoscopic jejunostomy in cancer patients with previous gastric resection. Gastrointest Endosc 1987;33: 372–4.

42. Baron TH. Direct percutaneous endoscopic jejunostomy. Am J Gastroenterol 2006;101:1407–9.

43. Varadarajulu S, DeLegge MH. Use of a 19-guage injection needle as a guide for direct jejunostomy tube placement. Gastrointest Endosc 2003;57:942–5.

44. Zhu Y, Shi L, Tang H, et al. Current considerations in direct percutaneous jejunostomy. Can J Gastroenterol 2012;26:92–6.

45. Despott EJ, Gabe S, Tripoli E, et al. Enteral access by double balloon enteroscopy: an alternative method of direct percutaneous endoscopic jejunostomy placement. Dig Dis Sci 2011;56:494–8.

46. Maple JT, Petersen BT, Baron TH, et al. Direct percutaneous endoscopic jejunostomy: outcomes in 307 consecutive attempts. Am J Gastroenterol 2005;100: 2681–8.

47. Gerndt SJ, Orringer MB. Tube jejunostomy as an adjunct to esophagectomy. Surgery 1994;115:164–9.

48. Rombeau JL, Caldwell MD, Forlaw L, et al. Atlas of nutrition support techniques. Boston: Little Brown; 1989. p. 167–74.

49. Meyers JG, Page CP, Stewart RM, et al. Complications of needle catheter jejunostomy in 2022 consecutive applications. Am J Surg 1995;170:547–50.

50. Haun JL, Thompson JS. Comparison of needle catheter versus standard jejunostomy. Am Surg 1985;55:466–9.

51. Holmes JH, Brundage SI, Yeun PC, et al. Complications of surgical feeding jejunostomy in trauma patients. J Trauma 1999;47:1009–12.

52. van Overhagen H, Schipper J. Percutaneous jejunostomy. Semin Intervent Radiol 2004;21:199–204.

53. Yang ZQ, Shin JH, Song HY, et al. Fluoroscopically guided direct percutaneous jejunostomy: outcomes in 25 consecutive patients. Clin Radiol 2007;62:1061–5.

54. Ponsky JL, Aszodi A. Percutaneous endoscopic jejunostomy. Am J Gastroenterol 1984;79:113–6.

55. DeLegge MH, Patrick PG, Gibbs R. Percutaneous endoscopic gastrojejunostomy with a tapered tip, unweighted jejunal feeding tube: improved placement success. Am J Gastro 1996;91:1130–4.

56. Berger WL, Shaker R, Dean RS. Percutaneous endoscopic gastrojejunal tube placement. Gastrointest Endosc 1996;43:63–6.

57. Adler DG, Gostout CJ, Baron TH. Percutaneous transgastric placement of jejunal feeding tubes with an ultrathin endoscope. Gastrointest Endosc 2002;55:106–10.

58. Sibille A, Glorieux D, Fauville J-P, et al. An easier method for percutaneous endoscopic gastrojejunostomy tube placement. Gastrointest Endosc 1998;48:514–7.

59. Zopf Y, Rabe C, Bruckmoser T, et al. Percutaneous endoscopic jejunostomy and jejunal extension tube through percutaneous endoscopic gastrostomy; a retrospective analysis of success, complications and outcome. Digestion 2009;79: 92–7.

60. Alzate GD, Coons HG, Elliott J, et al. Percutaneous gastrostomy for jejunal feeding: a new technique. AJR Am J Roentgenol 1986;147:822–5.

61. Santos-Antunes J, Corte-Real Nunes A, Jose Rosas M, et al. First long-term prospective case series of percutaneous endoscopic gastrostomy with jejunal extension for drug administration. Acta Gastroenterol Belg 2016;79:511–2.

Parenteral Nutrition
Indications, Access, and Complications

Brian M. Lappas, MD, MPH[a], Dhyanesh Patel, MD[b], Vanessa Kumpf, PharmD, BCNSP[b],
Dawn Wiese Adams, MD, MS[b], Douglas L. Seidner, MD[b],*

KEYWORDS

- Parental nutrition • Intestinal failure • Malnutrition • Central venous catheter
- Complications

KEY POINTS

- Parenteral nutrition (PN) is indicated in patients who are malnourished and have intestinal failure.
- Initiation and monitoring of PN is best done by a multidisciplinary team composed of physicians, nutritionists, pharmacists, and nurses who are specially trained in PN prescribing and compounding methods.
- Tunneled central venous catheters are the preferred access for delivery of long-term PN.
- Patients on PN need close monitoring to reduce the risk of thromboembolic, infectious, and metabolic complications.

INTRODUCTION

Parenteral nutrition (PN) is a mixture of solutions that include dextrose, amino acids, electrolytes, vitamins, minerals, trace elements, and lipid emulsions. The formulation is delivered via a catheter device placed directly into the venous system of patients with intestinal failure. The modern PN was clinically implemented in the 1960s, with a recent study estimating that approximately 25,000 patients receive home PN (HPN) in the United States.[1] This article reviews the indications and complications of PN and discusses the various types and indications for devices.

Disclosure: The authors have nothing to disclose.
[a] Department of Internal Medicine, Vanderbilt University Medical Center, Nashville, TN, USA;
[b] Division of Gastroenterology, Hepatology and Nutrition, Vanderbilt University Medical Center, Nashville, TN, USA
* Corresponding author. Division of Gastroenterology, Hepatology and Nutrition, Vanderbilt University Medical Center, 1211 21st Avenue South, 514 Medical Arts Building, Nashville, TN 37232.
E-mail address: Douglas.seidner@vanderbilt.edu

Gastroenterol Clin N Am 47 (2018) 39–59
https://doi.org/10.1016/j.gtc.2017.10.001
0889-8553/18/© 2017 Elsevier Inc. All rights reserved.

PARENTERAL NUTRITION INDICATIONS

PN is indicated in patients who are malnourished and cannot tolerate enteral nutrition (EN). Malnutrition is defined as "an acute, subacute or chronic state of nutrition, in which a combination of varying degrees of over nutrition or under nutrition with or without inflammatory activity have led to a change in body composition and diminished function."[2] The European Society for Clinical Nutrition and Metabolism (ESPEN) released a consensus statement in 2015 further defining malnutrition as either a body mass index (BMI) less than or equal to 18.5 kg/m^2 or the combined findings of weight loss greater than 10% of habitual weight, greater than 5% over 3 months, and 1 of the following: (1) reduced BMI less than 20 kg/m^2, or less than 22 kg/m^2 in adults older than 70 years; or (2) reduced fat-free mass index, of less than 15 kg/m^2 in females or less than <17 kg/m^2 in men.[3]

Malnutrition may be from starvation or an acute or chronic disease state. The inflammatory response in acute disease or injury may cause high cytokine levels resulting in metabolic alterations; specifically, increased energy expenditure, muscle catabolism, fluid shifts, and hyperglycemia. All patients being admitted to the hospital or diagnosed with a chronic disease should be assessed for malnutrition risk and severity. The assessment should consider factors such as weight loss, muscle loss, subcutaneous fat loss, diminished hand-grip strength or another measure of functional status, visceral protein levels, albumin and/or prealbumin levels, and inflammatory markers such as C-reactive protein and/or interleukin-6 (IL-6). Multiple assessment tools have been validated to classify patients into low-risk and high-risk malnutrition groups, such as the Nutritional Risk Screening (NRS 2002) and Nutrition Risk in the Critically Ill (NUTRIC) score.

The NRS 2002 tool was developed from the retrospective review of 128 randomized controlled trials (RCTs) of hospitalized patients who were at risk for malnutrition.[4] Patients were included if they had at least 1 of the following: BMI less than 20.5 kg/m^2, weight loss within the last 3 months, reduced dietary intake during the last week, or severe illness. The degree of weight loss, impaired food intake, and severity of disease were all used to create a scale of 0 to 10 points. Patients were then classified into a high-risk group (score $\geq$3) that would benefit from supplemental nutrition.

The NUTRIC score was validated by a prospective, observational study in Europe of 597 patients in the intensive care unit (ICU) to classify critically ill patients into a low-risk or high-risk malnutrition group.[5] The NUTRIC score includes age, Acute Physiology And Chronic Health Evaluation (APACHE II) score, Sequential Organ Failure Assessment (SOFA) score, number of comorbidities, days from hospital admission, and IL-6 level. Score greater than or equal to 5 (without using IL-6) was associated with increased mortality and longer ventilation times and patients with those scores were most likely to benefit from aggressive nutrition therapy including PN.

Patients who are identified at high risk should be started on a nutrition care plan under the direction of a certified nutrition specialist who will assess enteral or parenteral supplementation. EN is always preferred to PN unless there is a contraindication to its use. Absolute contraindications to EN include bowel trauma, intestinal obstruction, active gastrointestinal hemorrhage, and ischemic bowel with hemodynamic instability. Other conditions that may limit EN include gastrointestinal inflammation or infection, severe malabsorption, and small bowel fistulas. If PN is used, the nutrition team should reassess the patient at regular intervals to consider initiating EN and oral feeding when clinically appropriate. PN can usually be discontinued when at least 60% of the patient's nutrition needs are met via EN or oral feeding.[6]

Patients who require PN may be classified as having intestinal failure. This term was recently redefined by ESPEN as "the reduction of gut function below the minimum necessary for the absorption of macronutrients and/or water and electrolytes, such that intravenous supplementation is required to maintain health and/or growth."[7] Intestinal failure can be grouped into 3 different classification schemes: functional, pathophysiologic, and clinical. The functional classification includes types I, II, and III based on the onset, metabolic, and expected outcomes of the illness (**Box 1**). There are 5 different groups in the pathophysiologic classification of intestinal failure: short bowel, intestinal fistula, intestinal dysmotility, mechanical obstruction, and extensive small bowel mucosal disease. Diseases within pathophysiologic classifications can shift between functional types over the course of an illness. The clinical classification scheme stratifies patients into one of 16 groups based on the average daily parenteral fluid (<1 L, 1–2 L, 2–3 L, and >3 L) and energy (0 kcal, 1–10 kcal, 11–20 kcal, >20 kcal) requirements to sustain health. The rationale for these classification schemes is to improve the categorization of patients recruited for clinical trials, standardize language, and to guide effective diagnosis and therapy with respect to individual patients. The designation of a subtype may not influence the decision to initiate PN but may provide a framework for the patient's long-term needs and potential complications.

Acute Disease Indications

Critically ill patients

Optimizing overall nutrition improves morbidity and mortality in critically ill patients, patients with trauma, and surgical patients.[6] Critically ill patients are inherently at greater risk for malnutrition given the increased hypermetabolic or catabolic state. These patients should be evaluated with a malnutrition screening tool. As previously discussed, the NRS 2002 and NUTRIC scores have been validated in the critically ill population and stratify patients into high-risk and low-risk groups for the development of complications associated with malnutrition.[5,8]

PN is only indicated when the enteral route fails or cannot be safely accessed to meet daily nutritional requirements. Early EN, which is defined as the initiation of EN within 24 to 48 hours of ICU admission, has been shown to decrease the risk of infectious complications and ICU length of stay, although few studies have shown differences in mortality.[6,9] Early RCTs indicated a mortality benefit between early EN

Box 1
Summary of intestinal failure by functional and pathophysiologic definition

Intestinal failure by functional type:

- Type I
  - Acute and short-term. Usually self-limiting condition. Often seen in perioperative setting, abdominal surgery, or critical illness requiring PN for days to weeks.

- Type II
  - Prolonged acute condition causing metabolic unstable patients. Requires PN over weeks to months. Often seen in intra-abdominal catastrophe (eg, mesenteric ischemia, volvulus, trauma) with massive enterectomy and often a need for enterocutaneous fistula.

- Type III
  - Chronic condition in metabolic stable patients, requiring PN more than months to years. May be reversible of irreversible and often seen in short bowel syndrome, radiation enteritis, or malignancy.

Data from Pironi L, Arends J, Bozzetti F, et al. ESPEN guidelines on chronic intestinal failure in adults. Clin Nutr 2016;35(2):247–307.

compared with early PN in the critically ill.[10] This finding may have been affected by excessive caloric delivery in the PN groups (>40 kcal/kg/d) and permissive hyperglycemia. Several other RCTs have shown no mortality difference between EN and PN when the caloric intake was reduced to 15 to 28 kcal/kg (approximating energy expenditure) and tighter glucose control was maintained[11–13] A large meta-analysis in 2016 evaluated 18 RCTs of critically ill patients found no difference in mortality (relative risk [RR] 1.04; 95% confidence interval [CI], 0.82–1.33; $P = .75$).[14] The meta-analysis also confirmed an overall decrease in infectious complications when including all 11 trials that followed mortality (RR 0.64; 95% CI, 0.48–0.87; $P = .004$). A subgroup analysis found no difference in infectious complications when the caloric delivery was similar between EN and PN groups.

"One multicenter RCT showed that ICU patients with an absolute contraindication to EN, who were started on PN on day 3 were less likely to be discharged alive than those started on day 8".[15] Therefore, PN should be withheld for the first 7 days in patients at low nutritional risk (NRS 2002 <3 or NUTRIC score <5) if EN is not feasible. In contrast, patients who are at high risk for nutritional deficiency (NRS 2002 ≥3 or NUTRIC score ≥5) or severely malnourished (defined as recent weight loss 10%–15% of their previous weight, or weight <90% of their ideal body weight) should start PN at presentation if EN is not feasible or inadequate.[6] **Fig. 1** shows a proposed evidence-based algorithm that can be used by clinicians to determine when to initiate PN in critically ill patients.

Surgical patients

Patients with abdominal trauma or gastrointestinal surgery may not tolerate EN and are at increased risk for malnutrition. The perioperative period is usually associated with an increase in proinflammatory mediators that increase catabolism of glycogen,

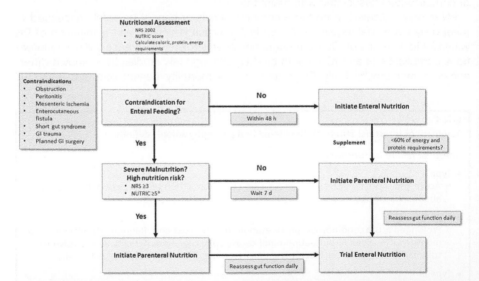

Fig. 1. Proposed algorithm of when to initiate parenteral nutrition in critically ill patients. [a] Not including IL-6. GI, gastrointestinal. (*Data from* McClave SA, Taylor BE, Martindale RG, et al. Guidelines for the provision and assessment of nutrition support therapy in the adult critically ill patient: Society of Critical Care Medicine (SCCM) and American Society for Parenteral and Enteral Nutrition (A.S.P.E.N.). JPEN J Parenter Enteral Nutr 2016;40(2):159–211; with permission.)

fat, and protein with release of glucose, free fatty acids, and amino acids into the circulation. Furthermore, undernutrition is an independent risk factor for increased mortality, infectious complications, length of hospital stay, and increased cost in this population.[16]

PN should only be considered in preoperative patients who are severely malnourished and unable to tolerate EN or maintain greater than 50% of oral intake for more than 7 days. Several studies have shown that 7 to 10 days of preoperative PN improves outcomes in severely undernourished patients but has no benefit and might increase morbidity in well-nourished patients.[17–19] One meta-analysis has shown that PN in severely malnourished surgical patients may have a lower mortality[20]; however, these results were not confirmed in another meta-analysis, with an expert group recommending EN when feasible.[21,22]

Chronic Disease Indications

There are many chronic disease states that may eventually progress to type III or chronic intestinal failure. These patients are often hemodynamically stable and have little or no inflammation but require PN for months to years. These patients can clearly benefit from HPN because this therapy has been shown to prolong life and improve quality of life. However, there are many complications that have been associated with long-term PN administration, which underscores the importance of proper patient selection, training, and monitoring of this treatment so that beneficial clinical outcomes are maximized.

Conditions that require HPN include inflammatory bowel disease, intestinal pseudo-obstruction, scleroderma, and gastrointestinal cancers. Radiation enteritis is a condition that is an important indication for HPN and is discussed later. It is important to remember that the condition is not the sole criterion for PN administration. A full assessment is necessary to determine whether PN is indicated and includes appraisal of nutritional status; evaluation of the functional status of the bowel, which is affected by the remaining bowel length; functional status of the upper gastrointestinal tract and integrity of the intestinal mucosa; and whether the patient is able to consume a well-balanced diet of an adequate amount.

Radiation enteritis

Radiation therapy in the region of the abdomen and pelvis can result in chronic radiation enteritis. This condition affects one-fifth of all patients undergoing abdomen/pelvic radiation therapy and may present as early as 6 to 12 months or as late as 1 to 2 decades after treatment.[23] A multicenter survey in 1998 found that 8% of patients on HPN had radiation enteritis as an indication for PN. Acute radiation injury, which causes edema and neutrophilic infiltration of all 3 layers of the bowel wall, subsides in nearly all patients. Patients with chronic radiation enteritis have histologic changes of mononuclear infiltrates, fibrosis and vasculitis that may result in stenosis, ulcerations, necrosis, and possibly perforation of the bowel. Surgery is indicated for segmental strictures with bowel obstruction, refractory or severe gastrointestinal bleeding, and bowel perforation. Most patients have intestinal dysmotility that can be managed with an oral diet and medications to provide symptomatic relief of diarrhea and abdominal pain. A small subset of patients may require supplemental EN and an even smaller group may need PN. The prognosis of patients with radiation enteritis in large HPN programs is quite good, with a 5-year survival rate of nearly 90%.[24] Importantly, the possibility of EN should be reassessed frequently because an observational study in 2006 found that one-third of patients were able to resume oral intake after chronic HPN.[25]

PARENTERAL NUTRITION FORMULATION

A multidisciplinary team of experienced clinicians, including physicians, dietitians, pharmacists and nurses, is recommended to ensure the prescribing of a complete and balanced PN formulation.[26] The PN formulation contains protein (amino acids), carbohydrate (dextrose), fat (intravenous lipid emulsion [ILE]), electrolytes, minerals, vitamins, trace elements, and water. It should be individualized to the needs of the patient and typically involves sterile compounding of 10 to 15 components. A total nutrient admixture (TNA), or 3-in-1 formulation, refers to all 3 macronutrients (amino acid, dextrose, ILE) included in the same bag. When ILE is administered separately, it is referred to as a 2-in-1 formulation. Advantages of a TNA compared with 2-in-1 formulation include convenience, reduced cost, and reduced risk of microbial growth. However, there are certain factors that limit emulsion stability that should be considered, such as mixture with neonatal amino acid solutions or addition of iron. Regulations are in place to foster safe and accurate compounding of sterile products and it is the pharmacist's duty to review the PN formulation for appropriate stability and compatibility.[27] Automated compounding devices are available that provide computer-assisted commands and incorporate safety features into the compounding process of individual PN formulations. Alternatively, standardized premixed PN formulations are commercially available in a variety of fixed nutrient doses that are designed to meet standard nutrient requirements in non–critically ill patients but not necessarily for patients with nutrient requirements outside a standard range.

Standard ranges for protein and energy requirements are age specific and incorporate metabolic demand and dosing weight, adjusted for obesity (**Table 1**). The usual distribution of nonprotein calories is 70% to 85% as carbohydrate and 15% to 30% as fat. This distribution may be adjusted based on tolerance and to minimize potential immune-suppressive effects of soybean oil–based ILE. Use of intermittent ILE administration (eg, 2–3 times weekly) instead of daily administration is a strategy that allows for provision of estimated essential fatty acid requirements while minimizing potential adverse effects. Standard ranges for electrolytes and minerals are age specific and based on normal organ function and normal losses but may also be limited by compatibility issues. A parenteral multivitamin preparation that contains 13 vitamins should be added daily. Guidelines for trace element content are provided in **Table 1**; however, variations may exist among individual patients on long-term PN and in patients with chronic cholestatic liver disease and renal insufficiency.[28] Our approach is to monitor blood levels of trace elements in all HPN patients every 6 months and to modify dosing as needed. In addition, nearly every component of the PN formulation has been and continues to be affected by product shortages that expose patients to risk of harm related to nutrient deficiency. Practice recommendations for dealing with PN product shortages are available from the American Society for Parenteral and Enteral Nutrition (ASPEN) that incorporate measures to ration supply and identify alternative therapeutic options.[29] Initiation of PN should occur in a hospital setting where daily monitoring of fluid intake/output along with laboratory monitoring (serum electrolytes, glucose, calcium, magnesium, and phosphate) can be accurately measured. Special circumstances, like major electrolyte imbalances or refeeding syndrome, may require more frequent and prolonged laboratory monitoring. Once electrolytes and nutrient levels have stabilized, the intervals of monitoring may be increased. **Table 2** shows a schedule of proposed monitoring needs for patients on long-term PN. This article briefly reviews some special considerations of PN formulations in different disease states.

Table 1
Estimated daily fluid, electrolyte, carbohydrate, protein, and lipid requirements in hospitalized patients receiving parenteral nutrition

Nutritional Requirement	Dose
Protein (catabolic)	1.2–2 g/kg/d
Calories	25–30 kcal/kg/d

Fluid and Electrolytes	Dose
Water	25–35 mL
Sodium	1–2 mEq/kg
Potassium	1–2 mEq/kg
Chloride	As needed to maintain acid-base balance
Phosphorus	20–40 mmol
Magnesium	8–20 mEq
Calcium	10–15 mEq

Trace Elements	Dose
Zinc	2.5–5 mg
Copper	0.3–0.5 mg
Manganese	60–100 µg
Chromium	10–15 µg
Selenium	20–60 µg
Iron	Not routinely added

Vitamins	Dose
Vitamin A	3300 IU
Vitamin E	10 IU
Vitamin K	150 µg
Vitamin D	200 IU
Vitamin B_1	6 mg
Vitamin B_2	3.6 mg
Vitamin B_6	6 mg
Niacin	40 mg
Folic acid	600 µg
Vitamin B_{12}	5 µg
Biotin	60 µg
Vitamin C	200 mg

Data from Refs.[7,27,37]

Pulmonary Failure

Macronutrient metabolism can adversely affect respiratory function in mechanically ventilated patients with acute or chronic respiratory failure. Excess amino acid and glucose infusion may increase minute ventilation and carbon dioxide production, whereas soybean oil–based ILE may adversely affect immune function. Current clinical guidelines recommend using indirect calorimetry to determine energy requirements or, if this equipment is not available, to prescribe 25 to 30 kcal/kg/d.[6] They also recommend 1.2 to 2.0 g/kg/d of protein, withholding or limiting soybean oil–based ILE to 100 g in a divided dose during the first week of critical illness. This group also

Table 2		
Recommended laboratory monitoring for patients receiving parenteral nutrition		
	Frequency	
Parameter	Initiation of Therapy (Acute Care)	Long-term Therapy
Capillary glucose	Every 6 h until advanced to goal and as needed to maintain 140–180 mg/dL	Not routine As needed basis to coordinate with PN infusion cycle
Basic metabolic panel Phosphorus, magnesium	Daily, until advanced to goal and stable; then 1–2 times/wk	Weekly, then decrease frequency as stable
CBC (with differential)	Baseline; then 1–2 times/wk	Monthly, then decrease frequency as stable
Liver function: ALT, AST, ALP, total bilirubin	Baseline; then weekly	Monthly, then decrease frequency as stable
Serum triglycerides	Baseline if at risk; then as needed	Not routine As needed
Iron studies, 25-OH vitamin D	Not routine	Baseline, then every 3–6 mo
Zinc, copper, selenium, manganese	Not routine	Baseline, then every 6 mo

Abbreviations: ALP, alkaline phosphatase; ALT, alanine transaminase; AST, aspartate transaminase; CBC, complete blood count; 25-OH vitamin D, 25-hydroxyvitamin D.

recommends close monitoring of serum phosphorous because up to 30% of patients in the ICU may develop phosphorous deficiency, which may result in diaphragmatic weakness and increased ventilator time.[30] Strict monitoring of intake and output is also important in pulmonary failure to reduce the risk of pulmonary edema.

Renal Failure

Protein goals in patients with renal failure should be based on the degree of renal insufficiency, the use of renal replacement therapy, and the degree of illness. The recommended dose of protein is 0.6 to 0.8 g/kg/d for patients with chronic kidney disease (CKD) who are not receiving hemodialysis (HD), 1.2 g/kg/d for patients with CKD on maintenance HD, and 1.5 g/kg/d for non–critically ill patients with acute kidney injury (AKI) on intermittent HD. In critically ill patients with AKI, the recommended protein amount is 1.2 to 2 g/kg/d. This amount should be increased to 1.8 to 2.5 g/kg/d during continuous renal replacement therapy because of increased losses of amino acids and protein with this treatment modality.[6,31] In most cases, a standard 10% amino acid PN solution is appropriate in critically ill patients with renal failure. If excess fluid is a management challenge, a 15% amino acid concentrated formulation should be considered. Because of electrolyte imbalances, initiating PN in malnourished patients with renal failure increases the risk of refeeding syndrome; thus, serum potassium, magnesium, calcium, and phosphorus levels should be monitored closely. In addition, energy requirements for critically ill patients with renal failure are similar to those without, ranging from 25 to 30 kcal/kg/d.[6]

Hepatic Failure

PN should be started immediately for patients with alcoholic steatohepatitis or cirrhosis with moderate to severe malnutrition and in those with acute liver failure who may not be able to start EN within 5 to 7 days. The recommended protein goal for alcoholic steatohepatitis and cirrhosis is 1.2 to 1.5 g/kg/d, whereas for acute or sub-acute liver failure it should be reduced slightly to 0.8 to 1.2 g/kg/d.[32] Patients with hepatic encephalopathy (HE) should be given protein at the lower end of this range until the causes of encephalopathy have been identified and treated. Once patients show signs of improvement, protein intake should be increased as tolerated to goals as noted earlier to help maintain nitrogen balance and promote recovery.[33] In nearly all patients with liver disease, standard amino acid solutions should be used. Concentrated formulas with 15% amino acids may be used in the management of patients who need fluid restriction. Branched chain amino acid (BCAA)–enriched formulas for patients with liver disease consist of an 8% amino acid solution with 36% of total amino acids provided as BCAAs (eg, valine, isoleucine, and leucine) and 2% as aromatic amino acids (eg, tryptophan, phenylalanine, and tyrosine). These formulas have been shown to reduce symptoms of HE but are no better than standard medical intervention.[34] The authors therefore reserve the use of BCAA formulas in PN solutions to patients with greater than or equal to grade III HE who do not improve after 48 hours of medical therapy and 0.8 g/kg/d of standard amino acids. Energy requirements are similar to amounts used for patients with pulmonary and renal disease.[6]

VASCULAR ACCESS

PN is delivered via a catheter that is placed directly into the venous system. The choice of vascular access location, catheter type, site of the vein entry, and routine care are vital for patient safety and quality of life. The choices of vascular access location and catheter type are based on multiple factors and should be decided by a multidisciplinary team of PN specialists. Anticipated duration of administration, PN formulation, and patient-specific factors are the main determinants of access choice. Special attention to wounds, systemic illness, social situation, and the ability of the patient to care for the access is needed when making this decision. There are few RCTs that directly compare venous access type in PN patients. In general, tunneled catheters are the preferred method for home or long-term (>3 months) PN delivery, especially for patients requiring daily access to a catheter device. **Table 3** highlights the limitations and advantages of different types of vascular catheter access.

Peripheral Venous Access

The safest and easiest way to access the vascular system is through a small-caliber peripheral venous catheter. These devices are often inserted into a readily accessible forearm vessel but may also be placed in the upper extremity or neck. The fragility of such vessels limits the duration and formulation of PN. They are generally used for less than 6 days in patients who are not fluid restricted because formulations must be diluted to avoid the development of phlebitis, which often limits the total number of calories that can be delivered. Peripheral PN is compounded with a final concentration of amino acids less than 5%, glucose less than 10%, and an osmolarity of less than 900 mOsm/L.[35,36] Peripheral venous catheters have the highest risk of thrombophlebitis compared with other access methods. However, they have the lowest risk of catheter-related infections, which may be related to their limited duration.[36]

Midline catheters are becoming an increasingly popular way to administer PN in the hospital setting. PN through a midline catheter may be administered over a period longer than 6 days, although the same formulation restrictions as for short cannula devices apply. Although convenient, midline catheters are not appropriate for HPN administration. They also carry a significant risk for thrombophlebitis, which may be

Table 3
Comparison of insertion site, duration, advantages, and limitations of various types of vascular access

Type of Access	Insertion Site	Duration	Limitations	Advantages
Short peripheral catheter	Superficial upper extremity or neck vein	Days	Fragile, solutions <600 mOsm/L, high phlebitis risk, hospital use only	Ease of access and placement, cost, lowest infection risk
PICC	Basilic, cephalic, or brachial vein	Weeks to months	Difficult access for self-care, uncomfortable, placed by trained technician only	Central access with lowest risk of pneumothorax or arterial damage, acute or home setting
Nontunneled CVC	Jugular, subclavian, femoral vein	1 wk	Hospital setting only, highest infectious risk, uncomfortable, placement complications operator dependent	Quick procedure, cost, easy to remove
Tunneled CVC	Subclavian or jugular vessels	Months to years	Requires placement in procedure room by trained radiologist or surgeon	Long-term home use, self-care easy, decreased infection risk
Implanted CVC	Subclavian or jugular vessels	Months to years	—	—

Abbreviations: CVC, central venous catheter; PICC, peripherally inserted central catheter.

From Kryzyda EA, Andris DA, Edmiston CE. Parenteral access devices. In: Mueller CM, editor. The A.S.P.E.N. adult nutrition support core curriculum. 2nd edition. Silver Spring (MD): American Society for Parenteral and Enteral Nutrition; 2012. p. 265–83; with permission.

reduced by ultrasonography placement in the basilic or brachial veins. Midline catheters have an average life span of 2 to 6 weeks.

Centrally Placed Venous Catheters

Central venous access is the preferred delivery of medium-term and long-term PN. The most common insertion sites include the subclavian, internal jugular, cephalic, and basilic veins. The catheter tip should terminate near the junction of the superior vena cava (SVC) and right atrium. The advantages of central venous catheter (CVC) use include that they are not limited by the type, pH, osmolarity, or volume of the PN infusion. Percutaneous CVCs placed in the subclavian or jugular venous systems are usually indicated for short-term use because they are often placed in urgent or emergent conditions. Because of the higher risk of infection compared with other CVCs, they are not appropriate for home PN administration.

Peripherally inserted central catheters (PICCs) are CVCs that are typically placed by a trained nurse and interventional radiologist using ultrasonography guidance into the basilic, cephalic, or brachial vein. Because of the location of the insertion site, PICC placement is associated with a significantly lower risk of thoracic placement complications such as pneumothorax, uncontrolled bleeding, and arterial puncture. PICCs are ideal for administration of PN in the hospital, rehabilitation facility, and the home setting when therapy is indicated for less than 3 months.[37] Although most studies have shown that the incidence of central line–associated bloodstream infection (CLABSI) is greater with PICCs compared with tunneled CVCs, a nonrandomized prospective trial of patients with a cancer receiving HPN found a significant decrease in infections in patients with PICCs compared with those with tunneled CVCs or portacaths.[38] Other advantages include lower overall cost compared with tunneled central lines.[36,39,40] Difficulties include home care and convenience of the antecubital placement, which may be a barrier to patient quality of life.

Tunneled CVCs are the preferred method of HPN delivery in patients requiring this therapy for 3 months or more. With proper care, they may be safely used for years. Most often, the skin insertion site is on the upper chest with the venipuncture occurring in the right internal jugular vein. Tunneled catheters are placed by trained interventional radiologists or vascular surgeons in the operating room and also require a procedure for removal. The decrease in risk of CLABSI is attributed to the barrier of soft tissue that separates the vein entrance site from the catheter exit site. Importantly, tunneled catheters provide a discrete catheter option that is easy to access and maintain for patients on long-term PN.

Another type of tunneled CVC is an implanted portacath. These devices have a catheter attached to a self-sealing silicone elastomer septum that is placed into a subcutaneous pocket in the anterior chest wall and must be accessed with a noncoring needle that is intermittently placed percutaneously. The advantage of these CVCs is that they require minimal maintenance aside from routine cleaning during access and monthly heparin flushes if they are not in use. When they are not accessed, patients can maintain normal activities with minimal restriction, including bathing. Although these devices may be accessed 2000 to 3000 times, they are better suited for intermittent use as opposed to daily access. As a result, they are used infrequently for the administration of PN.

PARENTERAL NUTRITION COMPLICATIONS

Some of the common and most serious complications associated with PN are discussed here, which we have arbitrarily categorized as either acute or chronic. It should be noted that complications associated with PN can be avoided or mitigated through selection of the most appropriate CVC; careful preparation and monitoring of the PN formula; and, in patients requiring long-term PN, training of the patient or caregiver on the catheter care and PN delivery. Many hospitals have pharmacists and dietitians with expertise in nutrition support to assist in the management of patients in the acute care setting. Referral to a multidisciplinary team at a tertiary center that specializes in the management of intestinal failure should be considered for patients requiring HPN for greater than 3 to 6 months.

Acute Complications

Vascular access
Placing a catheter, whether peripherally or centrally, has inherent risks that can arise immediately or postprocedure. Peripherally placed catheters have the lowest risk of complications compared with CVC placement. CVC placement results in pneumothorax, arterial puncture, and line malposition in approximately 1% to 4% of attempts. One large multicenter trial in 2015 compared complication rates of internal jugular, subclavian, and femoral nontunneled central venous access. Pneumothorax requiring chest tube insertion occurred in 1.5% of subclavian insertions compared with 0.5%

of the internal jugular attempts.[41] Femoral central access is generally not recommended for administration with PN because of sanitary challenges and increased infection risk.[42] Jugular and subclavian CVCs should be placed using ultrasonography and this is now standard of practice in the United States. Multiple RCTs and meta-analyses have confirmed that ultrasonography-guided techniques have a higher first-attempt rate and a decrease in bleeding and pneumothorax rates.[43] The number of unsuccessful insertion attempts is the most powerful predictor of immediate complications.[44]

Hyperglycemia

Hyperglycemia is a common occurrence in hospitalized patients initiated on PN. One observational study found that up 50% of hospitalized patients on PN experienced an episode of hyperglycemia.[45] The development of hyperglycemia during PN in the hospital is independently associated with higher rates of mortality, infections, organ dysfunction, and length of hospital stay.[45–48] Patients with acute illness, surgery, or trauma have an increased risk of developing hyperglycemia because of increased hepatic glucose production and increased peripheral insulin resistance with reduced glucose use. There are no specific clinical trials to evaluate the effect of glucose levels on hospitalized patients on PN; however, ASPEN recommends a blood glucose target of 140 to 180 mg/dL.[49]

Hyperglycemia tends to occur more frequently during the initiation of PN as the dextrose infusion is being titrated to goal and need for supplemental insulin is being determined. PN formulations are typically initiated with 2 g/kg/d of glucose to limit gluconeogenesis derived from protein catabolism. One study showed that PN formulations with a lower glucose load (1.8 ± 1.3 g/kg/d compared with 2.6 ± 1.4 g/kg/d) had decreased incidence of hyperglycemia and improved mortality in ICU patients.[50] Dextrose administration of more than 4 mg/kg/min is a significant predictor of hyperglycemia.[51] In average-sized adults the authors follow the current guidelines and limit the initial glucose load to between 150 and 200 g/d[6] Hyperglycemia should be treated with scheduled divided insulin doses or a continuous inulin infusion in critical ill patients. If a moderate dose of insulin is required, then a portion of this is typically added to the PN formulation. A prospective cohort study in 2012 showed that initiating PN with insulin at a dose of 1 U/20 g of glucose in hyperglycemic patients resulted in improved glycemic control compared with a sliding-scale replacement method.[52]

Refeeding syndrome

Malnourished patients who undergo rapid nutritional repletion are at risk for refeeding syndrome, which is characterized by cardiac, respiratory, and neurologic symptoms caused by hypophosphatemia, hypokalemia, and hypomagnesemia. Patients with anorexia, alcoholism, prolonged starvation, bariatric surgery, and chronic illnesses (such as cancer or cirrhosis) are at higher risk for this condition. In starvation, insulin concentrations decrease and permit a shift in metabolism from using glucose as a primary source of fuel to ketones and free fatty acids to help spare nitrogen. During this catabolic process, total-body phosphorus, magnesium, and potassium levels are depleted as these electrolytes are released from intracellular sources. When sufficient dietary or nutrition support is provided to these patients, insulin concentrations increase, especially in response to glucose, and to a lesser extent protein, and lead to cellular uptake of phosphorus, magnesium, and potassium. This process may result in dangerously low concentrations of these electrolytes in the serum and lead to symptoms associated with refeeding syndrome. Hypophosphatemia is especially dangerous because it may result in respiratory failure, cardiac dysfunction, and arrhythmias, as well as hematologic, endocrine, and neuromuscular dysfunction. The risk of refeeding syndrome can be tempered by decreasing the number of calories provided while PN is initiated. Our approach has been modeled on the recommendations of the United Kingdom National Institute for Health and Care Excellence (NICE) on nutrition support in adults who are at high risk for developing refeeding problems [www.nice.org.uk/guidance/cg32]. The authors provide 45% to 50% of total dextrose calories for the first 24 to 48 hours, based on initial total energy goals in the ICU of 25 kcal/kg/d (30 kcal/kg/d for ambulatory patients), where the patients' current body weight is used up to a BMI of 25 kg/m^2 and an adjusted body weight is used in overweight and obese individuals. A basic metabolic panel with magnesium and phosphorus should be monitored daily and electrolyte abnormalities should be corrected immediately. We slowly advance the formula to goal over 5 to 7 days if the patient is metabolically stable. We also provide supplemental thiamine 100 mg and folate 1 mg daily over this time frame.

Chronic Complications

Thromboembolic complications
Cather-related venous thrombosis can result in patient discomfort, emergency room visits, hospital admissions, and delays in PN administration. One large multicenter study of 50,470 patients on HPN found a thrombosis rate of 0.23 per 1000 catheter days.[53] Another recent retrospective cohort study found an incidence of catheter-related venous thrombosis of 11.4% within the first year of HPN use.[54] PICC lines also have higher rates of thromboembolic events, up to 5%, as shown by one study of 102 hospitalized patients.[39] In general, shorter peripherally placed catheters have higher rates of thrombophlebitis than CVCs. This risk can be reduced by using aseptic placement techniques, smaller-gauge catheters, avoiding Teflon cannulas, and proper fixation techniques.

Using ultrasonography-guided placement for CVCs and confirming catheter tip placement in the cavoatrial junction with a chest radiograph reduces the rates of thromboembolic complications. Comparing types of CV access, subclavian CVC had lower risks of symptomatic deep vein thrombosis compared with jugular and femoral access. Femoral access has the highest rates of thromboembolism and should be avoided in HPN administration.[41]

Multiple RCTs and meta-analyses have determined that intermittent prophylaxis with flushing of catheters with heparin is no more beneficial than flushing with normal saline alone.[51,55–57] Many manufacturers of portacaths or open-ended catheter lumens recommend a heparin flush when locking the device. This method may be helpful when devices are scheduled to remain closed for more than 8 hours. However, heparin should not be flushed immediately before or after lipid-containing PN because of the risk of lipid precipitation. This problem is generally avoided because patients who use heparin as a lock solution are instructed to administer it with saline before and after medication administration (saline, administer medication, saline, heparin [SASH]). Closed-ended valve catheters should be flushed and locked with saline only.

Infectious complications
Infections remain a common and serious complication of PN that is inherent to both the type of PN formulation and CVC line that is selected for the administration of this therapy. CLABSI remains the most morbid complication of PN. For our purposes, CLABSI is defined by the Centers for Disease Control and Prevention (CDC) as a laboratory-confirmed bloodstream infection in a patient with a central line more than 48 hours from symptom onset and unrelated to an infection from another site.[58] The CDC estimates that 30,100 cases of CVC-associated bloodstream infections occur

annually in United States.[58] A large systematic review showed that PN rates of infections range from 0.38 to 4.58 episodes per 1000 catheter days.[59] An additional multi-center observational study in 2016 followed 1046 patients on HPN in the United States and found that 10.7% experienced a CLABSI event over 3 years, totaling 0.87 episodes per 1000 PN days.[60] Patients on PN, compared with intravenous fluid and other parenteral therapies, have inherently higher rates of CLABSI. A large single-center study showed an odds ratio of 2.65 (95% CI 2.20–3.19; $P<.0001$) of CLABSI with PN compared with patients with CVC not receiving PN.[61] Patients also had higher odds of developing CLABSI if they had longer line duration, renal failure, human immunodeficiency virus, or malignancy.[61]

The most prevalent organisms cultured include coagulase-negative staphylococci, *Staphylococcus aureus*, and *Klebsiella pneumoniae*.[60] There are many techniques to decrease CLABSI incidence, and these are summarized in **Box 2** based on the ESPEN guidelines of 2009. Tunneled catheters and implanted venous access devices have the lowest rates of CLABSI, especially for patients with long-term PN administration.[62] PICC lines may also be considered for short-term and medium-term access because they have decreased rates of CLABSI compared with temporary percutaneous CVCs placed in the jugular, subclavian, or femoral vein.[36] Single-lumen CVCs are preferred to multilumen catheters, as shown in multiple RCTs, although recent quantitative meta-analysis has found the difference in CLABSI rates to be nonsignificant.[63,64] Precautions taken during the insertion of CVC access greatly decrease the rates of CLABSI. In a multicenter prospective study, a bundle including hand washing, full-barrier precautions during insertion, chlorhexidine antisepsis, removing unnecessary catheters, and avoiding the femoral site resulted in up to a 66% reduction in CLABSI incidence.[65] The use of antimicrobial locking solutions to prevent CLABSI is controversial.[7] Antibiotic locks have not been shown to reduce the incidence of CLABSI in HPN and may result in the development of antibiotic resistance.[62] Ethanol (70%) lock has been shown to reduce the rate of CLABSI from 10.1 to 2.9 per 1000 catheter days in a series of 31 HPN patients.[66] However, its regular use has not been endorsed because there is concern that this solution may increase the risk of catheter occlusion and venous thrombosis.[67] If these solutions are used, then ethanol lock is only

---

Box 2
Techniques that can be used to reduce risk of central line–associated bloodstream infections

Summary of techniques used to decrease risk of CLABSI
- Appropriate choice of the insertion site
- Using tunneled and implanted catheters (value only confirmed in long-term use)
- Using antimicrobial coated catheters (value only shown in short-term use)
- Using lowest number of lumens possible; single-lumen catheters preferred
- Using peripheral access (PICC) when possible
- Ultrasonography-guided venipuncture for all central line placements
- Use of maximal barrier precautions during insertion
- Proper education and specific training of staff
- An adequate policy of hand washing
- Use of 2% chlorhexidine as skin antiseptic; let dry completely before applying
- Appropriate dressing of the exit site
- Disinfection of hubs, stopcocks, and needle-free connectors; change weekly
- Regular change of administration sets

From Pittiruti M, Hamilton H, Biffi R, et al. ESPEN guidelines on parenteral nutrition: central venous catheters (access, care, diagnosis and therapy of complications). Clin Nutr 2009;28(4):365–77; with permission.

appropriate for tunneled silicone catheters because it is not compatible with polyurethane, which is used to manufacture most of the infusion devices.

Other infectious complications of long-term vascular access devices (VADs) include exit site and tunnel infections. These infections present with localized signs and symptoms and are generally not accompanied by systemic inflammation and bacteremia. Localized exit site infections of tunneled catheters can usually be managed with local care and oral antibiotics. Exit site infections of PICCs and pocket infections of implanted portacaths should be managed with line removal and, in some instances, antibiotics to prevent systemic infection. Infections limited to the tunneled segment of a CVC are very difficult to clear with antibiotics and often necessitate removal of the device.

Hepatic complications

Hepatobiliary disease associated with PN includes intestinal failure–associated liver disease (IFALD) and biliary tract disease. IFALD (previously referred to as parenteral nutrition-associated liver disease) includes PN factors that adversely affect metabolism or direct injury of the liver, in addition to liver injury attributed to the primary disease for which PN is being used.[68] PN factors that may contribute to liver injury include excess glucose calories, phytosterols contained in plant-based lipid emulsions, essential fatty acid deficiency, taurine deficiency, and hypermanganesemia. Factors unrelated to PN include inflammation associated with the patient's underlying disease, bacterial infection, bacterial overgrowth, and bile acid deficiency or toxicity. These factors generally lead to either steatosis or cholestasis. Excessive glucose calories result in steatosis through a combination of factors including hyperglycemia, increased insulin to glucagon ratio, and perhaps choline and carnitine deficiency. It can be prevented by avoiding overfeeding, is often reversible, and rarely leads to steatohepatitis or cirrhosis. Cholestasis is more common in children than in adults, often presents after long-term PN use, and is more likely than steatosis to progress to cirrhosis. The incidence of end-stage liver disease in adults on long-term PN is unknown but estimates range from 15% to 30%.[69,70] In contrast, mild increase of liver enzyme levels is common in adults during the first few weeks of PN and often resolves as long as patients are not overfed.

Management of increased liver enzyme levels includes the avoidance of overfeeding after the patient's nutritional status is replete. The infusion of soybean oil–based ILE should not be greater than 1 g/kg/d.[70] If a formula that is predominantly glucose based can be tolerated, then soybean oil–based ILE can be reduced to 100 g/wk to meet essential fatty acid requirements. If appropriate, a diet should be initiated in patients who are nil per os. Other actions should include maintenance of good glycemic control, discontinuation of hepatotoxic drugs, avoidance of alcohol consumption, and control of any underlying infection or inflammatory process. If available, alternative ILEs that contain lower concentrations of soybean oil may be considered if enzyme improvement does not occur. Evaluation for other causes of liver disease should be undertaken if enzyme levels remain chronically increased, especially for treatable causes of liver disease. If possible, restoration of intestinal continuity should be considered if the increase in liver enzyme levels is moderate or severe. Referral to a center that performs intestinal transplants may be considered for patients with impending liver failure, defined as a total bilirubin level greater than 3 to 6 mg/dL, or symptomatic liver failure.[7]

Biliary complications

Long-term PN is associated with biliary complications including cholelithiasis, biliary sludge, and acalculous cholecystitis. These complications may result in pain or infection requiring percutaneous cholecystostomy tube or surgical cholecystectomy. Biliary sludge is very common in long-term PN. One observational study showed that 50% of participants on PN developed sludge after 4 weeks and 100% developed sludge after 6 weeks.[71] A lack of enteral feeding prevents the release of cholecystokinin (CCK), which is required to stimulate gallbladder contraction and emptying. A small, prospective study found that no patients developed biliary sludge or cholelithiasis after 4 weeks of continuous enteral tube feeds.[72] In addition, Messing and colleagues[71] found that patients who developed biliary sludge on PN had resolution after 4 weeks of enteral feeding. Methods to decrease the incidence of biliary sludge and therefore cholelithiasis formation are challenging but early oral intake should always be encouraged. Some studies have shown that empiric CCK injections may reduce biliary sludge by inducing gallbladder contractions.[73] However, CCK injections are not routine practice because of increased rates of flushing, nausea, and cholecystitis.

Metabolic bone disease

Metabolic bone disease (MBD) was first described in the 1980s after large studies reported symptoms of bone pain, weakness, hypercalciuria, and hypercalcemia in long-term HPN patients. Originally, bone biopsies from these patients reported findings of both osteoporosis and osteomalacia.[74] MBD remains prevalent in patients on long-term HPN, with a large survey in Europe showing a prevalence of at least osteopenia in 84% of participants who had been on PN for an average of 61 months.[75] Up to one-third of patients experience symptoms of bone pain, fractures, or weakness, whereas most patients with MBD are asymptomatic. In the early 1980s, MBD was likely related to increased levels of aluminum in formulations containing casein hydrolysate as the primary nitrogen source.[76] Decreased serum 1,25-dihydroxyvitamin D levels, reduced bone formation, and osteomalacia are typical features of aluminum toxicity. However, MBD persists in long-term HPN patients despite limiting aluminum by switching to crystalline free amino acid–based PN formulas.[77]

The pathogenesis of MBD associated with long-term PN is poorly understood and may be related to various components of PN formulations and the patient's underlying risk factors and medical conditions. Sufficient amounts of protein, energy, calcium, phosphorus, magnesium, and vitamins D and K are needed for adequate bone development and turnover. Increased amounts of amino acid in PN formulations in combination with sulfate, acid, and insulin can cause hypercalciuria and a negative total calcium balance. PN formulation should have 1:2 calcium to phosphorus ratio with at least 15 mEq/d of calcium to avoid excessive calcium excretion.[78,79] Vitamin D deficiency (as defined by <20 ng/mL of serum 25-hydroxyvitamin D) may be inadequate to stimulate osteoblast formation as part of the bone remodeling process. Excess vitamin D may also contribute to MBD because one study showed that removal of vitamin D from PN formulations had benefits on bone remodeling.[80] Current formulations contain 200 IU daily of vitamin D.

Few controlled trials have evaluated strategies proposed to prevent and treat long-term PN–associated MBD. Patients should be counseled in lifestyle changes to stop smoking, limit alcohol consumption, and participate in weight-bearing exercise and careful sunlight exposure. PN formulation should have less than 25 µg/L of aluminum, the calcium to phosphorus ratio should be less than 1:2, and vitamin D infusion should be 200 IU/daily. Sodium should be dosed to meet renal, diarrheal, and other nonrenal losses because excessive infusion can induce hypercalciuria. Amino acid dosing should be reduced to a maintenance level (1–1.2 g/kg) after patients recover from hospitalization because doses given during repletion (1.5–2.0 g/dL) can induce hypercalciuria as well. Dual energy x-ray absorptiometry scan is the gold standard for diagnosing osteoporosis and should be performed every 2 years. Vitamin D levels should be checked if symptomatic bone pain, fracture, or previous diagnosis of osteoporosis, osteomalacia, or osteopenia is known.

Renal

Although uncommon, PN-associated nephropathy may occur with long-term PN characterized by a decrease in creatinine clearance and impaired tubular function with a potential for glomerular sclerosis. Renal disorders such as hyperoxaluria, hypercalciuria, and tubular renal defects may occur. Risks for renal dysfunction include higher amino acid loads, concurrent nephrotoxic drugs, and previous bloodstream infections.[81] Hyperoxaluria and hypercalciuria occur in adult PN patients but are not directly related to an increased incidence of nephrolithiasis.[82] The incidence of hyperoxaluria is probably related to the vitamin C content in PN formulations.

SUMMARY

PN is a safe and effective means of providing nutrition in patients with intestinal failure who are unable to tolerate EN or in whom the enteral route cannot be safely accessed. The optimal timing of PN initiation depends on the level of nutrition risk and should factor both disease severity and nutritional status. Type and location of the VAD should be meticulously evaluated based on type of PN, length of therapy, and risk of infection. Measures should be taken to minimize risk of infection, and thromboembolic and mechanical complications associated with the VAD. Initiation of PN should typically occur in the hospital setting to allow for close monitoring of fluid and electrolyte status and glucose control. Metabolic complications associated with long-term use of PN may include MBD, renal disease, and hepatobiliary disease. A multidisciplinary team of experienced clinicians is recommended to promote safe use of PN and minimize risk of complications.

REFERENCES

1. Mundi MS, Pattinson A, McMahon MT, et al. Prevalence of home parenteral and enteral nutrition in the United States. Nutr Clin Pract 2017. 0884533617718472. [Epub ahead of print].
2. Soeters PB, Schols AM. Advances in understanding and assessing malnutrition. Curr Opin Clin Nutr Metab Care 2009;12(5):487–94.
3. Cederholm T, Barazzoni R, Austin P, et al. ESPEN guidelines on definitions and terminology of clinical nutrition. Clin Nutr 2017;36(1):49–64.
4. Kondrup J, Rasmussen HH, Hamberg O, et al. Nutritional risk screening (NRS 2002): a new method based on an analysis of controlled clinical trials. Clin Nutr 2003;22(3):321–36.
5. Heyland DK, Dhaliwal R, Jiang X, et al. Identifying critically ill patients who benefit the most from nutrition therapy: the development and initial validation of a novel risk assessment tool. Crit Care 2011;15(6):R268.
6. McClave SA, Taylor BE, Martindale RG, et al. Guidelines for the provision and assessment of nutrition support therapy in the adult critically ill patient: Society of Critical Care Medicine (SCCM) and American Society for Parenteral and Enteral Nutrition (A.S.P.E.N.). JPEN J Parenter Enteral Nutr 2016;40(2):159–211.
7. Pironi L, Arends J, Bozzetti F, et al. ESPEN guidelines on chronic intestinal failure in adults. Clin Nutr 2016;35(2):247–307.

8. Rahman A, Hasan RM, Agarwala R, et al. Identifying critically-ill patients who will benefit most from nutritional therapy: further validation of the "modified NUTRIC" nutritional risk assessment tool. Clin Nutr 2016;35(1):158–62.

9. Peter JV, Moran JL, Phillips-Hughes J. A metaanalysis of treatment outcomes of early enteral versus early parenteral nutrition in hospitalized patients. Crit Care Med 2005;33(1):213–20 [discussion: 260–1].

10. Doig GS, Heighes PT, Simpson F, et al. Early enteral nutrition, provided within 24 h of injury or intensive care unit admission, significantly reduces mortality in critically ill patients: a meta-analysis of randomised controlled trials. Intensive Care Med 2009;35(12):2018–27.

11. Doig GS, Simpson F, Sweetman EA, et al. Early parenteral nutrition in critically ill patients with short-term relative contraindications to early enteral nutrition: a randomized controlled trial. JAMA 2013;309(20):2130–8.

12. Harvey SE, Parrott F, Harrison DA, et al. A multicentre, randomised controlled trial comparing the clinical effectiveness and cost-effectiveness of early nutritional support via the parenteral versus the enteral route in critically ill patients (CALORIES). Health Technol Assess 2016;20(28):1–144.

13. Heidegger CP, Berger MM, Graf S, et al. Optimisation of energy provision with supplemental parenteral nutrition in critically ill patients: a randomised controlled clinical trial. Lancet 2013;381(9864):385–93.

14. Elke G, van Zanten AR, Lemieux M, et al. Enteral versus parenteral nutrition in critically ill patients: an updated systematic review and meta-analysis of randomized controlled trials. Crit Care 2016;20(1):117.

15. Casaer MP, Mesotten D, Hermans G, et al. Early versus late parenteral nutrition in critically ill adults. N Engl J Med 2011;365(6):506–17.

16. Correia MI, Caiaffa WT, da Silva AL, et al. Risk factors for malnutrition in patients undergoing gastroenterological and hernia surgery: an analysis of 374 patients. Nutr Hosp 2001;16(2):59–64.

17. Bozzetti F, Arends J, Lundholm K, et al. ESPEN guidelines on parenteral nutrition: non-surgical oncology. Clin Nutr 2009;28(4):445–54.

18. Detsky AS, McLaughlin JR, Abrams HB, et al. Quality of life of patients on long-term total parenteral nutrition at home. J Gen Intern Med 1986;1(1):26–33.

19. Veterans Affairs Total Parenteral Nutrition Cooperative Study Group. Perioperative total parenteral nutrition in surgical patients. N Engl J Med 1991;325(8):525–32.

20. Braunschweig CL, Levy P, Sheean PM, et al. Enteral compared with parenteral nutrition: a meta-analysis. Am J Clin Nutr 2001;74(4):534–42.

21. Heyland DK, Montalvo M, MacDonald S, et al. Total parenteral nutrition in the surgical patient: a meta-analysis. Can J Surg 2001;44(2):102–11.

22. Weimann A, Braga M, Carli F, et al. ESPEN guideline: clinical nutrition in surgery. Clin Nutr 2017;36(3):623–50.

23. Miller AR, Martenson JA, Nelson H, et al. The incidence and clinical consequences of treatment-related bowel injury. Int J Radiat Oncol Biol Phys 1999; 43(4):817–25.

24. Gavazzi C, Bhoori S, Lovullo S, et al. Role of home parenteral nutrition in chronic radiation enteritis. Am J Gastroenterol 2006;101(2):374–9.

25. Bozzetti F, Staun M, Gossum Av. Home parenteral nutrition. 2006.

26. Ayers P, Adams S, Boullata J, et al. A.S.P.E.N. parenteral nutrition safety consensus recommendations. JPEN J Parenter Enteral Nutr 2014;38(3):296–333.

27. Mirtallo J, Canada T, Johnson D, et al. Safe practices for parenteral nutrition. JPEN J Parenter Enteral Nutr 2004;28(6):S39–70.

28. Vanek VW, Borum P, Buchman A, et al. A.S.P.E.N. position paper: recommendations for changes in commercially available parenteral multivitamin and multitrace element products. Nutr Clin Pract 2012;27(4):440–91.
29. Available at: http://www.nutritioncare.org/public-policy/product-shortages. Accessed September 26, 2017.
30. Alsumrain MH, Jawad SA, Imran NB, et al. Association of hypophosphatemia with failure-to-wean from mechanical ventilation. Ann Clin Lab Sci 2010;40(2):144–8.
31. Scheinkestel CD, Kar L, Marshall K, et al. Prospective randomized trial to assess caloric and protein needs of critically Ill, anuric, ventilated patients requiring continuous renal replacement therapy. Nutrition 2003;19(11–12):909–16.
32. Plauth M, Cabre E, Campillo B, et al. ESPEN guidelines on parenteral nutrition: hepatology. Clin Nutr 2009;28(4):436–44.
33. Amodio P, Bemeur C, Butterworth R, et al. The nutritional management of hepatic encephalopathy in patients with cirrhosis: International Society for Hepatic Encephalopathy and Nitrogen Metabolism Consensus. Hepatology 2013;58(1): 325–36.
34. Gluud LL, Dam G, Les I, et al. Branched-chain amino acids for people with hepatic encephalopathy. Cochrane Database Syst Rev 2015;(9):CD001939.
35. Palmer D, Macfie J, Bradford IM, et al. Administration of peripheral parenteral nutrition: a prospective study comparing rotation of venous access sites with ultrafine cannulas. Clin Nutr 1996;15(6):311–5.
36. Ryder M. Evidence-based practice in the management of vascular access devices for home parenteral nutrition therapy. JPEN J Parenter Enteral Nutr 2006; 30(1 Suppl):S82–93, s98–9.
37. Staun M, Pironi L, Bozzetti F, et al. ESPEN guidelines on parenteral nutrition: home parenteral nutrition (HPN) in adult patients. Clin Nutr 2009;28(4):467–79.
38. Cotogni P, Pittiruti M, Barbero C, et al. Catheter-related complications in cancer patients on home parenteral nutrition: a prospective study of over 51,000 catheter days. JPEN J Parenter Enteral Nutr 2013;37(3):375–83.
39. Cowl CT, Weinstock JV, Al-Jurf A, et al. Complications and cost associated with parenteral nutrition delivered to hospitalized patients through either subclavian or peripherally-inserted central catheters. Clin Nutr 2000;19(4):237–43.
40. Raad I, Davis S, Becker M, et al. Low infection rate and long durability of nontunneled Silastic catheters. A safe and cost-effective alternative for long-term venous access. Arch Intern Med 1993;153(15):1791–6.
41. Parienti JJ, Mongardon N, Megarbane B, et al. Intravascular complications of central venous catheterization by insertion site. N Engl J Med 2015;373(13): 1220–9.
42. Ukleja A, Romano MM. Complications of parenteral nutrition. Gastroenterol Clin North Am 2007;36(1):23–46, v.
43. Shekelle PG, Wachter RM, Pronovost PJ, et al. Making health care safer II: an updated critical analysis of the evidence for patient safety practices. Evid Rep Technol Assess (Full Rep) 2013;(211):1–945.
44. Kusminsky RE. Complications of central venous catheterization. J Am Coll Surg 2007;204(4):681–96.
45. Gosmanov AR, Umpierrez GE. Management of hyperglycemia during enteral and parenteral nutrition therapy. Curr Diab Rep 2013;13(1):155–62.
46. Cheung NW, Napier B, Zaccaria C, et al. Hyperglycemia is associated with adverse outcomes in patients receiving total parenteral nutrition. Diabetes Care 2005;28(10):2367–71.

47. Lin LY, Lin HC, Lee PC, et al. Hyperglycemia correlates with outcomes in patients receiving total parenteral nutrition. Am J Med Sci 2007;333(5):261–5.
48. Ziegler TR. Parenteral nutrition in the critically ill patient. N Engl J Med 2009; 361(11):1088–97.
49. McMahon MM, Nystrom E, Braunschweig C, et al. A.S.P.E.N. clinical guidelines: nutrition support of adult patients with hyperglycemia. JPEN J Parenter Enteral Nutr 2013;37(1):23–36.
50. Lee H, Koh SO, Park MS. Higher dextrose delivery via TPN related to the development of hyperglycemia in non-diabetic critically ill patients. Nutr Res Pract 2011;5(5):450–4.
51. Ahrens CL, Barletta JF, Kanji S, et al. Effect of low-calorie parenteral nutrition on the incidence and severity of hyperglycemia in surgical patients: a randomized, controlled trial. Crit Care Med 2005;33(11):2507–12.
52. Jakoby MG, Nannapaneni N. An insulin protocol for management of hyperglycemia in patients receiving parenteral nutrition is superior to ad hoc management. JPEN J Parenter Enteral Nutr 2012;36(2):183–8.
53. Moureau N, Poole S, Murdock MA, et al. Central venous catheters in home infusion care: outcomes analysis in 50,470 patients. J Vasc Interv Radiol 2002; 13(10):1009–16.
54. Barco S, Heuschen CB, Salman B, et al. Home parenteral nutrition-associated thromboembolic and bleeding events: results of a cohort study of 236 individuals. J Thromb Haemost 2016;14(7):1364–73.
55. Goode CJ, Titler M, Rakel B, et al. A meta-analysis of effects of heparin flush and saline flush: quality and cost implications. Nurs Res 1991;40(6):324–30.
56. Peterson FY, Kirchhoff KT. Analysis of the research about heparinized versus non-heparinized intravascular lines. Heart Lung 1991;20(6):631–40.
57. Randolph AG, Cook DJ, Gonzales CA, et al. Benefit of heparin in peripheral venous and arterial catheters: systematic review and meta-analysis of randomised controlled trials. BMJ 1998;316(7136):969–75.
58. Centers for Disease Control and Prevention. National and state healthcare-associated infections progress report. 2014. Available at: http://www.cdc.gov/HAI/pdfs/progress-report/hai-progress-report.pdf. Accessed July 29, 2017.
59. Dreesen M, Foulon V, Spriet I, et al. Epidemiology of catheter-related infections in adult patients receiving home parenteral nutrition: a systematic review. Clin Nutr 2013;32(1):16–26.
60. Ross VM, Guenter P, Corrigan ML, et al. Central venous catheter infections in home parenteral nutrition patients: outcomes from sustain: American Society for Parenteral and Enteral Nutrition's National Patient Registry for Nutrition Care. Am J Infect Control 2016;44(12):1462–8.
61. Fonseca G, Burgermaster M, Larson E, et al. The relationship between parenteral nutrition and central line-associated bloodstream infections. JPEN J Parenter Enteral Nutr 2017. 148607116688437. [Epub ahead of print].
62. Pittiruti M, Hamilton H, Biffi R, et al. ESPEN guidelines on parenteral nutrition: central venous catheters (access, care, diagnosis and therapy of complications). Clin Nutr 2009;28(4):365–77.
63. Dezfulian C, Lavelle J, Nallamothu BK, et al. Rates of infection for single-lumen versus multilumen central venous catheters: a meta-analysis. Crit Care Med 2003;31(9):2385–90.
64. Zurcher M, Tramer MR, Walder B. Colonization and bloodstream infection with single- versus multi-lumen central venous catheters: a quantitative systematic review. Anesth Analg 2004;99(1):177–82.

65. Pronovost P, Needham D, Berenholtz S, et al. An intervention to decrease catheter-related bloodstream infections in the ICU. N Engl J Med 2006;355: 2725–32.

66. John BK, Khan MA, Speerhas R, et al. Ethanol lock therapy in reducing catheter related bloodstream infections in adult home parenteral nutrition patients: results of a retrospective study. JPEN J Parenter Enteral Nutr 2012;36:603–10.

67. Mermel LA, Alang N. Adverse effects associated with ethanol catheter lock solutions: a systematic review. J Antimicrob Chemother 2014;69(10):2611–9.

68. Buchman A. Total parenteral nutrition-associated liver disease. JPEN J Parenter Enteral Nutr 2002;26(5):543–8.

69. Chan S, McCowen KC, Bistrian BR, et al. Incidence, prognosis, and etiology of end-stage liver disease in patients receiving home total parenteral nutrition. Surgery 1999;126(1):28–34.

70. Cavicchi M, Beau P, Crenn P, et al. Prevalence of liver disease and contributing factors in patients receiving home parenteral nutrition for permanent intestinal failure. Ann Intern Med 2000;132(7):525–32.

71. Messing B, Bories C, Kunstlinger F, et al. Does total parenteral nutrition induce gallbladder sludge formation and lithiasis? Gastroenterology 1983;84(5 Pt 1): 1012–9.

72. Douard H, Cosnes J, Sebag A, et al. Ultrasonic study of gallbladder motility during exclusive continuous enteral feeding. Gastroenterol Clin Biol 1987;11(10): 643–7 [in French].

73. Doty JE, Pitt HA, Porter-Fink V, et al. Cholecystokinin prophylaxis of parenteral nutrition-induced gallbladder disease. Ann Surg 1985;201(1):76–80.

74. Klein GL, Targoff CM, Ament ME, et al. Bone disease associated with total parenteral nutrition. Lancet 1980;2(8203):1041–4.

75. Pironi L, Labate AM, Pertkiewicz M, et al. Prevalence of bone disease in patients on home parenteral nutrition. Clin Nutr 2002;21(4):289–96.

76. Ott SM, Maloney NA, Klein GL, et al. Aluminum is associated with low bone formation in patients receiving chronic parenteral nutrition. Ann Intern Med 1983; 98(6):910–4.

77. Vargas JH, Klein GL, Ament ME, et al. Metabolic bone disease of total parenteral nutrition: course after changing from casein to amino acids in parenteral solutions with reduced aluminum content. Am J Clin Nutr 1988;48(4):1070–8.

78. Sloan GM, White DE, Murray MS, et al. Calcium and phosphorus metabolism during total parenteral nutrition. Ann Surg 1983;197(1):1–6.

79. Wood RJ, Sitrin MD, Cusson GJ, et al. Reduction of total parenteral nutrition-induced urinary calcium loss by increasing the phosphorus in the total parenteral nutrition prescription. JPEN J Parenter Enteral Nutr 1986;10(2):188–90.

80. Verhage AH, Cheong WK, Allard JP, et al. Harry M. Vars Research Award. Increase in lumbar spine bone mineral content in patients on long-term parenteral nutrition without vitamin D supplementation. JPEN J Parenter Enteral Nutr 1995; 19(6):431–6.

81. Moukarzel AA, Ament ME, Buchman A, et al. Renal function of children receiving long-term parenteral nutrition. J Pediatr 1991;119(6):864–8.

82. Buchman AL, Moukarzel AA, Ament ME. Excessive urinary oxalate excretion occurs in long-term TPN patients both with and without ileostomies. J Am Coll Nutr 1995;14(1):24–8.

Nutritional Therapy in Adult Short Bowel Syndrome Patients with Chronic Intestinal Failure

Palle Bekker Jeppesen, MD, PhD*, Kristian Asp Fuglsang, MD

KEYWORDS

- Nutrition • Diet • Enteral nutrition • Short bowel syndrome • Intestinal insufficiency
- Intestinal failure

KEY POINTS

- Nutritional therapy is described as one of the cornerstones of intestinal rehabilitation in patients with intestinal failure (IF), but the evidence base for general recommendations is weak.
- Due to the heterogeneity of the IF population and due to significant effect heterogeneity an individualized approach on nutritional management is mandated.
- Successful nutritional interventions defined by the ability to maintain or wean off parenteral support are most likely to be achieved in patients located in the borderline between severe intestinal insufficiency and mild intestinal failure.
- Ideally, the effects of nutritional therapy should be evaluated by objective measures, and the interventions should respect patient autonomy to achieve best compliance and quality of life in patients with IF.

INTRODUCTION

Multiple factors should to be taken into considerations when discussing nutritional therapy in adult patients with chronic, type 3 intestinal failure (IF). As a large patient heterogeneity exists within this group of rare patients, this article provides a brief introduction with suggestions of definitions and concepts in the field of interest that may be relevant before the discussion of the potential effects of nutrition interventions.

Disclosure Statement: The authors have nothing to disclose.
Department of Medical Gastroenterology, University Hospital of Copenhagen, Rigshospitalet, Blegdamsvej 9, Copenhagen 2100, Denmark
* Corresponding author. Department of Medical Gastroenterology, University Hospital of Copenhagen, Rigshospitalet, CA 2-12-1, Blegdamsvej 9, Copenhagen 2100, Denmark.
E-mail address: bekker@dadlnet.dk

Gastroenterol Clin N Am 47 (2018) 61–75
https://doi.org/10.1016/j.gtc.2017.10.004
0889-8553/18/© 2017 Elsevier Inc. All rights reserved.

gastro.theclinics.com

Classification of Intestinal Failure

The hallmark of IF is the reduction in intestinal function below a minimum necessary for absorption of fluid, electrolytes, and/or macronutrients to maintain health and/or growth.[1] Consequently, supplemental or even total parenteral support (PS) is mandated. The European Society for Clinical Nutrition and Metabolism (ESPEN) recently defined 5 major pathophysiological conditions causing IF: short bowel, intestinal fistula, intestinal dysmotility, mechanical obstruction, and extensive mucosal disease.[1] Based on the convalescence outcome following the event leading to IF, IF can be classified as an acute (Type 1), prolonged acute (Type 2), or chronic condition (Type 3).[2] In adults, the most common cause of IF is short bowel syndrome (SBS),[3–5] in which the small bowel length by definition is less than 200 cm.[1] Frequently, patients with SBS are subdivided into 3 anatomic groups: *jejunostomy* or *ileostomy* (group 1), *jejuno-colonic anastomosis* (group 2), and *jejuno-ileo-colonic anastomosis* (group 3).[6] Regarding a classification according to diagnosis, in most cases, SBS occurs as a consequence of extensive surgery related to inflammatory bowel disease, mesenteric vascular disease, cancer, and complications of other surgery. In the pediatric population, intestinal malformation, Hirschprung disease, necrotizing enterocolitis, volvulus, and rare conditions may be the cause of surgery.[1]

Anatomically, in adults, the patients at greatest risk of IF and dependence on PS are those with an end-jejunostomy and less than 115 cm of residual, functional small bowel; those with a jejuno-colic anastomosis and less than 60 cm of residual small intestine (absent ileocecal valve); and those with a jejuno-ileal anastomosis and less than 35 cm of residual small intestine (but presence of ileocecal valve and colon).[7,8] However, because a relatively poor correlation exists between remnant bowel anatomy and remnant bowel function, it has been suggested that patients with suspected "dys-homeostasis in the nutritional equilibrium" should be categorized based on results obtained in metabolic balance studies within a spectrum ranging from mild, moderate, and severe intestinal insufficiency, coping without need for PS, across a borderline to mild, moderate, and severe IF.[9,10] By these balance studies, in clinical practice, the borderline between intestinal insufficiency and failure has been defined as an energy absorption of 81% of the calculated basal metabolic rate (BMR) and a wet weight absorption of 21 g/kg body weight per day equaling findings in research settings (84% of BMR and 23 g/body weight per day, respectively).[9,10]

Because the access to performing metabolic balance studies is limited even in most centers of experience in providing care for patients with IF, the provision of PS has been suggested as an indirect measure of intestinal function.[11] However, it should be noted that in instable patients, in whom PS may be used to accelerate recovery from nutritional deficits, this may not be valid. Furthermore, the net intestinal absorptive capacity may not be stationary over time, as the bowel is able to adapt to endogenous and exogenous stimulations. Thus, the residual absorptive capacity of the intestine is dynamic and highly coordinated, and it does not only depend on oral intake, but also on multiple neuro-endocrine regulations of digestive and absorptive mechanisms, mucosal growth, motility, and blood flow. The adaptive potential of the gastrointestinal tract is illustrated by the finding that some patients with Type 3 SBS-IF may eventually regain intestinal autonomy several years after the diagnosis even without restorative surgery.[3,4,12] The likelihood of gradually regaining intestinal autonomy by gaining the adaptive effects on top on those achieved by the conventional dietary and pharmacologic therapies seem to be best in patients with a preserved segment of the ileum and colon in continuity, whereas improvements in intestinal absorption over time seem to be less predominant in patients with end-jejunostomies.[13,14]

The Aims and Challenges of Nutritional Therapy in Intestinal Failure

The ultimate aim in IF treatment is to maximize remnant intestinal function, minimizing IF-associated symptoms, weaning from PS, regaining intestinal autonomy, and thereby providing patients with IF with the best possible quality of life.[15] Although potentially life-saving by preventing malnutrition-related complications, PS and the concomitant need for a central line is related to morbidity and even mortality due to catheter-related complications, such as catheter infections and thrombosis.[16] In addition, IF and the need for long-term PS also may contribute to various comorbidities and even mortality related to organ dysfunction, such as IF-associated liver disease and renal failure. Thus, IF and PS dependence may not only restrict the spontaneous lifestyle of the patients, it also may reduce their ability to be reintegrated into working life and reduce their quality of life and ultimately their life expectancy.[17] In addition, the overall, direct and indirect, health-associated costs are significant in patients with IF.[18]

When considering alternatives for PS, the route for dietary interventions through conventional regular food, oral supplements or enteral feedings should be considered. Enteral feeding requires a placement of tubes (eg, nasogastric or percutaneous endoscopic gastrostomy tubes). They are invasive and hold significant disadvantages, potential risks, and in general the long-term acceptance and compliance are low.[19] Oral supplements are convenient, but costs and palatability may be a problem. When considering dietary advice for patients with IF, the psychological, social, and cultural benefits related to normal consumption of regular food should not be neglected. The long-term compliance eventually will be the key to a potential success. Therefore, an individualized approach, weighing the clinical benefit of rigorous dietary advice on nutritional parameters, like diet restriction, use of unpalatable diets, or the use of enteral access, should be balanced against the potential inconveniences on socialization, identity, and the feeling of pleasure. Dietary interventions also may affect the sense of appetite and satiety, which may compromise the overall dietary intake and thereby jeopardize the anticipated overall benefits. Likewise, dietary interventions may aggravate gastrointestinal symptoms related to IF (eg, abdominal pain, bloating, passing of wind, urgency, and incontinence). Finally, cost needs to be considered. Coping strategies and acceptance of inconveniences related to dietary interventions may differ among patients. Some patients cope with the challenges of regular oral hyperphagia and even supplemental enteral feedings, passing of large stool volumes, fatigue, and chronic dehydration to avoid a life dominated by the central line and a need for PS. Others see PS as a place of refuge, escaping the demands of constant hyperphagia, the inconveniences of enteral feedings, and the concomitant large stool volumes and potential abdominal discomfort. Therefore, the individual patient management and treatment strategy should rely on a discussion between the patient and the health care provider.[11] In the ideal world, the short-term and long-term experiences and effects of the dietary interventions should be evaluated in the individual patients with IF in metabolic balance studies, whereby physiologic effects on energy, fluid and electrolyte balances, PS requirements, and the well-being of the patients could be demonstrated. In reality, in most centers, general dietary advice is provided, but the true effects of these recommendations in the individual patients are often difficult to objectivize, poorly documented, or remain unknown.

As illustrated by the suggested multiple classifications of patients with IF, a large interpatient heterogeneity exists. In addition, results from the current literature suggest that even in studies in which subgroups of patients with IF are included into studies based on the suggested IF classifications, a large interpatient heterogeneity effect in relation to interventions may exist. The lack of a solid evidence basis for the recommendation of dietary interventions in patients with IF is also evident in the guideline published by ESPEN in 2016.[20] Among the statements focusing on dietary advice in patients with IF, the grade of evidence was low in 14 statements related to patients with SBS, very low in 2 statements related to patients with chronic intestinal pseudo-obstruction, and very low in 1 statement related to patients with radiation enteritis. This clearly indicates that the amount and quality of scientific studies in this area is low. Because evidence is very scarce in areas other than in adult patients with SBS-IF, the following section will mainly focus on this condition.

The evidence for dietary therapy in patients with intestinal failure

Conceptually, the absorptive ability of the bowel would mainly be dependent on the oral intake, intestinal anatomy, and intestinal mucosal surface area. However, intestinal assimilation is a highly coordinated process also integrating various digestive secretions, motility, and blood flow. This complex neuroendocrine coordination is affected by the nutrient exposure of entero-endocrine sensor cells throughout the gastrointestinal tract.[21] Under normal conditions, tightly regulated feedback loops will ensure the optimal nutrient intake and assimilation. The intact and healthy gastrointestinal tract has a considerable reserve capacity for nutrient, fluid, and electrolyte assimilation.[22] Thus, even under conditions of massive hyperphagia, less than 5% of dietary energy intake is lost in the feces, and fecal wet weight excretion normally is less than 300 g/d.[23] In patients with inadequate oral intake, intestinal diseases, or increased metabolic needs, the nutritional homeostasis may be jeopardized, and malnutrition, dehydration, or other deficiencies may develop.[24]

When instituting nutritional therapy in patients with IF, it is important to be aware that the dependence of PS may be related to either energy or fluid/electrolytes, or both. It is also important to realize that intestinal diseases or resection may disturb the highly co-ordinated process of nutrient, fluid, and electrolyte absorption by interruption of the complex neural signaling or removal of enteroendocrine sensor cells in the gastrointestinal tract. Thus, whereas increasing nutrient intake or changing diet composition may be beneficial for macronutrient absorption, it could detrimentally stimulate various hypersecretions, potentially aggravating the overall fluid and electrolyte losses. Likewise, excessive oral fluid intake may negatively affect energy absorption.

Oral Compensation/Hyperphagia

As a group, patients with IF due to eating and motility disorders (radiation enteritis, mechanical obstruction, and dysmotility) have been demonstrated to consume calories equivalent to only half of their basal energy expenditure (BEE).[25] In general, malabsorption is relatively small in these patients. However, a large interpatient heterogeneity exists. In contrast, in patients with SBS-IF, hyperphagia seems to be present even shortly after surgery.[26] In the long-term stable phase after surgery, some patients with SBS with intestinal insufficiency have a remarkable ability to compensate for malabsorption and thereby eventually avoid the need for PS by increasing their oral energy intakes by up to 4 times their BEE.[9,27] Even some patients with SBS-IF who are chronically confined to PS energy support consume energy in an amount equaling 2.5 times their BEE.[9,25,28] The nature of this compensatory behavioral effort remains to be established. Although dietary advice from health care professionals may be involved, it is also likely that physiologic changes in the neuroendocrine signaling involving increases in the sense of thirst and appetite could contribute. The effect and compliance of advising hyperphagia on top of the increased spontaneous oral dietary intake in patients with SBS is poorly scientifically evaluated. Clinically, oral nutrient supplements and more rarely enteral feedings are used in the borderline patients located in the "gray zone" between intestinal insufficiency and failure. It is likely, that the effect of oral nutrient supplements would be largest in those patients who tend to have a low ability to orally compensate for malabsorption but who have a high percentage absorption of what they consume. In patients who have fully "stretched their ability to compensate for malabsorption" and who already have low percentage absorption, the effort may be in vain.

Based on the idea that intestinal absorption is maximized in patients with SBS ensuring just the right nutrient amount, avoiding "overwhelming of the intestine," and providing a timewise prolonged exposure of the mucosal surface area to macronutrients, patients are often advised to eat frequent meals. It has also been recommended that the timing of nutrient and beverage intake should be separated.[29] Although conceptually appealing, the scientific evidence to illustrate an effect of this is lacking.

Animal studies suggest that the absence of nutrition in the lumen causes bowel atrophy with decrease of the villus height, whereas hyperphagia increases hyperplasia and villus height.[30,31] However, the evidence for the nature of adaptive effects of oral or enteral nutrients is far less solid in humans.[32] It is currently unknown if a more constant exposure of the intestinal mucosa by increasing the supply of nutrients would increase the overall absolute energy absorption by improving adaptation and the relative nutrient absorption. It has been suggested that a time-confined "window of opportunity" following surgery for gaining such hyperadaptation should exist, but the compliance to such intervention and the consequent duration of the effect of the "hyperadaptive dietary intervention" is still speculative.[33] Likewise, in humans, the macronutrient (fat, carbohydrate, or protein) with the most profound effect on intestinal adaptation has not been identified.

Effect of Manipulation of the Macronutrient Energy-Ratio in Oral Diets in Patients with Short Bowel Syndrome–Intestinal Failure

When considering dietary management of the patients with short bowel, clarification of the remnant intestinal anatomy is crucial. As mentioned previously, it is recommended that patients with SBS-IF are divided into 3 groups based on the absence or presence of the terminal ileum and the colon. The importance of the colon in the fluid and electrolyte absorption and its role in ileal-resection diarrhea has been known for decades.[34] Because diarrhea is associated with steatorrhea,[35–40] a low-fat diet has been recommended in the symptomatic treatment of patients with short bowel with a preserved colon. A low-fat diet also would increase the absorption of calcium, magnesium, and zinc in these patients.[41,42] Several herbivorous and omnivorous animals meet a considerable proportion of their energy requirements from the anaerobic bacterial breakdown of complex carbohydrates not hydrolyzed and absorbed in the upper digestive tract. In many hindgut-fermenting animals this bacterial degradation of carbohydrates to the easily absorbed short-chain fatty acids (SCFAs) contributes to more than 50% of their maintenance energy requirements. In humans, this was studied in patients subjected to jejunal bypass operations, and Bond and colleagues[43] found that an appreciable fraction of carbohydrate was removed during colonic transit. Likewise, Royall and colleagues[44,45] described the colonic fermentation and suggested the energy-salvaging role of the colon in humans. The significance of colon on energy absorption in human patients with SBS was indirectly demonstrated by Nightingale and colleagues,[13] who found that patients with equal length of small intestine did better, not only with respect to fluid absorption but also with regard to the needs for parenteral supply of energy, if the patients had a colon in continuity. The preservation of at least half of the large bowel was equivalent to approximately 50 cm of the small intestine in terms of the need for parenteral supplements. The significance of a preserved colon in patients with short bowel receiving home parenteral nutrition (HPN) was also described in a cross-sectional study of the parenteral support given to the total cohort of 73 patients.[46] The number of patients receiving HPN with a substantial remnant colon ($\geq$50%) was compared with the number with no colonic function (0%) in subgroups of patients with remnant small bowels. Eight of 20 patients with less than 100 cm of small bowel (group 1) had $\geq$50% colon in function, in contrast to 2 of 23 patients with 100 to 200 cm small bowel (group 2) (Fisher exact test, $P = .028$). In patients in group 1, the need for parenteral energy in percentage of BEE (HPN/BMR%, mean $\pm$ SD) was 110% $\pm$ 31% in patients with no colon and 59% $\pm$ 31% in patients with a preserved colon ($P = .001$). In patients without a colon in groups 2 (100–200 cm) and 3 (>200 cm small bowel) HPN/BMR% was 58% $\pm$ 45% and 33% $\pm$ 47%, respectively. Thus, dependency of HPN was rarely seen in patients with a substantial colonic function ($\geq$50%) combined with greater than 100-cm remnant small bowel, and in patients with less than 100 cm small bowel a substantial colon remnant was associated with a reduction of parenteral energy requirements of approximately 3 MJ/d (51% of BMR). These data added to the reports of the colon as an energy-salvaging organ ($\sim$3–4 MJ/d), which renders HPN unnecessary in most patients in whom small bowel length is sufficient to absorb another 3 to 4 MJ/d.[47]

Bearing in mind the energy-salvaging effect of a preserved colon, the clinical effect of changing from a high-fat diet to a high-carbohydrate diet was investigated by Nordgaard and colleagues[48] in patients with short bowel with a preserved colon. Eight patients with SBS who all managed without PS and therefore by definition did not suffer from IF, received 2 isoenergetic diets (10.7 MJ/d) for two 4-day periods in a crossover balance study. The high-carbohydrate–low-fat diet reduced fecal loss of energy by 2.0 MJ/d compared with the low-carbohydrate high-fat diets and absorption of energy increased significantly from 49% to 69%. Fecal excretions of carbohydrates were low and not influenced by alterations in intake of carbohydrates, whereas excretions of fat were dependent on the amount of fat ingested and accounted for the differences in loss of energy in feces. No changes in fecal volume were observed between the 2 study periods, but the amount of water included in the high-carbohydrate diet was approximately 1000 mL higher than in the high-fat diet, thereby providing a better overall fluid absorption.

Thus, theoretically, based on these physiologic experiments, a low-fat carbohydrate-rich diet is recommended in patients with short bowel intestinal insufficiency with a preserved colon. However, carbohydrates have a lower energy density than fat (17 kJ/g vs 37 kJ/g), and therefore carbohydrate-rich meals need to be more voluminous to contain equal amounts of energy and will likely give a higher satiety. Furthermore, foods containing less fat may be less palatable and tasty, and in the nature of fermentation, surplus gas is produced, which may cause bloating. Hence, implementing a low-fat diet in the everyday life of the patients is not without disadvantages and may reduce the overall spontaneous dietary energy intake. Therefore, patients tend to find their own balance, maximizing energy intake and absorption, reducing the social disability of bloating and the bulky offensive stools provoked by carbohydrates and fats, respectively.

With complex carbohydrates suggested to be an important dietary carbohydrate for patients with SBS with a preserved colon in continuity, it was investigated if soluble fiber supplements such as pectin (4 g 3 times a day for 2 weeks) could be used to enhance intestinal absorption through an increased production of SCFAs and effects on intestinal transit. However, a pectin supplement did not increase macronutrient or energy absorption (1768 vs 1477 kcal/d, $P = .15$), fecal wet weight (1582 vs 1689 g/d,

$P = 1.00$), or urine production (1615 vs 1610 mL/d, $P = 1.00$).[49] Patients with SBS with a colon in continuity may experience the beneficial effects of ispaghula husk and calcium on stool viscosity and consistency, which may ameliorate the sensation of urgency.[50] Some patients with an end ostomy also report benefit from the use of fiber supplements, as they help to gelatinize the ostomy effluent.

In the spectrum between the easy absorbable SCFAs and the nonabsorbable long-chain fatty acids, the medium-chain fatty acids could potentially serve as an alternative source of energy absorbed from the large bowel in patients with short bowel. Replacement of normal fat with medium-chain triglycerides (MCTs) has been advocated for many years in the dietary treatment of patients with short bowel, but the effect on energy absorption and stool volume was initially not fully evaluated by using the right techniques.[51–53] Therefore, Jeppesen and Mortensen[54] investigated this issue in an open, randomized controlled study. Nine patients with resected small bowel without and 10 with a colon in continuity with a fecal energy excretion between 2 and 6 MJ/d were randomized and crossed over between 2 high-fat diets (approximately 10,000 kJ/d, 50% as fat), based on either long-chain triglycerides (LCTs) alone or equal quantities of LCTs and MCTs. Four of the 9 patients with SBS jejunostomy received PS. In patients with a preserved colon, in which 2 patients received PS, the absorption of medium-chain C8 to C18 fatty acids gradually decreased as the length of the fatty acid chain increased. Fecal excretion of medium-chain fatty acids was negligible, and MCT absorption was almost complete even in patients who malabsorbed 90% to 100% of dietary LCTs. Patients with a colon absorbed C8 to C10 fatty acids better than patients without a colon. In contrast, a preserved colon did not improve the absorption of long-chain C14 to C18 fatty acids. On average, a 30% MCT diet increased fat (MCT + LCT) absorption from 23% to 58% ($P<.001$) in patients with a colon, and increased energy absorption from 46% to 58% ($P<.05$). The short-term clinical consequence of replacement of LCTs with MCTs in patients with small bowel resection and a jejunostomy or ileostomy was a small increase in fat absorption, which was counterbalanced to the level of no effect on the overall energy balance due to a negative effect on the absorption of carbohydrate and nitrogenous substances. The absence of an effect observed in patients with a jejunostomy or ileostomy may be explained by a trend toward an increase in the stoma effluents observed in these patients. The weight of the stoma effluent tended to increase 25% from 2177 ± 1455 g/d to 2729 ± 1543 g/d ($P = .07$) when patients were changed from the LCT diet to the L/MCT diet. In the patients with jejunostomy with intestinal insufficiency near the borderline toward IF, the use of MCTs may be the cause of increase in the stomal output and cause dehydration and lead to a need for parenteral fluid and electrolyte support. In contrast, the increase in the fecal volumes was only 12% in patients with short bowel with a colon. The fecal volumes during the LCT and L/MCT diet was 981 ± 379 g/d and 1114 ± 622 g/d, respectively ($P = .32$); however, the large effect of heterogeneity illustrated by the large SDs suggests that attention should be paid in the individual borderline patients, in whom a desirable increase in energy absorption may be counterbalanced by a detrimental effect on wet weight absorption.

It also should be noted that the effect of a replacement of dietary LCTs with MCTs in patients with short bowel on the total intestinal energy absorption is conditioned on a difference between the absorption of LCTs and MCTs, respectively, and the amount of MCTs given. Thus, a difference in the level of absorption between MCTs and LCTs of 20%, 40%, and 80% would result in an increase in the energy absorption of 5%, 10%, and 20% (corresponding to 0.5, 1, and 2 MJ/d on a diet containing 10 MJ/d), if 25% of the total energy in the diet based on LCTs was replaced by MCTs, as was done in the study of Jeppesen and colleagues.[54] Thus, large quantities of MCT replacements of diet LCTs are needed, which may result in poor long-term tolerability with respect to taste preferences. In patients with a preserved colon, the average increase in the total energy absorption was approximately 1.3 MJ/d. It is also important to emphasize that replacement of LCTs with MCTs leads to a reduction in the supply of essential fatty acids. Consequently, more severe signs of essential fatty acid deficiency may be encountered during MCT treatment. Thus, when treating patients with short bowel with a preserved colon, focus should not only be directed toward improved overall energy absorption, but also on the potential for promoting deficiencies of nutrients normally absorbed in the small bowel when changing the diet composition.

Most studies dealing with fat absorption after small bowel resection have stressed the clinical sign of fat malabsorption. As increasing amounts of fat in the diet leads to a greater amount of fat in the stool, high-carbohydrate–low-fat diets have been recommended for decades for all patients with small bowel resection. However, a positive linear relationship has been proven in the normal intestine between the concentration of lipids in the aqueous phase in the intestinal lumen and proportion of lipids absorbed by the small intestine.[55,56] Thus, a high-carbohydrate–low-fat diet decreases the concentration of dietary fat offered to the intestine. Patients with short bowel without a colon, who do not experience the deleterious effects of malabsorbed fatty acids in the colon, thereby may not use their full capacity of the remaining small intestine for fat absorption. Simko and colleagues[57] proved the effect of increasing amounts of dietary fat on absolute fat absorption in a patient with jejunostomy. They found that an increase in the dietary fat from 64 to 200 g/d led to an increase in absolute fat absorption from 44 to 133 g. This would correspond to an increase in energy absorption of more than 3 MJ/d. No changes in transit time, ostomy dry weights, or fluid outputs could be detected.

Using bomb calorimetry, McIntyre and colleagues[58] compared the absorption of a chemically defined liquid diet consisting mainly of small peptides, oligosaccharides, and little fat (half of which was MCTs) with absorption of a polymeric diet in patients with short residual intestine (<150 cm) ending in a stoma. Furthermore, 3 solid diets with various amounts of fiber and fat were compared. In these short-term experiments, no therapeutic benefit was gained from any of the high-fat or low-fat diets or in the chemically defined diet compared with the polymeric diet. The relative specific absorption of nitrogen, fat, and energy was unchanged in each patient from each diet, neither of which significantly reduced the weight of stoma effluent, when compared with the other. A high-fat diet did lead to increased fat excretion but not to increased jejunostomy effluent or mineral losses. In line with the findings of Jeppesen and colleagues,[9] those patients who absorbed more than 50% of their total energy intake sustained normal health by an increased nutrient intake, whereas 2 of the 3 patients with energy absorption below 40% needed parenteral supplements.

Woolf and colleagues[59] studied the effect of a high-fat (~60%) versus a low-fat diet (high carbohydrate ~20%) on fecal excretion and energy absorption in 8 patients with short bowel in a randomized crossover design. Three of the patients had a jejuno-transverse anastomosis and a preserved rectum and 5 had a jejunostomy. Four of the patients received supplemental parenteral nutrition. Mean energy intake was approximately 6.9 MJ/d. Fecal water or dry weights were not different during the 2 study periods. The fecal fat excretion was 3 times higher on the high-fat than on the high-carbohydrate diet, but the proportion of ingested fat absorbed was not different between the 2 diets. There were no significant differences in the mean total energy, fat energy, and protein + carbohydrate energy absorbed, expressed as percentage of intake, between the high-fat and high-carbohydrate diet. The mean absorption percentages of fat and nonfat energy were similar and averaged 65% of intake. There were no significant differences in the absorption of calcium, magnesium, or zinc between the high-fat and high-carbohydrate diets. In all these studies, the patient SBS populations and effects were highly heterogeneous and therefore it cannot be ruled out that the inability to demonstrate effects may be due to type 2 errors.

Nordgaard and colleagues[48] studied the effect of a high-fat (60%) versus a low-fat diet (20%) on fecal excretion and energy absorption in a more homogeneous patient population consisting of 6 patients with short bowel with a jejunostomy in a randomized crossover design. Only 2 of the patients received parenteral supplements. The mean energy intake was 10.6 MJ/d. Fecal water or dry weight were not different during the 2 study periods and absorption of dietary energy was approximately 50% in both periods. A trend toward a reduced fecal energy excretion during the low-fat diet was seen. Absorption of divalent cations was not measured.

Ovesen and colleagues[60] compared the effect of 3 isoenergetic diets on jejunostomy output of fluid, fat, sodium, potassium, calcium, magnesium, zinc, and copper in 5 patients receiving HPN. One diet was low in fat (30%) but high in complex carbohydrate (55%), and 2 were high in fat (60%) but low in carbohydrate (25%). The polyunsaturated/saturated fatty acid ratios of the 2 high-fat diets were 1:4 and 1:1. Diets were eaten for 9 days each with collections of excreta the last 2 days. Mean energy intake was approximately 8.0 MJ/d. Although increasing the percentage of fat in the diet increased the amount of steatorrhea, altering the polyunsaturated/saturated fatty acid ratio had no clearly beneficial effect on the amount of fat absorbed. Neither the amount of fat, nor the type of fat, had any consistent influence on jejunostomy volume. The sodium and potassium concentration of the jejunostomy fluid stayed constant, and hence monovalent cation losses reflected jejunostomy volume rather than the fat:-carbohydrate content of the diet eaten. The high-fat diet increased the ostomy losses of divalent cations: calcium, magnesium, zinc, and copper. Most of the time, a net divalent cation secretion on the high-fat diet was converted into a net absorption on the low-fat–high-carbohydrate diet. Altering the polyunsaturated/saturated fatty acid ratio had no consistent effect on divalent cation losses. Again, the small patient numbers and large effect of heterogeneity make general recommendations difficult. However, based on these studies, it seems that a low-fat diet has no special benefit in stable patients with short bowel with a jejunostomy concerning energy, fluid, or monovalent electrolyte absorption. A constant proportion of dietary fat is absorbed, and more is absorbed if more is taken. As described earlier, dietary fat has a role in providing essential fatty acids and fat-soluble vitamins and increases both diet palatability and energy density, which is of major importance, encouraging patients to eat more.[61] When recommending changes in the carbohydrate:fat ratio in the diet, the potential changes in the excretion of divalent cations should be considered.

Other dietary advice is up for debate. Regarding lactose intake in patients with SBS, in general, a diet containing 20 g/d of lactose is well tolerated in most patients, but it should be carefully titrated in case of previous intolerance.[62] In addition to restricting dietary choices, avoiding lactose potentially could diminish calcium intake and aggravate the development of osteoporosis commonly seen in these patients. In patients with a preserved colon, for the prevention of renal stones, a low oxalate, in addition to an increase of oral calcium, may be recommended to reduce the risk of oxalate stone formation. Currently, it is not recommended to add glutamine, probiotics, or other supplemental nutrients to the diet to promote the intestinal rehabilitation process. The ESPEN recommendation of limiting oral intake of low sodium, both hypotonic (eg, water, tea, coffee, or alcohol) and hypertonic (eg, fruit juices, colas) solutions to reduce output in patients with net secretion and high-output a jejunostomy relies on clinical experiences rather than scientific studies.[20]

Enteral Compensation

In contrast to regular oral consumption, tube feeding makes continuous feeding around the clock possible. Likewise, compared with bolus feeding or oral feeding, continuous enteral infusions have been suggested to ameliorate the detrimental effects on gastrointestinal hypersecretions and accelerated gastrointestinal transit time most frequently seen in patients with distal bowel resections. However, the requirements for an enteral tube adds another layer of complexity to the care of these challenging patients.

In 1985, Cosnes and colleagues[26] were able to stabilize most of 25 patients in a group of patients with severe SBS (fat malabsorption between 31% and 93% and fecal wet weight ranging from 2005 to 6188 g/d) by continuous enteral alimentation (CEA) and provision of approximately 3500 kcal and 2640 mL/d. Fourteen patients in 1 subgroup (group 1) suffered from intestinal failure evidenced by their need for PS. In the remaining 11 patients (group 2), a provisional jejunostomy was present, and they were evaluated before reestablishment of intestinal continuity. The patients were allowed to eat unrestrictedly in excess of the infused formula diet. Adjunctive oral medications included loperamide, tincture of opium, and cimetidine. CEA was maintained for 4 to 8 weeks. In patients in group 1, CEA was discontinued in all cases, and PS was withdrawn in 11 patients under this regimen. In group 1 patients, the decrease of caloric intake before discharge after withdrawal of CEA was accompanied by a decrease of mean fecal wet weight similar to that observed on admission, but at that time, the patients were receiving an unrestricted exclusively oral diet. This suggests that CEA could be used as a bridge to stimulate and promote spontaneous oral hyperphagia. In patients in group 2, CEA was continued in 8 patients until operation. Despite the increase in fecal losses in relation to enteral feedings, positive sodium and water balances could be achieved in most patients by increasing the enteral intake of sodium and water. The only noticeable side effect was an increased incidence of divalent cation (calcium and magnesium) deficiency as demonstrated previously by Ovesen and collelagues.[60] The hypocalcemia and hypomagnesemia, potentially induced by a high fat intake, were never life-threatening and were usually controlled without PS. Because a control arm was not included in the study by Cosnes and colleagues,[26] it is difficult to evaluate the true benefit of CEA per se. CEA may both accelerate and increase the overall energy consumption in patients with SBS, but it is unclear if CEA affects the long-term adaptation and overall oral energy absorption once it is discontinued.

Levy and colleagues[63] investigated the feasibility of high-viscosity enteral nutrition in the early postoperative phase in 62 patients with SBS with 30 to 150 cm of remaining small bowel. All patients had persisting intra-abdominal complications. Twenty-nine patients had colon in continuity, 13 had a terminal jejunostomy and colonic mucous fistula, and 20 had a jejunostomy and an ileal mucosal fistula. Chyme was reinfused in patients with distal bowel out of continuity. Fecal volume during enteral nutrition showed a progressive decrease despite increase in the enteral volume infused. PS could be discontinued at a mean of 36 days and exclusive oral alimentation was obtained in 50 patients at a mean of 87 days. The beneficial effect of continuous enteral feeding was speculated to be attributable to an anti-inflammatory effect of enteral nutrition, and fewer detrimental effects on gastric emptying and secretion. Whereas a high tolerance and weaning from PS was demonstrated, comparison with conventional oral intake was not performed. In addition, reinfusion of succus entericus into the distal small bowel has been demonstrated to inhibit upper gastrointestinal secretions and thereby potentially increase nutrient, fluid, and electrolyte absorption.[64,65] Thus, by reinstituting feedback regulation from the distal intestine and by increasing absorption also from the excluded bowel, the true effect of enteral nutrition per se may have been overestimated by Levy and colleagues. The discomfort of the need for large-bore infusion tubes of at least 12-French diameter for nasogastric infusions and the challenges of chyme reinfusion were not discussed in the article. Although the results are not clearly presented, it is stated that "the theoretic advantage of providing readily absorbable nutrients (elemental diet) is offset by the high osmolality of these solutions."

Regarding enteral protein intake, Cosnes and colleagues[66] compared urinary and fecal excretions of fluid, electrolytes, and nutrients in 6 patients with a high jejunostomy during 3 randomized consecutive 3-day periods of total enteral nutrition with 3 diets differing only by the degree of hydrolysis of the protein moiety: whole proteins, their hydrolysate (63% nitrogen as small peptides with <1000 M), and the 2 mixed together. Daily nitrogen absorption was significantly enhanced with the small-peptide and mixed diets (14.3 ± 3.4 and 13.1 ± 2 g, respectively) compared with the whole protein diet (10.9 ± 2.4 g, $P = .012$). Concomitantly, blood urea nitrogen and urinary urea excretion increased with the small-peptide diet. However, apparent absorption of fat and calories, fecal weight, and urinary and fecal excretions of sodium, potassium, calcium, and magnesium remained unchanged. Thus, the true clinical benefit of a small-peptide–based diet in patients with SBS remains to be further examined.

Regarding supplemental enteral support, Joly and colleagues[67] completed a study in 15 adults with SBS (3–130 months from last surgery, 4 without a colon in continuity) that evidenced that continuous tube feeding for 7 days, alone or in combination with oral feeding, increased intestinal macronutrient absorption compared with oral feeding alone. The energy gain was in the magnitude of 400 kcal/d by increasing the oral energy intake by approximately 1000 kcal/d. Thus, this treatment could be recommended in patients on the borderline with a low level of HPN dependence and in whom the expected gain with tube feeding could allow them to wean off HPN and have the central catheter removed. Results on changes in abdominal symptoms, patient preferences, and fecal wet excretions were not reported in the study. This study did not examine the compliance and patient-reported outcomes, which will be of relevance in relation to longer-term tube feeding. Many patients may find it difficult to comply with long-term nasogastric feeding, unless the benefit could be related to the removal of the central catheter.

SUMMARY

In summary, the recommendations regarding dietary advice in patients with SBS is based on short-term observational studies of low quality and clinical experience rather than evidence-based data. The presentation of research findings related to dietary interventions is also hampered by a large patient and effect heterogeneity. Thus, it is difficult to generalize findings and give general recommendations in relation to dietary interventions in patients with SBS. Based on these reservations, in general, in the post-resection period, regular oral diet should be introduced as soon as possible in patients with SBS. Oral supplements or even enteral feeding may be required in selected patients to accelerate the resumption of conventional oral intake following surgery. Bearing in mind the psychological and social pleasures related to eating, dietary advice, as well as pharmacologic management, should be tailored based also on the individual preferences in light of the objective outcome of interventions. One of the primary goals of dietary interventions should be to reduce or even eliminate the need for PS (nutrients and/or fluid and electrolytes) in patients with SBS-IF, thereby avoiding the need for a central venous catheter. If that is achievable by hyperphagia, a fat-restricted or even enteral nutrition, some patients may accept the adverse events potentially associated with most of these interventions, but long-term compliance may be an issue. In general, the optimal dietary fat intake varies among patients with SBS. It is frequently based on the remnant functional intestinal anatomy and absence or presence of a stoma. In general, patients with an end-jejunostomy can tolerate a higher proportion of energy from dietary fat than patients with a colon in continuity. Overall, the true effect of manipulation of the dietary macronutrient composition, the effect of pushing hyperphagia, or introducing enteral nutrition on the reduction or elimination of PS, is unknown. In the attempt of increasing intestinal energy absorption, intestinal absorption of fluids and electrolytes may suffer. Thus, the overall effects of interventions need to be addressed. Because most patients with SBS are prone to deficiencies in fluid, electrolytes, and macronutrients and micronutrients, a close clinical, anthropometric, and biochemical monitoring of the patients is recommended. A more careful short-term and long-term monitoring should be considered when introducing new dietary therapies. In addition, positive patient-reported outcomes should be ensured. In essence, the science behind dietary advice in patients with SBS is still in its infancy. Future research should focus on the effect of an individualized patient education to empower patients to subjectively report and objectively evaluate the effects of dietary interventions, which may promote their rehabilitation and reduce patient PS dependency and dependency on health care professionals, thereby enabling patients to achieve their optimal quality of life.

REFERENCES

1. Pironi L, Arends J, Baxter J, et al. ESPEN endorsed recommendations. Definition and classification of intestinal failure in adults. Clin Nutr 2015;34:171–80.
2. Shaffer J. Definition and service development. Clin Nutr 2002;21(Supplement 1): 144–5.
3. Brandt CF, Tribler S, Hvistendahl M, et al. A single-center, adult chronic intestinal failure cohort analyzed according to the ESPEN-endorsed recommendations, definitions, and classifications. JPEN J Parenter Enteral Nutr 2015;41: 566–74.
4. Dibb M, Teubner A, Theis V, et al. Review article: the management of long-term parenteral nutrition. Aliment Pharmacol Ther 2013;37:587–603.
5. Dibb M, Soop M, Teubner A, et al. Survival and nutritional dependence on home parenteral nutrition: three decades of experience from a single referral centre. Clin Nutr 2017;36:570–6.
6. Messing B, Crenn P, Beau P, et al. Long-term survival and parenteral nutrition-dependency of adult patients with nonmalignant short bowel. Transplant Proc 1998;30:2548.
7. Carbonnel F, Cosnes J, Chevret S, et al. The role of anatomic factors in nutritional autonomy after extensive small bowel resection. JPEN J Parenter Enteral Nutr 1996;20:275–80.
8. Messing B, Crenn P, Beau P, et al. Long-term survival and parenteral nutrition dependence in adult patients with the short bowel syndrome. Gastroenterology 1999;117:1043–50.
9. Jeppesen PB, Mortensen PB. Intestinal failure defined by measurements of intestinal energy and wet weight absorption. Gut 2000;46:701–6.

10. Prahm AP, Brandt CF, Askov-Hansen C, et al. The use of metabolic balance studies in the objective discrimination between intestinal insufficiency and intestinal failure. Am J Clin Nutr 2017;106:831–8.

11. Jeppesen PB. Short bowel syndrome–characterisation of an orphan condition with many phenotypes. Expert Opin Orphan Drugs 2013;1:515–25.

12. Amiot A, Messing B, Corcos O, et al. Determinants of home parenteral nutrition dependence and survival of 268 patients with non-malignant short bowel syndrome. Clin Nutr 2013;32:368–74.

13. Nightingale JM, Lennard Jones JE, Gertner DJ, et al. Colonic preservation reduces need for parenteral therapy, increases incidence of renal stones, but does not change high prevalence of gall stones in patients with a short bowel. Gut 1992;33:1493–7.

14. Hill GL, Mair WS, Goligher JC. Impairment of 'ileostomy adaptation' in patients after ileal resection. Gut 1974;15:982–7.

15. Jeppesen PB. The non-surgical treatment of adult patients with short bowel syndrome. Expert Opin Orphan Drugs 2013;1:527–38.

16. Brandt CF, Tribler S, Hvistendahl M, et al. Home parenteral nutrition in adult patients with chronic intestinal failure: catheter-related complications over 4 decades at the main Danish tertiary referral center. JPEN J Parenter Enteral Nutr 2016. [Epub ahead of print].

17. Jeppesen PB, Langholz E, Mortensen PB. Quality of life in patients receiving home parenteral nutrition. Gut 1999;44:844–52.

18. Schalamon J, Mayr JM, Hollwarth ME. Mortality and economics in short bowel syndrome. Best Pract Res Clin Gastroenterol 2003;17:931–42.

19. McClave SA, DiBaise JK, Mullin GE, et al. ACG clinical guideline: nutrition therapy in the adult hospitalized patient. Am J Gastroenterol 2016;111:315–34.

20. Pironi L, Arends J, Bozzetti F, et al. ESPEN guidelines on chronic intestinal failure in adults. Clin Nutr 2016;35:247–307.

21. Furness JB. Integrated neural and endocrine control of gastrointestinal function. Adv Exp Med Biol 2016;891:159–73.

22. Kasper H. Faecal fat excretion, diarrhea, and subjective complaints with highly dosed oral fat intake. Digestion 1970;3:321–30.

23. Jeejeebhoy KN. Symposium on diarrhea. 1. Definition and mechanisms of diarrhea. Can Med Assoc J 1977;116:737–9.

24. O'Keefe SJ, Buchman AL, Fishbein TM, et al. Short bowel syndrome and intestinal failure: consensus definitions and overview. Clin Gastroenterol Hepatol 2006;4:6–10.

25. DiCecco S, Nelson J, Burnes J, et al. Nutritional intake of gut failure patients on home parenteral nutrition. JPEN J Parenter Enteral Nutr 1987;11:529–32.

26. Cosnes J, Gendre JP, Evard D, et al. Compensatory enteral hyperalimentation for management of patients with severe short bowel syndrome. Am J Clin Nutr 1985;41:1002–9.

27. Rodrigues CA, Lennard Jones JE, Thompson DG, et al. Energy absorption as a measure of intestinal failure in the short bowel syndrome. Gut 1989;30:176–83.

28. Messing B, Pigot F, Rongier M, et al. Intestinal absorption of free oral hyperalimentation in the very short bowel syndrome. Gastroenterology 1991;100:1502–8.

29. Matarese LE, O'Keefe SJ, Kandil HM, et al. Short bowel syndrome: clinical guidelines for nutrition management. Nutr Clin Pract 2005;20:493–502.

30. Altmann GG. Influence of starvation and refeeding on mucosal size and epithelial renewal in the rat small intestine. Am J Anat 1972;133:391–400.

31. Menge H, Grafe M, Lorenz Meyer H, et al. The influence of food intake on the development of structural and functional adaptation following ileal resection in the rat. Gut 1975;16:468–72.
32. Buchman AL, Moukarzel AA, Ament ME, et al. Effects of total parenteral nutrition on intestinal morphology and function in humans. Transplant Proc 1994;26:1457.
33. Jeppesen PB. Growth factors in short-bowel syndrome patients. Gastroenterol Clin North Am 2007;36:109–21.
34. Cummings JH, James WP, Wiggins HS. Role of the colon in ileal-resection diarrhoea. Lancet 1973;1:344–7.
35. Kellock TD, Pearson JR, Russell RI, et al. The incidence and clinical significance of faecal hydroxy fatty acids. Gut 1969;10:1055.
36. Binder HJ. Editorial: fecal fatty acids-mediators of diarrhea? Gastroenterology 1973;65:847–50.
37. Ammon HV, Phillips SF. Inhibition of ileal water absorption by intraluminal fatty acids. Influence of chain length, hydroxylation, and conjugation of fatty acids. J Clin Invest 1974;53:205–10.
38. Ammon HV, Phillips SF. Inhibition of colonic water and electrolyte absorption by fatty acids in man. Gastroenterology 1973;65:744–9.
39. James AT, Webb JPW. The occurrence of unusual fatty acids in faecal lipids from human beings with normal and abnormal fat absorption. Biochem J 1961;78:333–9.
40. Spiller RC, Brown ML, Phillips SF. Decreased fluid tolerance, accelerated transit, and abnormal motility of the human colon induced by oleic acid. Gastroenterology 1986;91:100–7.
41. Andersson H. The use of a low-fat diet in the symptomatic treatment of ileopathia. World Rev Nutr Diet 1982;40:1–18.
42. Hessov I, Andersson H, Isaksson B. Effects of a low-fat diet on mineral absorption in small-bowel disease. Scand J Gastroenterol 1983;18:551–4.
43. Bond JH, Currier BE, Buchwald H, et al. Colonic conservation of malabsorbed carbohydrate. Gastroenterology 1980;78:444–7.
44. Royall D, Wolever TM, Jeejeebhoy KN. Clinical significance of colonic fermentation. Am J Gastroenterol 1990;85:1307–12.
45. Royall D, Wolever TM, Jeejeebhoy KN. Evidence for colonic conservation of malabsorbed carbohydrate in short bowel syndrome. Am J Gastroenterol 1992;87:751–6.
46. Jeppesen PB, Mortensen PB. Significance of a preserved colon for parenteral energy requirements in patients receiving home parenteral nutrition. Scand J Gastroenterol 1998;33:1175–9.
47. Nordgaard I, Hansen BS, Mortensen PB. Importance of colonic support for energy absorption as small-bowel failure proceeds. Am J Clin Nutr 1996;64:222–31.
48. Nordgaard I, Hansen BS, Mortensen PB. Colon as a digestive organ in patients with short bowel [see comments]. Lancet 1994;343:373–6.
49. Atia A, Girard-Pipau F, Hebuterne X, et al. Macronutrient absorption characteristics in humans with short bowel syndrome and jejunocolonic anastomosis: starch is the most important carbohydrate substrate, although pectin supplementation may modestly enhance short chain fatty acid production and fluid absorption. JPEN J Parenter Enteral Nutr 2011;35:229–40.
50. Qvitzau S, Matzen P, Madsen P. Treatment of chronic diarrhoea: loperamide versus ispaghula husk and calcium. Scand J Gastroenterol 1988;23:1237–40.
51. Bochenek W, Rodgers JB Jr, Balint JA. Effects of changes in dietary lipids on intestinal fluid loss in the short-bowel syndrome. Ann Intern Med 1970;72:205–13.

52. Zurier RB, Campbell RG, Hashim SA, et al. Use of medium-chain triglyceride in management of patients with massive resection of the small intestine. N Engl J Med 1966;274:490–3.
53. Tandon RK, Rodgers JB Jr, Balint JA. The effects of medium-chain triglycerides in the short bowel syndrome. Increased glucose and water transport. Am J Dig Dis 1972;17:233–8.
54. Jeppesen PB, Mortensen PB. The influence of a preserved colon on the absorption of medium chain fat in patients with small bowel resection. Gut 1998;43: 478–83.
55. Borgström B. Studies on intestinal cholesterol absorption in the human. J Clin Invest 1960;39:809 15.
56. Hofmann AF, Borgström B. The intraluminal phase of fat digestion in man: the lipid content of the micellar and oil phases of intestinal content obtained during fat digestion and absorption. J Clin Invest 1964;43:247–57.
57. Simko V, McCarroll AM, Goodman S, et al. High-fat diet in a short bowel syndrome. Intestinal absorption and gastroenteropancreatic hormone responses. Dig Dis Sci 1980;25:333–9.
58. McIntyre PB, Fitchew M, Lennard Jones JE. Patients with a high jejunostomy do not need a special diet. Gastroenterology 1986;91:25–33.
59. Woolf GM, Miller C, Kurian R, et al. Diet for patients with a short bowel: high fat or high carbohydrate? Gastroenterology 1983;84:823–8.
60. Ovesen L, Chu R, Howard L. The influence of dietary fat on jejunostomy output in patients with severe short bowel syndrome. Am J Clin Nutr 1983;38:270–7.
61. Jeppesen PB, Christensen MS, Hoy CE, et al. Essential fatty acid deficiency in patients with severe fat malabsorption. Am J Clin Nutr 1997;65:837–43.
62. Arrigoni E, Marteau P, Briet F, et al. Tolerance and absorption of lactose from milk and yogurt during short-bowel syndrome in humans. Am J Clin Nutr 1994;60: 926–9.
63. Levy E, Frileux P, Sandrucci S, et al. Continuous enteral nutrition during the early adaptive stage of the short bowel syndrome. Br J Surg 1988;75:549–53.
64. Picot D, Layec S, Dussaulx L, et al. Chyme reinfusion in patients with intestinal failure due to temporary double enterostomy: a 15-year prospective cohort in a referral centre. Clin Nutr 2017;36:593–600.
65. Thibault R, Picot D. Chyme reinfusion or enteroclysis in nutrition of patients with temporary double enterostomy or enterocutaneous fistula. Curr Opin Clin Nutr Metab Care 2016. [Epub ahead of print].
66. Cosnes J, Evard D, Beaugerie L, et al. Improvement in protein absorption with a small-peptide-based diet in patients with high jejunostomy. Nutrition 1992;8: 406–11.
67. Joly F, Dray X, Corcos O, et al. Tube feeding improves intestinal absorption in short bowel syndrome patients. Gastroenterology 2009;136:824–31.

Nutritional Aspects of Acute Pancreatitis

Kristen M. Roberts, PhD, RDN, LD[a], Marcia Nahikian-Nelms, PhD, RDN, LD, FAND[b],
Andrew Ukleja, MD, CNSP[c], Luis F. Lara, MD[d],*

KEYWORDS

- Nutrition • Acute pancreatitis • Enteral • Parenteral

KEY POINTS

- Acute pancreatitis is associated with a catabolic and hypermetabolic state.
- Nutrition support is critical in severe acute pancreatitis (SAP).
- Early enteral nutrition is safe and beneficial in SAP and its use is linked to better glycemic control, reduced infectious complications, and reduced multiorgan failure and mortality.
- Enteral nutrition may be provided by the gastric or jejunal route in patients with SAP.
- Nasogastric tube feeding seems to be feasible in SAP; however, further randomized controlled trials are needed.

INTRODUCTION

Acute pancreatitis (AP) is often a self-limited inflammation of the pancreas with an excellent prognosis. Most patients with AP have mild or moderately severe pancreatitis that is associated with low morbidity and mortality, thus patients recover within a few days, and usually do not require nutritional support.[1] Historically, most of the patients admitted with a diagnosis of AP were kept nil per os to avoid further stimulation of an already inflamed organ.[2] This concept has been challenged and does not apply to cases of AP unless there is significant gastrointestinal tract dysfunction present. Depending on disease severity, maintaining hemodynamic and respiratory stability, preventing and treating end-organ damage, and treating infection are prioritized more highly than nutritional needs.[3]

Disclosure: The authors have nothing they wish to disclose.
[a] Division of Gastroenterology, Hepatology and Nutrition, School of Health and Rehabilitation Sciences, The Ohio State University, 453 West 10th Avenue, Columbus, OH 43210, USA; [b] School of Health and Rehabilitation Sciences, College of Medicine, The Ohio State University, 453 West 10th Avenue, Columbus, OH 43210, USA; [c] Department of Gastroenterology, Digestive Disease Institute, 2950 Cleveland Clinic Florida, Weston FL 33331, USA; [d] Division of Gastroenterology, Hepatology and Nutrition, Wexner Medical Center, The Ohio State University, 395 West 12th Avenue, 2nd Floor Office Tower, Columbus, OH 43210, USA
* Corresponding author.
E-mail address: Luis.Lara@osumc.edu

Gastroenterol Clin N Am 47 (2018) 77–94
https://doi.org/10.1016/j.gtc.2017.10.002
0889-8553/18/© 2017 Elsevier Inc. All rights reserved.

There is scientific evidence that enteral nutrition (EN) is beneficial in critically ill patients with sepsis, trauma, burns, and severe pancreatitis, with demonstrable improvement in total and intensive care unit (ICU) length of stay, infectious complications, and multiorgan failure compared with patients who receive parenteral nutrition (PN) or are kept NPO.[4-7] In contrast, early initiation of PN in critically ill patients, usually within 24 hours, has been associated with an improved nitrogen balance but increased risk of infection complications and length of hospitalization even compared with patients in whom EN was started later.[8-10] Early EN may be more beneficial because it attenuates the catabolism associated with sepsis by maintaining the gut barrier integrity and reducing the translocation of bacteria and bacteria-derived endotoxin into the systemic circulation.[11,12]

AP is a highly metabolic disease process with activation of an inflammatory cascade that leads to catabolic stress, formation of reactive oxygen species, and activation of immune responses that can rapidly overwhelm innate immune regulation and inherent antioxidant capacity.[13-15] Approximately 20% of AP cases are severe, manifesting as the systemic inflammatory response syndrome (SIRS) associated with multiorgan dysfunction (MOD) and a 15% to 40% mortality.[16,17] The exaggerated, uninhibited, and self-perpetuating inflammatory response is the cause of early mortality in severe AP (SAP), defined as within the first week of presentation. Infection of peripancreatic fluid and/or pancreas or other organs and necrosis of the pancreas is associated with late mortality (after the first week of presentation).[4,18-23]

For AP, resting the pancreas has been advocated to help resolve inflammation, and oral feeding was usually held until the patient was free of pain and nausea. Most cases of mild and moderately severe acute pancreatitis are self-limited, and patients recover within a few days, thus nutrition support is not necessary because oral feeding can be started as soon as the patient can tolerate it.[24-26]

Predicting the severity of AP, and thus patients in whom therapeutic interventions including nutrition could prove helpful, has been difficult.[27] Severity scores can help identify patients at risk for increased morbidity, prolonged hospitalizations, and mortality who could be targets for institution of early treatment, including nutrition, but the scores are limited as predictors of disease severity because most patients, even with a high score, usually survive.[8,27-29] Nonoperative supportive care and delay of procedures are strongly recommended for patients with SAP, because early surgery is associated with a substantial increase in morbidity and mortality; thus, nutritional support becomes an important part of the patient's care, because prolonging the time to any invasive intervention decreases mortality.[26,30,31]

In AP, the initial insult, which has been called the sentinel AP event, causes a liberation of proinflammatory cytokines and chemokines; increased levels of reactive oxygen species; activation and recruitment of neutrophils and macrophages; and vascular and lymphatic dilation mediated by cathepsin 3, intracellular calcium, tumor necrosis factor, nuclear factor kappa-B, platelet activating factor, heat shock protein, and others that contribute to disease severity, possibly determined by associated genetic mutations, epigenetic events, and the native oxidative stress response.[8,9,32,33] Ultimately, the complex inflammatory cascade, which the pancreas can self-regulate up to a point, leads to acinar cell death by apoptosis or necrosis, the latter associated with SAP.[34] Extra-acinar inflammation is modulated by neuropeptidases and oxidative stress that cause vascular permeability and stimulate neutrophil infiltration, with associated gland ischemia and reperfusion injury because nitrous oxide production is affected, and leakage of reactive oxygen species and proinflammatory cytokines to the systemic circulation, which leads to the local and systemic complications associated with SAP.[35-37]

Bacterial translocation across the intestinal barrier to the mesenteric lymph nodes and then to the systemic circulation has been well described in critically ill patients, and is a major cause of local and systemic complications, and the morbidity and mortality seen in SAP.[4,21,38,39] Oxidative stress leads to the formation of thiobarbituric acid reactive substances (a by-product of lipid peroxidation), downregulation of the heat shock protein, and a lack of commensal flora caused by NPO status, decreased intestinal motility caused by SAP-associated ileus, the use of systemic antibiotics, and decreased intestinal short chain fatty acid levels caused by fasting promote enteropathogen proliferation and bacterial endotoxemia as measured by the presence of systemic antiendotoxin immunoglobulin (Ig) M and IgG antibodies, which are markers of increased intestinal barrier permeability.[2,17,21,40,41] The proinflammatory state that started with the acinar injury is enhanced by altered intestinal blood flow and augmented inflammation that promotes intestinal permeability. Some studies suggest lower than expected levels of endotoxemia for the severity of the disease process in SAP, and that a proliferation of virulent intestinal lumen bacteria that stimulate the activation of inflammatory cytokines such as interleukin-1, tumor necrosis factor alpha (TNF-α), and interleukin-8 ultimately spills into the systemic circulation, causing the subsequent complications.[8]

The understanding of the inflammatory progression has led to the institution of treatment using antiinflammatory cytokines, inflammatory factor inhibitors, and even antioxidants with poor to no clinical results as shown by a recent Cochrane Systemic Review that found low-quality studies and no clinical benefit of direct pharmacologic interventions for AP.[42]

However, nutritional therapy (EN) for SAP, which functions as immunonutrition, merits further discussion. As described byMcClave,[8] "the strongest evidence for impact of nutrition therapy on patient outcome is in severe acute pancreatitis."

MALNUTRITION IN ACUTE PANCREATITIS

All patients with pancreatitis should be classified as having a moderate to high nutritional risk because of the complex disease process and the subsequent impact on nutritional status.[1,43] Prolonged nil per os status and/or delay in specialized nutrition support (SNS) initiation and/or advancement of feeding regimens also contribute to the nutritional risk for patients with AP. Furthermore, in those individuals with concurrent alcoholism, there is an even higher risk of malnutrition. These patients require supplementation of both thiamin and folate to prevent Wernicke encephalopathy and anemia. Therefore, nutritional assessment of these patients within the first 24 to 48 hours of admission is required to formulate a plan for the appropriate nutritional intervention.

CHANGES IN ABSORPTION AND METABOLISM IN ACUTE PANCREATITIS

The pancreas is composed of 2 major types of tissues: the acini, exocrine tissue that is responsible for digestive secretions released into the duodenum; and the islets of Langerhans, which secrete the hormones insulin, glucagon, and somatostatin. The primary exocrine secretions include digestive enzymes and bicarbonate. Protein-digesting enzymes include trypsinogen, chymotrypsinogen, procarboxypeptidases, and elastase. Proteolytic enzymes are secreted as zymogens. When trypsinogen is activated to trypsin, the other zymogens are activated in a cascade phenomenon. Pancreatic amylase is the primary enzyme involved in carbohydrate digestion, and pancreatic lipase, colipase, phospholipase A2, and cholesterase are needed for lipid digestion. Gastric acid is the stimulus for the release of secretin from the duodenal mucosa (S cells), which in turn stimulates the secretion of water, electrolytes, and bicarbonate.

The extreme inflammatory response noted in AP can potentially impair both exocrine and endocrine functions. If this occurs, impaired synthesis or release of enzymes leads to maldigestion. Furthermore, the proposed pathophysiology of AP involves tissue damage from activated proteolytic enzymes. However, the extent of maldigestion is difficult to quantify and does not necessarily correlate with serum levels of lipase and amylase.

THE NIL PER OS CONUNDRUM IN ACUTE PANCREATITIS

Historically, individuals with AP were made NPO because oral intake increases the rate and synthesis of pancreatic enzymes, which vary with the dietary composition, and to avoid further stimulation of the pancreas until the pain subsided. This practice is no longer consistent with published data and the evidence-based guidelines that are explored here.[1,3] Fasting decreases pancreas exocrine output, but the understanding of the role that an intact gut barrier plays in critical illness, and especially in SAP, led to studies that revealed that enteral feeds distal to the papilla caused minimal exocrine pancreas stimulation in patients with SAP and healthy controls. Because EN has been shown to improve morbidity and possibly mortality in SAP (discussed later) there is no justification for keeping patients NPO; some studies even suggest that gastric feeding, in contrast with direct jejunal feeding, is as beneficial and well tolerated in patients with SAP, supporting the view that the maintenance of gut integrity by EN is much more important than the mode of enteral delivery.[42,44–47]

NUTRITIONAL ASSESSMENT

During AP, the inflammatory cascade drives the increased metabolic demand requiring additional macronutrients and micronutrients to support the immune system and tissue regeneration after pancreatic injury. Nutritional intake supports intestinal integrity and prevents mucosal permeability and subsequent bacterial translocation, both of which can contribute to the infectious complications seen in AP. Nutrition therapy as EN is critical to maintain intestinal integrity and support the metabolic demand that ensues during the disease process and therefore plays a vital role in reducing the morbidity and mortality associated with AP.[43]

On admission to the hospital, a nutrition screening should identify all patients with AP having moderate to high nutritional risk. The nutrition assessment determines the presence and degree of malnutrition and allows a nutrition plan of care to be formed. For those patients admitted to the ICU, calculation of a Nutritional Risk in Critically Ill (NUTRIC) score to determine nutritional risk can assist in determining the appropriate nutrition therapy for the patient. Patients with a NUTRIC score of greater than or equal to 5, should start EN and meet the energy and protein goal within 24 to 48 hours.[48] In addition to determining risk of malnutrition, a malnutrition diagnosis can be confirmed by the presence of greater than or equal to 2 of the following criteria[49]:

- Insufficient energy intake
- Weight loss
- Loss of muscle mass
- Loss of subcutaneous fat
- Presence of edema or fluid accumulation
- Diminished functional status as measured by handgrip strength or reduction in activities of daily living

These criteria can be ascertained by completing a nutrition-focused physical examination, assessing caloric intake before and during the hospital admission, and determining changes in body weight. This system of diagnosis has replaced the historical use of serum proteins (ie, albumin, prealbumin, transferrin, and retinol-binding protein) that more accurately describe the acute phase response and changes in body weight, which alone cannot identify malnutrition.

Determining Calorie and Protein Needs

Indirect calorimetry is the gold standard for measuring the resting metabolic rate of critically ill adults. When indirect calorimetry is not available, weight-based nomograms can be used to estimate energy and protein needs. In the ICU, it is recommended to have a reassessment of nutritional needs weekly as a minimum because the severity of disease can rapidly change (**Table 1**).[48]

Table 1
Monitoring nutrition care plans for hospitalized patients with acute pancreatitis

Parameters	Mild AP	Moderate to Severe AP
Intake/output	Weekly	Daily
Vitals	Daily	Daily
Anthropometrics		
Height	Baseline	Baseline
Weight	1–2 times/wk	Daily
Usual body weight	—	Admission
Nutritional Assessment		
Nutrition screening	Admission	Admission
Nutrition-focused physical examination	Weekly	Weekly or as needed
Abdominal examination	Weekly	Daily
Indirect calorimetry (when available)	—	2–3 times/wk
Nutrition-related History		
Food intolerances	Baseline	Baseline
Presence of nutrient deficiencies	As indicated	As indicated
Nutritional intake before admission	Baseline	Baseline
Laboratory Parameters		
White blood cell count	2–3 times/wk	Daily until stable
Hemoglobin/hematocrit	2–3 times/wk	Daily until stable
Triglycerides, serum	Weekly	Weekly
Lactic dehydrogenase	Weekly	Daily until stable
Liver-associated enzymes	2–3 times/wk	Daily until stable
Serum glucose	Daily	3 times daily
Serum amylase/lipase	2–3 times/wk	2–3 times/wk
C-reactive Protein	Weekly	Weekly
Blood urea nitrogen, creatinine	Daily	Daily until stable
Serum electrolytes	Daily until stable	Daily until stable
Arterial blood gas (when available)	—	As indicated
Vitamins/minerals/trace elements	As indicated	As indicated
Interleukin-6	—	As indicated
Nitrogen balance	—	As indicated
NUTRIC score		Admission

Using weight-based nomograms, determining caloric/protein requirements varies based on the severity of AP. In mild AP, 25 to 30 kcals/kg/d of energy, and 1.2 to 1.5 g/kg/d of protein can be used initially. If the disease progresses to moderate SAP, caloric demand is estimated to increase up to 35 kcals/kg/d.[50] Plasma glucose levels should be maintained less than or equal to 10 mmol/L (180 mg/dL) and plasma triglyceride levels maintained at less than or equal to 3 mmol/L (266 mg/dL).[51]

NUTRITION THERAPY IN ACUTE PANCREATITIS

Historically, on hospital admission, medical management evolved around minimizing pancreatic stimulation by keeping patients NPO. There is now a much better understanding of the role of nutrition (oral and tube-delivered nutrients) in minimizing the inflammatory cascade by the maintenance of gut barrier function and modulation of the immune and inflammatory responses.[52-54] Reduction in the duration of NPO and the use of aggressive nutrition support in severe pancreatitis has led to improved outcomes for this patient population. The degree of malnutrition and the severity of AP require customization and tailoring nutrition therapy for each patient. Patient with mild AP and who are not malnourished on diagnosis do not require SNS.[49] In contrast, malnourished patients with moderate AP, and certainly SAP, should start SNS within 24 to 48 hours of hospital admission.[50]

Because of the rapid disease progression seen in AP, establishing a plan for frequent monitoring is necessary to detect changes in the severity of pancreatitis. Mild pancreatitis might present at the onset of the inflammatory cascade and can rapidly progress to moderate to severe pancreatitis and thus may require more aggressive nutritional intervention. Some studies suggested that EN increases intestinal blood flow demands, which paradoxically could contribute to and enhance bacterial leak and translocation, and serve to highlight the importance of initiating enteral feeds before the gut barrier is disrupted.[25] It has also been described that target calories are reached 75% of the time, indicating the need for frequent nutritional reassessment[47] (see **Table 1**, which underscores the need for frequent monitoring of these patients).

NUTRITION IN MILD ACUTE PANCREATITIS

On admission with a diagnosis of mild AP, an oral diet is preferred. Approximately 80% of patients successfully transition to an oral diet within 7 days of hospital admission and experience minimal morbidities.[48] The optimal timing to initiate an oral diet and the type of oral diet prescribed are debatable. Numerous studies indicate that initiation of oral or enteral feeding in any form in mild AP decreases length of hospitalization, and a recent meta-analysis by Márta and colleagues[3,4,10,13,24,25,55-57] comparing EN with NPO in all types of AP found a general benefit of EN compared with fasting patients. Oral feeding with a low-fat regular diet is as well tolerated as, and nutritionally more beneficial than, a clear liquid diet (CLD) in this subset of patients. Eckerwall and colleagues[25] randomized 60 subjects with AP into a fasting group and an oral feeding group in which diet was advanced as tolerated. This study indicated that hospital length of stay (LOS) significantly decreased in the oral feeding group, suggesting that dietary prescription should be assigned at hospital admission to patients identified with mild AP (4 vs 6 days; $P<.05$). Various dietary patterns have been investigated, including the CLD, low-fat, soft, or regular diet. Jacobson and colleagues[58] pooled more than 350 subjects with mild AP to assess differences in hospital LOS and reoccurrence of abdominal pain after initiation of a liquid versus solid diet. Prescribing a solid diet, despite the percentage contribution of fat kilocalories, compared with a CLD was associated with a decreased hospital LOS (1.18 days; 95% CI, 0.82–1.55; P<.00001) without increased abdominal pain.[56–58] Monitoring and evaluation of dietary tolerance includes nausea, vomiting, and increased abdominal pain. An additional 2 randomized trials showed benefit of solid diet compared with liquid diet with shorter length of hospital stay with solids.[57,58] Therefore, patients with mild AP can be started on a low-fat oral diet after a short initial fasting period. Increased levels of amylase and lipase contribute to the overall assessment of the patient but are not required to drive decisions on advancing the diet.[48] For those patients whose disease progresses to moderate severe or severe pancreatitis or who are unable to advance to a regular diet within 7 days of hospital admission, the use of EN, as outlined later, should ensue.[48] Mild AP has an overall good prognosis and thus is less likely to benefit from or require interventions beyond supportive care.

IMPROVING TOLERANCE TO AN ORAL DIET

Although guidelines for the nutritional management of AP typically do not include a description of the size and timing of meals, extrapolation from other disease states leads clinicians to adjust to small, frequent meals to improve dietary tolerance, especially in patients experiencing nausea, vomiting, and early satiety.[59–61] Patient education should include the number and estimated kilocalories required per meal to better address adequate nutrient delivery.[61] Adjustment of the dietary fat content and consistency can also be considered to improve dietary tolerance.[62] If early satiety is present, increased dietary fat intake may result in delayed gastric emptying and ultimately decreasing oral intake. In this case, reducing the total amount of fat prescribed at each meal and/or converting to liquid fat sources might improve oral intake and promote gastric emptying.[62,63]

Tolerance to an oral diet is challenging because of the increased nausea, vomiting, and abdominal pain that are characteristic of AP. Various medications can be considered to treat symptoms associated with dietary intolerance. Antiemetic and prokinetic agents can combat nausea and vomiting by increasing peristalsis, blocking hormone signaling, and improving gastric emptying and have proved to be an effective strategy for improving gastrointestinal symptoms. Fiber supplementation is not routinely recommended for patients in the ICU because of the impact on delayed gastric emptying. For patients recovering from moderate to severe pancreatitis or with mild pancreatitis, consideration for initiating soluble fiber in those experiencing diarrhea as a result of the pancreatic inflammation may decrease nutrient loses. In addition, the use of antidiarrheals taken before meals can reduce the frequency of bowel movements and improve the consistency to promote absorption. **Table 2** provides an overview of medications to consider for improving enteral (oral and tube-delivered nutrients) tolerance.

NUTRITION IN MODERATELY SEVERE ACUTE PANCREATITIS

This subgroup of patients with AP have transient organ failure that usually subsides within 48 hours, and most have a good to excellent prognosis. Most studies group mild and moderate SAP together so it is difficult to know the impact of EN in this group of patients. As with all types of AP, EN support decreases hospital LOS, and is preferred to NPO or PN.[55] As described earlier, continuous monitoring for nutritional needs, supportive care, and deterioration to SAP is necessary.

Table 2
Medication management used in acute pancreatitis to improve enteral tolerance

Medication	Examples	Symptom	Mechanism	Administration
Pancreatic enzymes	Pancrelipase	Diarrhea, steatorrhea	Replaces pancreatic enzymes to improve fat, protein, and carbohydrate digestion	Take with meals
Prokinetic agents	Metoclopramide, erythromycin, bethanechol	Nausea, vomiting, early satiety	Increased peristalsis, improved gastric emptying	Take 10–15 min before meals
Antiemetic agents	Ondansetron, prochlorperazine	Nausea, vomiting, early satiety	Block dopamine and/or serotonin signaling	Take 30–45 min before meals
Soluble fiber	Guar gum, banana flakes, pectin	Diarrhea	Increases water absorption in the gastrointestinal tract. Thickens stool consistency	Mixed into hot or cold beverages/ foods
Antidiarrheals	Loperamide, diphenoxylate and atropine, codeine, opium tincture	Diarrhea	Decreases the number and frequency of bowel movements by slowing peristalsis	Take 30–60 min before meals

NUTRITION IN SEVERE ACUTE PANCREATITIS

The focus of nutritional therapy should be on patients with SAP, because they are more ill and are unable to tolerate oral feeds for a longer period of time. Aggressive fluid resuscitation is initially required to promote urinary output of 0.5 mL/kg/h and is linked to improved outcome.[51] The hypermetabolic and inflammatory state that characterizes SAP leads to rapid nutritional deterioration, increased caloric requirements, and rapid protein losses. These deficiencies are augmented by keeping the patients NPO, which leads to progressive nutrition deficit, and a negative nitrogen balance. The latter has been associated with increased morbidity and mortality, and a prolonged hospitalization and overall poor recovery.[1,13,15]

The use of SNS must be considered to meet the metabolic demand associated with the early phase of AP. A NUTRIC score indicating high nutrition risk can be calculated to support the initiation of early EN.[48] There is evidence for the therapeutic benefit of EN as treatment of SAP, and thus for effectively using enteral feeds as a form of immunonutrition as summarized from meta-analysis and a frequently revised Cochrane Review on the subject.[13] EN has been associated with decreased bacterial gut translocation and peripheral blood enterotoxin levels, and decreases TNF-α and C-reactive protein levels within 48 hours of its initiation.[4,64] Serum albumin level, an indirect measure of nutritional status, has been shown to improve with EN.[65] EN with an elemental diet containing omega-3 fatty acids, and possibly also omega-6 fatty acids, may also have a positive effect on neurogenic inflammation.[8] Individual studies and meta-analyses also indicate a significantly decreased relative risk of infection, and subsequent decreased need for surgical interventions as well as significant decrease in hospital and ICU LOS in patients with SAP on EN. In contrast, PN in patients with SAP was associated with poorer general outcomes, was more expensive than EN, and carried the inherent risks of infection and thrombosis.[1,55] Early peripheral

PN has been associated with a decreased risk of infection, but nutritional needs may not be met.

A few, but not all, meta-analyses show a significant decrease in multiorgan failure and mortality for EN, but all show a trend toward an improvement of these two important outcomes.[15,55,66-68] **Table 3** summarizes the impact of EN on clinical outcomes. Current guidelines support the use of a standard, polymeric formulas (see **Table 3**) delivered via a nasogastric and/or nasojejunal tube within the first 48 to 72 hours of hospital admission.[60] There may be a potential benefit for the use of specialized, immune-enhancing enteral formulations, but continued research in this area is warranted before changing current recommendations.[15]

IMMUNONUTRITION IN ACUTE PANCREATITIS

Various nutrients have been investigated to determine their effects on the immune response, inflammation, white blood cell recruitment, and disease outcome in AP.[69,70] Those that show some promise include omega-3 fatty acids, glutamine, and arginine.[48,71] Various micronutrients that are in demand during acute inflammation include vitamins A, C, E, B_6, folate, B_{12}, and pantothenic acid, in addition to iron and zinc. All of these nutrients have various roles in cell-mediated immunity and, when their levels are low, they can contribute to the poor/delayed immune response seen in AP.[71] Deficiencies of these nutrients are more common in chronic pancreatitis, but nutrition-focused physical examination can assist in identifying micronutrient deficiencies in patients with moderate to severe malnutrition.[72] If micronutrient deficiency is suspected, serum levels can be evaluated once inflammation has resolved, although the accuracy of these parameters as a reflection of total body stores is questionable.

Arginine

Arginine is a nonessential amino acid that plays a role in ureagenesis, immune function, wound healing, cell growth and differentiation, and vasodilation. The rationale for supplementing arginine in AP relates to the relative arginine deficiency that may occur during critical illness and sepsis. With supplementation of arginine, it is proposed that levels of nitric oxide would increase with subsequent improvement in blood flow and tissue perfusion. In contrast, there has been concern that the vasodilation mediated by nitric oxide could lead to hemodynamic instability by diverting blood flow.[67] Additional benefits include provision of substrate for collagen synthesis and enhanced T-cell function. Current American Society for Parenteral and Enteral Nutrition (ASPEN) guidelines do not routinely recommend immunonutrition in medical ICU patients, but it seems that a dose of 15 to 30 g of arginine is safe.[73]

Table 3
Effect of enteral nutrition compared with parenteral nutrition on clinical outcomes

	Infection	Organ Failure	LOS	SIRS	Mortality
McClave et al,[15] 2006	++	++	+	NR	None
Al-Omran et al,[13] 2010	NR	NR	+	None	++
Blaser et al,[3] 2017	++	NR	NR	None	NR
Petrov et al,[4] 2008	++	None	NR	NR	++

The plus symbols (+) indicate a nonsignificant difference; double plus (++) indicates a statistically significant difference.
Abbreviation: NR, not reported.

Glutamine

Glutamine is a nonessential amino acid under investigation for its antioxidant properties and the role in enhancing intestinal health and preventing bacterial translocation in critically ill patients. With mixed results on glutamine supplementation in the ICU and concern over safety in various critically ill patients, ASPEN does not endorse glutamine supplementation in patients with AP.[48]

Omega-3 Fatty Acid

Few studies have investigated the use of fish oil supplementation and/or the use of omega-3 fatty acids for modulating the inflammatory response in AP.[54,74] Although these studies show promise, the small sample sizes and heterogeneous methodologies make conclusions on the efficacy difficult at this time. Therefore, current recommendations do not support the use of oral, enteral, or parenterally delivered fish oil for treatment of AP at this time.[43,48] The potential benefits of immunonutrients are summarized in **Table 4**.

Improving tolerance to enteral nutrition

Intolerance to EN, such as abdominal pain, nausea, vomiting, and excessive gas production, is common in moderate AP to SAP. Strategies should be used to support tolerance before transitioning to PN. Tolerance can be improved through adjustments of the EN infusion rate, EN formula, and medications. Drug therapy can be used to optimize tolerance to diet and EN depending on the symptoms present and the underlying cause of these symptoms.

The first step in improving tolerance is to provide EN early as maintenance for intestinal integrity. In addition, the tip of the feeding tube can be advanced from the stomach into the small intestine in patients experiencing delayed gastric emptying and/or at risk for aspiration. Enteral formula changes from a standard, polymeric formula to a hydrolyzed formula can improve tolerance by improving the digestibility of nutrients in the gastrointestinal tract while pancreatic enzymatic action is insufficient (**Table 5**). An alternative to formula selection is for the infusion rate to be adjusted to improve tolerance. Typically, a slower infusion over a longer period of time (continuous) is better tolerated by individuals with compromised absorption. Selection of a

Table 4	
Effect of enteral nutrition, supplements, and immunonutrition in acute pancreatitis	
EN	Stimulates blood flow and intestinal microcirculation, inhibits bacterial overgrowth, and maintains integrity of the enteric barrier
L-Arginine	By nitric oxide pathway may improve intestinal blood flow, maintain the gut barrier, and improve pancreas blood flow
Glutamine	Antioxidant; stimulates release of heat shock protein, which controls intrapancreatic trypsin activation
Polyunsaturated fatty acids/ omega-3 fatty acids	Blunt inflammation by affecting chemotaxis and shunting to less aggressive inflammatory pathways, and regulates neurogenic inflammation
Docosahexaenoic acid	Inhibits intracellular signaling, stabilizes DNA and inhibits inflammatory cytokine activation, induces acinar apoptosis rather than necrosis
Zinc	Affects tight junctions, decreases permeability, indirectly affects glutathione production, and inhibits oxidative stress
Antioxidants	Replenish antioxidant capacity against reactive oxidant species

Table 5
Enteral nutrition formulations suggested for use in acute pancreatitis

Formulas	Indication	Characteristics
Polymeric formulas	Should be first trial if no indication of malabsorption and intact GI anatomy	Protein: intact protein lipid: triglycerides Carbohydrate: dextrin, oligosaccharides
Partially hydrolyzed	Indication of malabsorption, enteral feeding intolerance, or change in GI anatomy	Protein: peptides Lipid: medium-chain fatty acids, structured lipids, omega-3 fatty acids Carbohydrate: maltodextrin, oligosaccharides
Elemental	Indication of malabsorption, or change in GI anatomy	Protein: crystalline amino acids, dipeptides/tripeptides Lipid: medium-chain fatty acids, omega-3 fatty acids Carbohydrate: maltodextrin, <2% partially hydrolyzed cornstarch

Abbreviation: GI, gastrointestinal.

continuous infusion is preferred in the ICU to allow for delivery of a smaller volume into the gastrointestinal tract each hour. When these tactics have failed to improve EN tolerance, medication modifications can assist to improve tolerance.

EN delivery may have to be monitored more carefully in obese patients because nutritional goals may not be met as rapidly, and prolonging the time to reach them has been associated with poorer outcomes, including increased mortality.[16]

Nausea related to poor gastric and intestinal motility is commonly seen with the initiation of oral nutrition and EN in AP. Consideration should be given to the use of antiemetics and/or prokinetic agents to improve these symptoms and allowing the continuation and advancement of the diet and/or enteral feeding. As gastrointestinal function returns to baseline, these medications can often be discontinued.

Diarrhea is also commonly associated with AP. There is no role for pancreatic enzymes in interstitial pancreatitis but in necrotizing pancreatitis or in prolonged disease course it is prudent to provide them. Poor mixing of pancreatic enzymes with the food bolus leads to maldigestion and malabsorption.[59] Dosing guidelines vary worldwide, although most recommend monitoring for the presence of steatorrhea, clinical symptoms associated with fat maldigestion (ie, bloating, gas, essential fatty acid deficiency), and/or quantification of fecal fat.[75] None of the US Food and Drug Administration–approved pancreatic enzymes were used for EN until the recent release of an in-line digestive cartridge that allows mixing of lipase with the EN formula ex vivo. Although there are limitations to this product, its use seems superior to other methodologies for pancreatic enzyme delivery, with approximately 90% of fats being hydrolyzed within a 4-hour period.[75]

In addition to pancreatic enzymes, antidiarrheal medications slow the movement of the intestinal muscles through the opioid receptor to inhibit peristalsis, which promotes the contact of the enteral contents with the villi and microvilli lining of the gastrointestinal tract. The goal of antidiarrheal therapy is to decrease the number and frequency of bowel movements and ultimately improve intestinal absorption. Although use of antidiarrheal therapy is safe and effective, caution is needed in patients with hepatic injury or those who may have loperamide-induced AP.[76,77] **Table 3** provides a snapshot of the medications available that support improved tolerance to diet and EN. All EN parameters (formula, infusion rate, and tube location) and medications used to improve digestions and absorption must be considered before consideration of failure of enteral feeding and initiation of PN.

WHEN TO START ENTERAL NUTRITION

The best time to initiate EN is not clear, but the inflammatory response and cascade associated with SAP peaks at 72 hours, which is therefore considered the therapeutic window for any intervention[25,78] Most studies defined early nutrition as being within 24 to 48 hours of presentation. A recent prospective study of patients with moderately severe AP and SAP found that starting EN by day 3 of presentation was associated with a significant decrease of pancreatic and extrapancreatic infections.[79] A few studies have shown increased intestinal permeability after 72 hours or more in patients with mild AP, indicating that the mechanism for disease is more complex, and that the poorer outcomes are related to a host of factors that by then have become active and uncontrollable. This finding may explain why instituting EN within 24 to 48 hours of presentation improves patient outcome, and why starting it later may be less beneficial.[15,25,65,78,80]

Current nutrition practice guidelines support early initiation of EN in SAP within 24 to 48 hours from admission.[1,48]

PROBIOTICS

With basic science advancements in the area of metabolomics, tools are now available to understand the metabolic action of the gut microflora and its impact on gut permeability and modulation of the immune system. These data should help guide clinical investigations on the use of probiotics in patients with AP, focusing on strain-specific actions while clarifying the dose required for the biological actions intended from the use of probiotics. Initial experimental pancreatitis model trials with probiotics showed promising results by reducing the severity of pancreatitis, improving histopathologic scores, reducing bacterial translocation, and reducing late-phase mortality.[1–3] A randomized controlled trial of probiotics in AP was stopped early because of increased risk of mortality (increased rate of fatal bowel ischemia, multiorgan failure) in those who received a multispecies probiotic with Bifidobacterium.[81,82]

A more recent randomized trial by Cui and colleagues[83] involving 70 patients with SAP showed beneficial effects of probiotics in combination with EN by the significant reduction in upper gastrointestinal bleeding, infection, and abscess in the probiotic group. A systematic review of 6 randomized controlled trials of a total of 536 patients showed that probiotics had neither beneficial nor adverse effects on the clinical outcomes in SAP.[84] At present, probiotics should not be used in AP based on available clinical evidence.

ENTERAL NUTRITION SHOULD BE THE RULE, NOT THE EXCEPTION

The notion that the pancreas and/or the gastrointestinal tract need to be rested in cases of AP is not supported by data. Current guidelines for management of AP recommend immediate oral feeding in patients who tolerate it and have no contraindications, such as a risk of aspiration, and resolving abdominal pain.[1] There is no benefit to administering a liquid diet, and a low-fat regular diet can be prescribed to patients with mild AP.[1,14] In SAP, EN is preferred to PN, and the direct gastric and jejunal routes of feeding seem to be equivalent. Some studies also indicate that combination EN and PN improves outcomes compared with PN alone in matched cohorts, adding to the notion that maintenance of the gut barrier is how EN affects outcomes in AP.[85]

The nutritional practices in AP were addressed in a Dutch observational study in which 90% of the patients had mild AP.[45] Eighty percent of the patients were kept NPO for an average of 2 days, and 17% of the patients with mild AP were fed enterally using a nasojejunal feeding tube. Of the small group with SAP, only 3 patients were kept NPO, and 75% received PN with or without EN; 56% received EN only. It is encouraging to see the shift toward EN in the SAP group, but the practice of starving patients, which lasted more than 5 days in 5% of the cohort, and the use of PN is pervasive, which is highlighted by another study that found that only 2% of patients with SAP received EN alone but 64% were on combination EN plus PN.[66] This finding highlights the need to standardize treatment and to continuously educate and disseminate information, which can probably be done more effectively with multidisciplinary care including earlier consultation with the nutrition team.

LIMITATIONS

There are numerous limitations to the available data on nutrition therapy in AP. In most meta-analyses about 50% of the patient cohorts had mild to moderate SAP, or would be classified as such using the currently accepted diagnostic criteria. The role of EN in these two subgroups is not clear, but the prognosis is usually favorable so they are less likely to benefit from or require nutritional intervention. Based on the meta-analyses, selecting the patients with SAP who are most likely to benefit from immunonutrition is difficult, which makes generalization of even the most robust meta-analyses more difficult. The type of enteral formula that should be used, such as polymeric versus semielemental or elemental, is not clear. The studies also do not indicate how to treat acute exacerbations of chronic pancreatitis or idiopathic recurrent AP. A publication bias of studies showing a positive impact of EN also needs to be considered.

SUMMARY

The goal of nutritional support in AP is to reduce inflammation, prevent nutritional depletion, correct a negative nitrogen balance, and improve outcomes. EN in SAP has a positive impact on disease burden, and should be preferred to PN, which has a negative impact on patient outcomes. It maintains the integrity of the gut barrier, decreases intestinal permeability, downregulates the systemic inflammatory response, maintains intestinal microbiota equilibrium, and reduces the complications of the early phase of SAP (first week of the disease), improving morbidity and possibly improving mortality, and it is less expensive.[55,66,86] EN should be initiated within 24 hours in patients with SAP or predicted SAP, so practitioners who are taking care of them need to have a good knowledge of severity scoring systems and nutrition guidelines.[27,45] Nutritional practices for AP are widely variable and need to be aligned with the current evidence-based recommendations. The role of EN for mild or moderately SAP is not clear, but in most cases oral feeds with a low-fat regular diet can be started as soon as tolerated, because a CLD is not superior. PN should be reserved only for patients in whom EN is not tolerated or is contraindicated because PN is associated with a higher rate of infectious and metabolic complications, and greater morbidity and length of hospitalization.[16,87–89] Further studies to understand optimal timing for initiation of nutrition, route of delivery of EN, and the type of nutrition and nutrients are necessary.

REFERENCES

1. Tenner S, Baillie J, DeWitt J, et al. American College of Gastroenterology guideline: management of acute pancreatitis. Am J Gastroenterol 2013;108:1400–15.
2. Gupta R, Patel K, Calder PC, et al. A randomised clinical trial to assess the effect of total enteral and total parenteral nutritional support on metabolic, inflammatory and oxidative markers in patients with predicted severe acute pancreatitis (APACHE II ≥6). Pancreatology 2003;3:406–13.
3. Blaser AR, Starkopf J, Alhazzani W, et al. Early enteral nutrition in critically ill patients: ESICM clinical practice guidelines. Intensive Care Med 2017;43:380–98.
4. Petrov MS, van Santvoort HC, Besselink MGH, et al. Enteral nutrition and the risk of mortality and infectious complications in patients with severe acute pancreatitis. Arch Surg 2008;143:1111–7.
5. Wang XD, Wang Q, Andersson R, et al. Alterations in intestinal function in acute pancreatitis in an experimental model. Br J Surg 1996;83:1537–43.
6. Juvonen PO, Alhava EM, Takala JA. Gut permeability in patients with acute pancreatitis. Scand J Gastroenterol 2000;35:1314–8.
7. Lehocky P, Sarr MG. Early enteral feeding in severe acute pancreatitis: can it prevent secondary pancreatic (super) infection? Dig Surg 2000;17:571–7.
8. McClave SA. Drivers of oxidative stress in acute pancreatitis: the role of nutrition therapy. JPEN J Parenter Enteral Nutr 2012;36:24–36.
9. Pandol SJ, Saluja AK, Imrie CW, et al. Acute pancreatitis: bench to the bedside. Gastroenterology 2007;132:1127–51.
10. McClave SA, Greene LM, Snider HL, et al. Comparison of the safety of early enteral versus parenteral nutrition in mild acute pancreatitis. J Parenter Enteral Nutr 1997;21:14–20.
11. Mochizuki H, Trocki O, Dominioni L, et al. Mechanisms of prevention of postburn hypermetabolism and catabolism by early enteral feeding. Ann Surg 1984;200:297–310.
12. Saito H, Trocki O, Alexander JW. The effect of rate of nutrient administration on the nutritional state, 1986 state, catabolic hormone secretion, and gut mucosal integrity after burn injury. J Parenter Enteral Nutr 1986;11:1–7.
13. Al-Omran M, AlBalawi ZH, Tashkandi MF, et al. Enteral versus parenteral nutrition for acute pancreatitis (review). Cochrane Database Syst Rev 2010;(1):CD002837.
14. Wu BU, Banks PA. Clinical management of patients with acute pancreatitis. Gastroenterology 2013;144:1272–81.
15. McClave SA, Chang WK, Dhaliwal R, et al. Nutrition support in acute pancreatitis: a systematic review of the literature. J Parenter Enteral Nutr 2006;30:143–56.
16. Hegazi R, Raina A, Graham T, et al. Early jejunal feeding initiation and clinical outcomes in patients with severe acute pancreatitis. J Parenter Enteral Nutr 2011;35:91–6.
17. Windsor AC, Kanwar S, Li AG, et al. Compared with parenteral nutrition, enteral feeding attenuates the acute phase response and improves disease severity in acute pancreatitis. Gut 1998;42:431–5.
18. Pezzilli R, Fantini L, Morselli-Labate AM. New approaches for the treatment of acute pancreatitis. JOP 2006;7:79–91.
19. Gloor B, Müller CA, Worni M, et al. Late mortality in patients with severe acute pancreatitis. Br J Surg 2001;88:975–9.
20. Johnson CD, Abu-Hilal M. Persistent organ failure during the first week as a marker of fatal outcome in acute pancreatitis. Gut 2004;53:1340–4.

21. Eckerwall GE, Axelsson JB, Andersson RG. Early nasogastric feeding in predicted severe acute pancreatitis: a clinical, randomized study. Ann Surg 2006; 244:959–65.
22. Buter A, Imrie CW, Carter CR, et al. Dynamic nature of early organ dysfunction determines outcome in acute pancreatitis. Br J Surg 2002;89:298–302.
23. Blum T, Maisonneuve P, Lowenfels AB, et al. Fatal outcome in acute pancreatitis: its occurrence and early prediction. Pancreatology 2001;1:237–41.
24. Pupelis G, Snippe K, Plaudis H, et al. Early oral feeding in acute pancreatitis: an alternative approach to tube feeding. Preliminary report. Acta Chir Belg 2006; 106:181–6.
25. Eckerwall GE, Tingstedt BB, Bergenzaun PE, et al. Immediate oral feeding in patients with mild acute pancreatitis is safe and may accelerate recovery–a randomized clinical study. Clin Nutr 2007;26:758–63.
26. Wig JD, Gupta V, Kochhar R, et al. The role of non-operative strategies in the management of severe acute pancreatitis. JOP 2010;11:553–9.
27. Papachristou GI, Muddana V, Yadav D, et al. Comparison of BISAP, Ranson's, APACHE-II, and CTSI scores in predicting organ failure, complications, and mortality in acute pancreatitis. Am J Gastroenterol 2010;105:435–41.
28. Nawaz H, Mounzer R, Yadav D, et al. Revised Atlanta and determinant-based classification: application in a prospective cohort of acute pancreatitis patients. Am J Gastroenterol 2013;108:1911–7.
29. Koutroumpakis W, Wu BU, Bakker OJ, et al. Admission hematocrit and rise in blood urea nitrogen at 24 h outperform other laboratory markers in predicting persistent organ failure and pancreatic necrosis in acute pancreatitis: a post hoc analysis of three large prospective databases. Am J Gastroenterol 2015; 110:1707–16.
30. Seifert H, Biermer M, Schmitt W, et al. Transluminal endoscopic necrosectomy after acute pancreatitis; a multicentre study with long-term follow-up (the GEPARD Study). Gut 2009;58:1260–6.
31. Mier J, Leon EL, Castillo A, et al. Early versus late necrosectomy in severe necrotizing pancreatitis. Ann Surg 1997;173:71–5.
32. Tsai K, Wang SS, Chen TS, et al. Oxidative stress: an important phenomenon with pathogenetic significance in the progression of acute pancreatitis. Gut 1998;42: 850–5.
33. Bhagat L, Singh VP, Song AM, et al. Thermal stress-induced HSP-70 mediates protection against intrapancreatic trypsinogen activation and acute pancreatitis in rats. Gastroenterology 2002;122:156–65.
34. Raraty MG, Murphy JA, Mcloughlin E, et al. Mechanisms of acinar cell injury in acute pancreatitis. Scand J Surg 2005;94:89–96.
35. Hegde A, Bhatia M. Neurogenic inflammation in acute pancreatitis. JOP 2005;6: 417–21.
36. Takeda K, Mikami Y, Fukuyama S, et al. Pancreatic ischemia associated with vasospasm in the early phase of human acute necrotizing pancreatitis. Pancreas 2005;30:40–9.
37. Kusterer K, Poschmann T, Friedemann A, et al. Arterial constriction, ischemia-reperfusion, and leukocyte adherence in acute pancreatitis. Am J Physiol 1993; 265:G165–71.
38. Ammori BJ, Leeder PC, King RF, et al. Early increase in intestinal permeability in patients with severe acute pancreatitis: correlation with endotoxemia, organ failure, and mortality. J Gastrointest Surg 1999;3:252–62.

39. Nettelbladt CG, Katouli M, Bark T, et al. Evidence of bacterial translocation in fatal hemorrhagic pancreatitis. J Trauma 2000;48:314–5.
40. Alverdy JC, Chang EB. The re-emerging role of the intestinal microflora in critical illness and inflammation: why the gut hypothesis of sepsis syndrome will not go away. J Leukoc Biol 2008;83:461–6.
41. Jensen GL, Miller RH, Talabiska D, et al. A double-blind, prospective, randomized study of glutamine-enriched compared with standard peptide-based feeding in critically ill patients. Am J Clin Nutr 1996;64:615–21.
42. Moggia E, Koti R, Belgaumkar AP, et al. Pharmacological interventions for acute pancreatitis (review). Cochrane Database Syst Rev 2017;(4):CD011384.
43. Pan LL, Li J, Shamoon M, et al. Recent advances on nutrition in treatment of acute pancreatitis. Front Immunol 2017;8:762.
44. O'Keefe SJ, Lee RB, Anderson FP, et al. Physiological effects of enteral and parenteral feeding on pancreaticobiliary secretion in humans. Am J Gastroenterol 2002;97:2255–62.
45. Kaushik N, Pietraszewski M, Holst JJ, et al. Enteral feeding without pancreatic stimulation. Pancreas 2005;31:353–9.
46. Spanier BW, Mathus-Vliegen EM, Tuynman HA, et al. Nutritional management of patients with acute pancreatitis: a Dutch observational study. Alimen Pharmacol Ther 2008;28:1159–65.
47. Eatock FC, Brombacher GD, Steven A, et al. Nasogastric feeding in severe acute pancreatitis may be practical and safe. Int J Pancreatol 2000;28:23–9.
48. McClave SA, Taylor BE, Martindale RG, et al. Guidelines for the provision and assessment of nutrition support therapy in the adult critically ill patient: Society of Critical Care Medicine (SCCM) and American Society for Parenteral and Enteral Nutrition (A.S.P.E.N.). J Parenter Enteral Nutr 2016;40:159–211.
49. Malone A, Hamilton C. The academy of nutrition and dietetics/the American Society for Parenteral and Enteral Nutrition consensus malnutrition characteristics: application in practice. Nutr Clin Pract 2013;28:639–50.
50. Mirtallo JM, Forbes A, McClave SA, et al. International consensus guidelines for nutrition therapy in pancreatitis. J Parenter Enteral Nutr 2012;36:284–91.
51. Meier R, Beglinger C, Layer P, et al. ESPEN guidelines on nutrition in acute pancreatitis. European Society of Parenteral and Enteral Nutrition. Clin Nutr 2002;21(2):173–83.
52. Marik PE, Zaloga GP. Early enteral nutrition in acutely ill patients: a systematic review. Crit Care Med 2001;29:2264–70.
53. Doig GS, Heighes PT, Simpson F, et al. Early enteral nutrition, provided within 24 h of injury or intensive care unit admission, significantly reduces mortality in critically ill patients: a meta-analysis of randomised controlled trials. Intensive Care Med 2009;35:2018–27.
54. Wang G, Wen J, Xu L, et al. Effect of enteral nutrition and ecoimmunonutrition on bacterial translocation and cytokine production in patients with severe acute pancreatitis. J Surg Res 2013;183:592–7.
55. Márta K, Farkas N, Szabó I, et al. Meta-analysis of early nutrition; the benefits of enteral feeding compared to nil per os diet not only in severe, but also in mild and moderate acute pancreatitis. Int J Mol Sci 2016;17:1691.
56. Moraes JM, Felga GE, Chebli LA, et al. A full solid diet as the initial meal in mild acute pancreatitis is safe and result in a shorter length of hospitalization: results from a prospective, randomized, controlled, double-blind clinical trial. J Clin Gastroenterol 2010;44:517–22.

57. Sathiaraj E, Murthy S, Mansard MJ, et al. Clinical trial: oral feeding with a soft diet compared with clear liquid diet as initial meal in mild acute pancreatitis. Aliment Pharmacol Ther 2008;28:777–81.

58. Jacobson BC, Vander Vliet MB, Hughes MD, et al. A prospective, randomized trial of clear liquids versus low-fat solid diet as the initial meal in mild acute pancreatitis. Clin Gastroenterol Hepatol 2007;5:946–51.

59. Banks PA, Freeman ML. Practice Parameters Committee of the American College of Gastroenterology, practice guidelines in acute pancreatitis. Am J Gastroenterol 2006;101:2379–400.

60. Working Group IAP/APA/Acute Pancreatitis Guidelines. IAP/APA evidence-based guidelines for the management of acute pancreatitis. Pancreatology 2013;13: e1–15.

61. Dashti HS, Mogensen KM. Recommending small, frequent meals in the clinical care of adults: a review of the evidence and important considerations. Nutr Clin Pract 2017;32:365–77.

62. Homko CJ, Duffy F, Friedenberg FK, et al. Effect of dietary fat and food consistency on gastroparesis symptoms in patients with gastroparesis. Neurogastroenterol Motil 2015;27:501–8.

63. Bevan MG, Asrani VM, Bharmal S, et al. Incidence and predictors of oral feeding intolerance in acute pancreatitis: a systematic review, meta-analysis, and meta-regression. Clin Nutr 2017;36:722–9.

64. Davies AR, Morrison SS, Ridley EJ, et al. Nutritional therapy in patients with acute pancreatitis requiring critical care unit management: a prospective observational study in Australia and New Zealand. Crit Care Med 2011;39:462–8.

65. Powell JJ, Murchison JT, Fearon KC, et al. Randomized controlled trial of the effect of early enteral nutrition on markers of the inflammatory response in predicted severe acute pancreatitis. Br J Surg 2000;87:1375–81.

66. Eatock FC, Chong P, Menezes N, et al. A randomized study of early nasogastric versus nasojejunal feeding in severe acute pancreatitis. Am J Gastroenterol 2005;100:432–9.

67. Doley RP, Yadav TD, Wig JD, et al. Enteral nutrition in severe acute pancreatitis. JOP 2009;10:157–62.

68. Meier R, Ockenga J, Pertkiewicz M, et al. ESPEN guidelines on enteral nutrition: pancreas. Clin Nutr 2006;25:275–84.

69. Cao Y, Xu Y, Lu T, et al. Meta-analysis of enteral nutrition versus total parenteral nutrition in patients with severe acute pancreatitis. Ann Nutr Metab 2008;53: 268–75.

70. Heyland DK, Novak F. Immunonutrition in the critically ill patient: more harm than good? J Parenter Enteral Nutr 2001;25:S51–5.

71. Koekkoek WA, van Zanten AR. Antioxidant vitamins and trace elements in critical illness. Nutr Clin Pract 2016;31:457–74.

72. Rasmussen HH, Irtun O, Olesen SS, et al. Nutrition in chronic pancreatitis. World J Gastroenterol 2013;19:7267–75.

73. Patel JJ, Miller KR, Rosenthal C, et al. When is it appropriate to use arginine in critical illness? Nutr Clin Pract 2016;31:438–44.

74. Lasztity N, Hamvas J, Biro L, et al. Effect of enterally administered n-3 polyunsaturated fatty acids in acute pancreatitis—a prospective randomized clinical trial. Clin Nutr 2005;24:198–205.

75. Freedman SD. Options for addressing exocrine pancreatic insufficiency in patients receiving enteral nutrition supplementation. Am J Manag Care 2017;23: S220–8.

76. Ericsson CD, Johnson PC. Safety and efficacy of loperamide. Am J Med 1990;88: 10S–4S.

77. Lee HM, Villa AF, Caudrelier S, et al. Can loperamide cause acute pancreatitis? Pancreas 2011;40:780–1.

78. Ziegler TR, Ogden LG, Singleton KD, et al. Parenteral glutamine increases serum heat shock protein 70 in critically ill patients. Intensive Care Med 2005;31: 1079–86.

79. Bhatia M. Novel therapeutic targets for acute pancreatitis and associated multiple organ dysfunction syndrome. Curr Drug Targets Inflamm Allergy 2002;1: 343–51.

80. Jin M, Zhang H, Lu B, et al. The optimal timing of enteral nutrition and its effect on the prognosis of acute pancreatitis: a propensity score matched cohort study. Pancreatology 2017;17:651–7.

81. Besselink MG, van Santvoort HC, Renooij W, et al. Intestinal barrier dysfunction in a randomized trial of a specific probiotic composition in acute pancreatitis. Ann Surg 2009;250:712–9.

82. Bongaerts GP, Severijnen RS. A reassessment of the PROPATRIA study and its implications for probiotic therapy. Nat Biotechnol 2016;34:55–63.

83. Cui LH, Wang XH, Peng LH, et al. The effects of early enteral nutrition with addition of probiotics on the prognosis of patients suffering from severe acute pancreatitis. Zhonghua Wei Zhong Bing Ji Jiu Yi Xue 2013;25:224–8.

84. Gou S, Yang Z, Liu T, et al. Use of probiotics in the treatment of severe acute pancreatitis: a systematic review and meta-analysis of randomized controlled trials. Crit Care 2014;18:R57.

85. Sun B, Gao Y, Xu J, et al. Role of individually staged nutritional support in the management of severe acute pancreatitis. Hepatobiliary Pancreat Dis Int 2004; 3:458–63.

86. Flint R, Winsor J. The role of the intestine in the pathophysiology and management of severe acute pancreatitis. Hepatobiliary 2003;5:69–85.

87. O'Keefe SJ, McClave SA. Feeding the injured pancreas. Gastroenterology 2005; 129:1129–30.

88. Sax H, Warner B, Talamini M, et al. Early total parenteral nutrition in acute pancreatitis: lack of beneficial effects. Am J Surg 1987;153:117–23.

89. Roberts KN, Conwell D. Acute pancreatitis: how soon should we feed patients? Ann Int Med 2017;166:903–4.

Nutritional Therapy in Chronic Pancreatitis

J. Enrique Domínguez-Muñoz, MD, PhD[a],*, Mary Phillips, RD[b]

KEYWORDS

- Pancreatic exocrine insufficiency • Fecal elastase • Vitamins • Proteins
- Nutritional markers • Anthropometry • Micronutrients
- Pancreatic enzyme replacement therapy

KEY POINTS

- Malnutrition is a frequent complication in patients with chronic pancreatitis that is associated with a high morbidity and increased mortality.
- Pancreatic exocrine insufficiency is the main cause of malnutrition in patients with chronic pancreatitis, supplemented by toxic habits (alcohol abuse), symptoms limiting food ingestion (abdominal pain), and complications (obstruction of the gastroduodenal tract).
- Patients with chronic pancreatitis must be screened for malnutrition and malnutrition-related complications with a nutritional evaluation that includes anthropometric parameters, biochemical markers, and imaging procedures.
- Pancreatic exocrine insufficiency may be diagnosed by pancreatic function tests and the evaluation of maldigestion-related symptoms (diarrhea, flatulence, abdominal distention and cramps, weight loss), nutritional status, and fecal elastase-1 concentration.
- Therapy for malnutrition in chronic pancreatitis includes a normal healthy diet with food fortification, and adequate pancreatic enzyme replacement therapy with nutritional supplements if needed.

INTRODUCTION

Chronic pancreatitis (CP) is a complex disease in which different factors, such as alcohol, smoking, autoimmune disorders, or obstruction of the main pancreatic duct, lead, in genetically predisposed patients, to acinar, ductal and islet cells damage, chronic inflammatory infiltration, and fibrosis. Although pain is the main symptom in

Disclosure: J. Enrique Domínguez-Muñoz has acted as advisor and has given lectures for Mylan Pharmaceuticals and Abbott laboratories.
Mary Phillips has received honoraria for teaching from Mylan Pharmaceuticals, Nutritia Clinical Care, Abbott Nutrition and Vitaflo.
a Department of Gastroenterology and Hepatology, University Hospital of Santiago de Compostela, C/ Choupana s/n, Santiago de Compostela 15706, Spain; b Department of Nutrition and Dietetics, Royal Surrey County Hospital NHS Foundation Trust, Egerton Road, Guildford GU2 7XX, UK
* Corresponding author.
E-mail address: enriquedominguezmunoz@hotmail.com

most patients, malnutrition is a major issue in patients with CP. Exocrine and endocrine pancreatic insufficiency and local alterations (eg, pseudocyst, biliary and duodenal obstruction, splenic and portal vein thrombosis, pancreatic cancer) are complications that frequently develop along the natural history of the disease. As a consequence, the mortality of CP is increased as compared with the general population.[1,2]

Alcohol is the single most common etiologic factor and accounts for 44% to 65% cases in the population.[3] In addition, smoking is the most frequent risk factor of CP that is often associated with alcohol consumption. These toxic habits and the social and psychological factors frequently associated with them play a relevant role in the development of malnutrition in patients with CP. Pancreatic exocrine insufficiency (PEI) is the main pancreatic cause of malnutrition in these patients. Its appropriate diagnosis and therapy, together with an adequate nutritional support, play a major role in the treatment of CP.

This article aims to review the risk factors of malnutrition and the nutritional evaluation and nutritional support in patients with CP. In addition, the diagnosis and therapy for PEI as the major cause of malnutrition in these patients is also discussed.

Risk Factors for Malnutrition in Chronic Pancreatitis

Malnutrition is multifactorial in CP, and the degree of malnutrition ranges from over-nourished obesity to severe malnutrition. Malnutrition may be macronutrient in nature leading to weight loss, sarcopenia, and poor quality of life[4] or micronutrient malnutrition, which causes osteopenia and osteoporosis,[5] vitamin A deficiency night blindness,[6] or other micronutrient deficiencies.[7,8] More recently, malnutrition has been shown to be associated with increased mortality in CP.[2]

Patients with CP may require surgery. A retrospective review of 313 patients who underwent surgery for CP found a higher incidence of infectious and intra-abdominal complications after surgery in those with more significant malnutrition.[9] In addition, pancreatic surgery may further impair digestive pancreatic function in patients with CP because of resection of the gland and anatomic changes of the gastrointestinal tract.[10]

Physical causes of malnutrition include food avoidance (secondary to pain) and maldigestion secondary to PEI. Duodenal stenosis or extrinsic compressions of the duodenum or stomach from pseudocysts result in delayed gastric emptying, causing nausea, vomiting, and poor oral intake.

Nutritional requirements are estimated at 25 to 35 kcal/kg energy and 1.2 to 1.5 g/kg protein[11,12]; however, there are concerns over the use of estimated weight-based nutritional requirements, as these do not adjust for malabsorption. There is limited research in this field, but an observational study of male patients with CP suggested a higher energy expenditure than healthy controls estimated from increased nutrient intake and lower nutritional markers.[13] The use of pancreatic enzyme replacement therapy (PERT) in 32 of 40 subjects confirmed the presence of exocrine dysfunction; but it remains unclear whether the nutritional deficit is from malabsorption of nutrients, increased energy expenditure, or a combination of both.

Furthermore, patients with CP often have a history of alcohol abuse and cigarette smoking; consequently, social and psychological factors, including poor compliance, financial constraints, and poor clinic attendance, often contribute significantly to malnutrition.

Nutritional Evaluation in Chronic Pancreatitis

Assessment of nutritional status is complex in CP, and no single isolated marker should be used.[14] Factors to consider when assessing nutritional status in CP are summarized in **Table 1**. **Fig. 1** summarizes the nutritional evaluation of patients

Table 1
Factors to consider when assessing nutritional status in chronic pancreatitis

Anthropometrics	Biochemical	Clinical
Height	Glucose and HbA$_{1c}$	Change in physical activity levels
Weight	Magnesium	Bone density
% Weight loss	Zinc	Oral intake: tolerance of solids
Hand grip strength	Vitamin D and parathyroid hormone	Oral intake: balanced diet
Midarm muscle circumference	Vitamin A and E	Oral intake: sufficient energy and protein
Triceps skinfold thickness	Vitamin K/clotting screen	Alcohol consumption
CT/US imaging of muscle mass	Iron studies, ferritin, and CRP	Prevalence of infections
—	Vitamin B12 and folate	Presence of nausea/vomiting/early satiety

Abbreviations: CRP, C-reactive protein; CT, computed tomography; HbA$_{1c}$, glycated hemoglobin; US, ultrasound.

diagnosed with CP in clinical practice. This evaluation should be done at the time of diagnosis of the disease and at regular intervals (eg, yearly) according to the nutritional status and clinical situation of the patients.

Anthropometric measurements
Persistent weight loss is universally considered as the most clinically significant marker of nutritional deterioration in surgical patients,[15] and the same criterion can also be useful in patients with CP, although specific data are limited.

A weight loss of greater than 10% in 6 months is a trigger for nutritional intervention[16] and grounds to delay surgery.[17] There are discrepancies in the classification of malnutrition for clinical study; some studies classify patients with more than 10% weight loss as mild/moderately malnourished, suggesting more significant differences in outcomes in patients with more severe malnutrition.[9] More recent work in pancreatic cancer has suggested sarcopenia may be an important consideration, especially in obese patients.[18,19] Although this is the subject of many studies in pancreatic cancer, there are not yet equivalent studies in CP, and it is an area for future study.

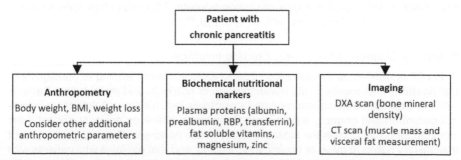

Fig. 1. Nutritional evaluation in patients diagnosed with CP. BMI, body mass index; CT, computed tomography; DXA, dual-energy x-ray absorptiometry; RBP, retinol-binding protein.

Weight loss should be considered over body mass index (BMI) as a stand-alone measurement, as although BMI changes over time. The widespread presence of obesity renders a single measurement of BMI clinically irrelevant. When BMI is used, changes in BMI should be considered in preference to a single measurement. Weight and BMI may be of use in monitoring patients with malnutrition or PEI.[14]

Other anthropometric parameters, such as grip strength, triceps skin-fold thickness, and mid–upper arm circumference, are frequently used for nutritional evaluation in different clinical scenarios. However, the information provided by these markers in patients with CP has not been properly investigated. Because of the well-known sex, age, intrainvestigator, and interinvestigator variability, longitudinal changes of these parameters in individual patients instead of single-point data should be used.[7]

Laboratory parameters

Several biochemical assessment tools are available to evaluate the nutritional status in patients with CP[8] (see **Table 1**). Deficiencies of micronutrients and macronutrients are well-known consequences of malnutrition and have been identified in patients with CP.[14] The prevalence of laboratory nutritional marker abnormalities, including vitamins, minerals, trace elements, and plasma proteins, in patients with CP has been investigated in several studies. In summary, low circulating levels of fat-soluble vitamins (A, D, E, K), proteins (albumin, prealbumin, retinol binding protein, transferrin), lipoproteins and apolipoproteins, and mineral trace elements (magnesium, zinc, calcium, iron, selenium) have been reported in patients with CP.[6–8,14,20] Most of these abnormalities are related to PEI; but other factors, such as toxic habits, deficient food intake, and complications, may play a relevant role.

Malnutrition should be assessed over time, as both malnutrition and PEI are progressive in CP. Monitoring of glucose and glycosylated hemoglobin levels is also relevant because of the high incidence of pancreatogenic (type 3c) diabetes in patients with CP, the frequent association of diabetes and PEI in these patients, and the impact of undiagnosed diabetes on their nutritional status,[14] which requires careful management.[21]

Imaging techniques

Imaging is gaining relevance in assessing body composition. This increasing relevance is mainly due to the acknowledgment that sarcopenia can occur in the presence of obesity and that it has a prognostic role in pancreatic diseases.[19,22]

Recently, sarcopenia and not visceral or subcutaneous fat, as evaluated by computed tomography (CT) scan, has been shown to be significantly associated with PEI in patients with different pancreatic diseases.[23] In addition, bone mineral density as evaluated by dual-energy x-ray absorptiometry (DXA) scan has been shown to be frequently altered in patients with CP and PEI.[24]

Nutritional Diagnosis of Pancreatic Exocrine Insufficiency

PEI in CP is defined as the alteration of pancreatic secretion leading to maldigestion. Maldigestion is associated with malabsorption of nutrients and malnutrition. Patients with PEI may have maldigestion-related symptoms (eg, diarrhea, flatulence, abdominal distention and cramps, weight loss). Symptoms, however, are only evident if the ingested food overcomes the digestive ability of the pancreas. Patients tend to adapt their dietary habits to avoid or minimize symptoms, and that explains why patients with PEI are often asymptomatic. PEI is usually diagnosed by the evaluation of pancreatic function tests, but the presence of nutritional deficiencies is a well-known consequence of PEI; therefore, a nutritional evaluation can be used to support the presence of PEI and to control for the efficacy of PERT in patients with pancreatic diseases.[14] **Fig. 2** summarizes the diagnostic approach to PEI in patients with CP in clinical practice.

Most of the nutritional markers mentioned earlier are more frequently altered in the presence of PEI. Anthropometric data have not been properly evaluated for the diagnosis of PEI in patients with CP. However, morphologic quantification of the bone mineral density and muscle mass by DXA and CT scan have shown a close relationship between PEI and the presence of bone mineral deficiency and sarcopenia.[23,24] These procedures cannot be considered as part of the diagnostic armamentarium of PEI in patients with CP but as methods to evaluate the clinical impact of PEI and its therapy In these patients.

Laboratory nutritional parameters have been evaluated as markers of PEI in patients with CP.[8,14,25] Fat-soluble vitamins are significantly reduced in patients with CP with PEI but not in those without PEI.[25,26] Vitamin D deficiency is associated with the risk of low bone mineral density in patients with CP,[24] but the clinical relevance of other fat soluble vitamin deficiencies in these patients is questionable. Water-soluble vitamins are rarely deficient in CP and they lack any diagnostic interest for PEI. Plasma proteins, such as albumin, prealbumin, retinol-binding protein (RBP), and transferrin, are frequently altered in patients with CP and PEI compared with patients with CP without PEI.[8] Finally, some mineral and trace elements, mainly magnesium, seem to be reduced in patients with PEI.[8]

An adequate nutritional evaluation in patients with CP can be used to support the presence of PEI. In fact, the absence of any nutritional deficiency allows excluding PEI in these patients, whereas the higher the number of deficient nutritional parameters is, the higher is the probability of PEI.[8] Given that only a small proportion of patients with PEI may have a deficiency in a particular parameter, the nutritional evaluation for PEI should comprise multiple nutritional markers and include at least circulating levels of fat-soluble vitamins (preferably vitamin E), prealbumin, RBP, zinc, and magnesium.[8,14] Further evidence is required to determine the optimal panel of markers for nutritional evaluation, and the utility, reliability, and accuracy of these markers in diagnosing PEI. It is important to point out that any nutritional deficiency is unspecific for PEI and other causes have to be considered in the individual patient with CP.

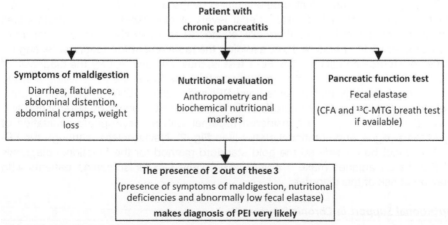

Fig. 2. Diagnosis of PEI in patients with CP. CFA, coefficient of fat absorption; ^{13}C-MTG, mixed ^{13}C-triglyceride.

Functional Diagnosis of Pancreatic Exocrine Insufficiency

PEI develops very frequently in patients with advanced CP, and more than 80% of patients with chronic calcifying pancreatitis present with PEI.[27] PEI may be diagnosed by means of tests evaluating fat digestion as well as tests measuring pancreatic secretion of enzymes. A third alternative is the evaluation of nutritional deficiencies as the consequence of PEI, as described earlier.

Tests evaluating fat digestion

Because the concept of PEI implies the presence of maldigestion, the quantification of the coefficient of fat absorption (CFA) after measurement of fecal fat concentration by the classic Van de Kamer test is still considered the gold standard for the diagnosis of PEI.[28] Despite that, this test has several important disadvantages limiting its clinical applicability. Patients must keep on a standard diet containing 100 g of fat daily for 5 consecutive days and collect all the feces produced over the last 3 days. This requirement is not easy to comply with for most patients. A strict control of fat intake and a 3-day stool collection are needed to reduce errors and variability. Quantification of fat in a small isolated stool sample lacks diagnostic ability.

A mixed ^{13}C-triglyceride (^{13}C-MTG) breath test has been developed and optimized as an alternative to CFA for the diagnosis of PEI in clinical routine.[29] A cumulative recovery of ^{13}C in breath over 6 hours less than 29% after oral intake of 250 mg of ^{13}C-MTG is an accurate marker of PEI. The ^{13}C-MTG breath test is also a reliable method to evaluate the efficacy of PERT in patients with CP.[30] The main advantage of the breath test in comparison with any other quantitative test is that of providing with a ^{13}C exhalation curve that qualitatively defines the dynamic of the digestive process in individual patients.

Tests evaluating pancreatic secretion

An alternative to digestion tests for the diagnosis of PEI is the quantification of pancreatic secretion. The concept is that the lower pancreatic secretion of enzymes and bicarbonate is, the higher is the probability of PEI. Direct tests of pancreatic secretion, mainly after intravenous secretin stimulation, have the highest accuracy for evaluating pancreatic secretion but are invasive, time consuming, and expensive. The main role of these tests in clinical practice is the diagnosis of CP in patients with indeterminate imaging findings.

Pancreatic secretion can also be evaluated by the quantification of the pancreatic elastase concentration in feces.[31] Fecal levels of elastase-1 (FE-1) correlate well with its pancreatic output. Furthermore, elastase-1 is highly stable in feces for up to 1 week at room temperature, thus, avoiding the requirement for specialist testing facilities or storage conditions. The FE-1 test is, thus, an easy test for the diagnosis of PEI.[31] FE-1 being a test of pancreatic secretion, the lower the FE-1 levels are, the higher the probability that patients have PEI and require PERT. Physicians should, thus, be aware that an exact cutoff of FE-1 levels for PEI cannot be established and that FE-1 levels should be considered together with an appropriate evaluation of symptoms, signs, and nutritional status (see **Fig. 2**). Nevertheless, although the FE-1 test cannot be considered the gold standard method for the functional diagnosis of PEI, its advantages make it a very appropriate test for screening patients who may be at risk of this disorder.

Nutritional Support in Chronic Pancreatitis

The need for nutritional support in patients with CP increases over time. In addition, many patients require counseling on healthy eating and positive lifestyle choices, including smoking and alcohol cessation, weight-bearing exercise, and sunlight exposure.

As oral intake diminishes high energy, high protein food fortification advice should be given, with oral nutritional supplements and enteral feeding when necessary. Where PEI is present, nutritional support must be used in conjunction with PERT.

Historically, patients have been advised to follow low-fat diets. However, a low-fat diet decreases pancreatic secretion of enzymes, renders endogenously secreted lipase unstable, and makes PERT less effective.[32–34] Some studies have shown that patients can tolerate 30% to 33% of their energy intake from fat[35] and that there is potential for significant malabsorption of both dietary carbohydrate[36] and protein.[37] Furthermore, dietary fat restriction will mask the onset of malabsorption by reducing steatorrhea.

Dietary fiber inhibits pancreatic lipase. A small study of 12 patients with CP found very-high-fiber diets were associated with significant increases in fecal fat[38]; consequently, very-high-fiber diets are not recommended in patients with CP and PEI.

Patients respond to the use of nutritional supplementation and food fortification provided by an experienced dietitian, and significant improvements were noted in anthropometric measurements and fat malabsorption.[35] In this randomized controlled trial of 60 patients with CP, a significant reduction in pain was also noted following both interventions.

In patients unable to tolerate a sufficient oral diet to prevent nutritional compromise, enteral nutrition (EN) should be provided via the best tolerated route. In patients with intractable pain or gastric stasis, jejunal feeding is indicated[39] and is well tolerated and effective at improving nutritional status in CP.[39,40] When EN is used, peptide semielemental products should be used to optimize absorption.[41]

In some patients with severe PEI, it may be necessary to use PERT alongside EN.[42] This supplementation is cumbersome[43]; although this has been examined in vitro,[44,45] there are no studies to report the efficacy of this in vivo.

A small number of patients may experience such severe uncontrollable malabsorption that parenteral nutrition is indicated.

Pancreatic Enzyme Replacement Therapy

Together with nutritional support, PERT is the cornerstone of PEI and malnutrition therapy in patients with CP. PERT should mimic postprandial exocrine pancreatic physiology as much as possible. With this aim, enzymes in microspheres or minimicrospheres, ideally of a size smaller than 2 mm, are preferred in order to facilitate an adequate dispersion and mixing with the food in the stomach and a coordinated gastric emptying with nutrients. Spheres should additionally be enteric coated to avoid the inactivation of enzymes by gastric acid. Duodenal pH should be as neutral as possible to ensure the release of enzymes from the enteric-coated pellets. Finally, the dose of enzymes should be high enough for food digestion.

A minimum lipase dose of 36,000 to 50,000 US Pharmacopeia (USP) units (1 USP unit equals 1 European Pharmacological Units) is recommended with main meals and 24,000 to 25,000 USP units with snacks to normalize digestion.[28,46] PERT has been shown to be effective in terms of fat and protein digestion, symptoms, quality of life, and nutritional status.[30,47,48]

The intake of oral pancreatic enzymes should be distributed along with meals and snacks.[46,49] Patient compliance is a key factor in the management of PEI with oral pancreatic enzymes. Patients should understand the importance of the therapy and the correct administration schedule.

Despite the use of modern pancreatic enzyme, preparations at the minimum recommended dose digestion does not revert to normal in almost half of the patients with CP and PEI. Acidic intestinal pH plays a major role in this lack of appropriate response. The abnormally low pancreatic secretion of bicarbonate in patients with PEI is associated with a limited buffering effect in the proximal intestine. A pH less than 4 is associated with an irreversible inactivation of endogenous and uncoated exogenous pancreatic lipase, as well as with precipitation of bile salts, contributing to fat maldigestion. In addition, enteric-coated pancreatic enzymes require a pH greater than 5 to be released, which may first occur in distal segments of the small intestine, thus, reducing the efficacy of the therapy. Because of that, the addition of a proton pump inhibitor before breakfast and dinner is recommended in cases of an unsatisfactory clinical response to the standard dose of PERT.[46] In addition, the enzyme dose should be increased (doubled or tripled) if needed to normalize digestion and the nutritional status of patients. If these strategies fail, another cause for maldigestion (eg, bacterial overgrowth) should be sought. **Fig. 3** summarizes the therapeutic approach of patients with CP and PEI in clinical practice.

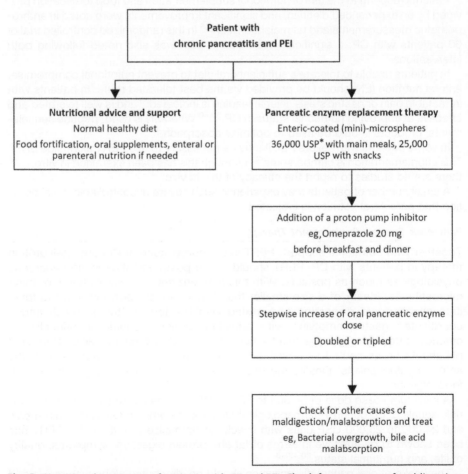

Fig. 3. Nutritional treatment of patients with CP and PEI. Check for symptoms of maldigestion and nutritional markers after each step. Maintain therapy if patients are asymptomatic and nutritional evaluation is normal. On the contrary, go to the next step. *1 USP unit equals 1 European Pharmacological Units.

In patients who have undergone surgery, there is a higher risk of bacterial overgrowth and bile acid malabsorption[50–52]; these differential diagnoses should be considered in patients failing to respond to routine nutritional intervention and PERT.

SUMMARY

Malnutrition is a frequent complication in patients with CP. Maldigestion as a consequence of PEI is the major cause of malnutrition in these patients. Together with that, toxic habits (alcohol abuse) and alterations of the gastroduodenal transit secondary to compression from pseudocysts or duodenal fibro-inflammatory involvement may play a relevant role. Malnutrition in CP is associated with osteoporosis, sarcopenia, poor quality of life, and increased mortality. An adequate nutritional evaluation, including anthropometric (weight loss, BMI) and biochemical nutritional markers (plasma levels of proteins, fat-soluble vitamins, and micronutrients) and imaging for body composition (DXA scan and CT scan), is recommended in these patients at diagnosis and over the follow-up. PEI may be diagnosed by the evaluation of maldigestion-related symptoms (diarrhea, flatulence, abdominal distention and cramps, weight loss), nutritional status and FE-1 concentration. Nutritional advice and support together with an adequate PERT are mandatory. A normal healthy diet should be recommended. Food fortification and oral nutritional supplements may be indicated in patients with limited food intake or severe malnutrition. EN and more rarely parenteral nutrition may be occasionally required. Together with nutritional support, PERT is the therapy of choice. A modern enzyme preparation in the form of enteric-coated mini-microspheres should be used at a minimum dose of 36,000 to 50,000 USP units with meals and 24,000 to 25,000 USP units with snacks. The addition of a proton pump inhibitor may be needed. The dose of oral pancreatic enzymes should be individualized according to the objective evaluation of the nutritional status.

REFERENCES

1. Bang UC, Benfield T, Hyldstrup L, et al. Mortality, cancer, and comorbidities associated with chronic pancreatitis: a Danish nationwide matched-cohort study. Gastroenterology 2014;146(4):989–94.
2. De la Iglesia D, Vallejo-Senra N, Iglesias-Garcia J, et al. Increased risk of mortality associated with pancreatic exocrine insufficiency in patients with chronic pancreatitis. J Clin Gastroenterol 2017. [Epub ahead of print].
3. Conwell DL, Lee LS, Yadav D, et al. American Pancreatic Association practice guidelines in chronic pancreatitis: evidence-based report on diagnostic guidelines. Pancreas 2014;43(8):1143–62.
4. Czako L, Takacs T, Hegyi P, et al. Quality of life assessment after pancreatic enzyme replacement therapy in chronic pancreatitis. Can J Gastroenterol 2003; 17(10):597–603.
5. Duggan SN, O'Sullivan M, Hamilton S, et al. Patients with chronic pancreatitis are at increased risk for osteoporosis. Pancreas 2012;41(7):1119–24.
6. Livingstone C, Davis J, Marvin V, et al. Vitamin A deficiency presenting as night blindness during pregnancy. Ann Clin Biochem 2003;40:292–4.
7. Duggan SN, Smyth ND, O'Sullivan M, et al. The prevalence of malnutrition and fat-soluble vitamin deficiencies in chronic pancreatitis. Nutr Clin Pract 2014; 29(3):348–54.
8. Lindkvist B, Dominguez-Munoz JE, Luaces-Regueira M, et al. Serum nutritional markers for prediction of pancreatic exocrine insufficiency in chronic pancreatitis. Pancreatology 2012;12(4):305–10.

9. Schnelldorfer T, Adams DB. The effect of malnutrition on morbidity after surgery for chronic pancreatitis. Am Surg 2005;71(6):466–72.
10. Sabater L, Ausania F, Bakker OJ, et al. Evidence-based guidelines for the management of exocrine pancreatic insufficiency after pancreatic surgery. Ann Surg 2016;264(6):949–58.
11. Duggan S, O'Sullivan M, Feehan S, et al. Nutrition treatment of deficiency and malnutrition in chronic pancreatitis: a review. Nutr Clin Pract 2010;25(4):362–70.
12. Mirtallo JM, Forbes A, McClave SA, et al. International consensus guidelines for nutrition therapy in pancreatitis. JPEN J Parenter Enteral Nutr 2012;36(3):284–91.
13. Vaona B, Armellini F, Bovo P, et al. Food intake of patients with chronic pancreatitis after onset of the disease. Am J Clin Nutr 1997;65(3):851–4.
14. Lindkvist B, Phillips ME, Dominguez-Munoz JE. Clinical, anthropometric and laboratory nutritional markers of pancreatic exocrine insufficiency: prevalence and diagnostic use. Pancreatology 2015;15(6):589–97.
15. Loh KW, Vriens MR, Gerritsen A, et al. Unintentional weight loss is the most important indicator of malnutrition among surgical cancer patients. Neth J Med 2012;70(8):365–9.
16. Stratton RJ, Hackston A, Longmore D, et al. Malnutrition in hospital outpatients and inpatients: prevalence, concurrent validity and ease of use of the 'malnutrition universal screening tool' ('MUST') for adults. Br J Nutr 2004;92(5):799–808.
17. Weimann A, Braga M, Harsanyi L, et al. ESPEN guidelines on enteral nutrition: surgery including organ transplantation. Clin Nutr 2006;25(2):224–44.
18. Peng P, Hyder O, Firoozmand A, et al. Impact of sarcopenia on outcomes following resection of pancreatic adenocarcinoma. J Gastrointest Surg 2012;16(8):1478–86.
19. Tan BH, Birdsell LA, Martin L, et al. Sarcopenia in an overweight or obese patient is an adverse prognostic factor in pancreatic cancer. Clin Cancer Res 2009;15(22):6973–9.
20. Montalto G, Soresi M, Carroccio A, et al. Lipoproteins and chronic pancreatitis. Pancreas 1994;9(1):137–8.
21. Duggan SN, Ewald N, Kelleher L, et al. The nutritional management of type 3c (pancreatogenic) diabetes in chronic pancreatitis. Eur J Clin Nutr 2017;71(1):3–8.
22. Engelen MP, Schroder R, Van der Hoorn K, et al. Use of body mass index percentile to identify fat-free mass depletion in children with cystic fibrosis. Clin Nutr 2012;31(6):927–33.
23. Shintakuya R, Uemura K, Murakami Y, et al. Sarcopenia is closely associated with pancreatic exocrine insufficiency in patients with pancreatic disease. Pancreatology 2017;17(1):70–5.
24. Sikkens EC, Cahen DL, Koch AD, et al. The prevalence of fat-soluble vitamin deficiencies and a decreased bone mass in patients with chronic pancreatitis. Pancreatology 2013;13(3):238–42.
25. Marotta F, Labadarios D, Frazer L, et al. Fat-soluble vitamin concentration in chronic alcohol-induced pancreatitis. Relationship with steatorrhea. Dig Dis Sci 1994;39(5):993–8.
26. Dutta SK, Bustin MP, Russell RM, et al. Deficiency of fat-soluble vitamins in treated patients with pancreatic insufficiency. Ann Intern Med 1982;97(4):549–52.
27. Domínguez-Muñoz JE, Alvarez-Castro A, Lariño-Noia J, et al. Endoscopic ultrasonography of the pancreas as an indirect method to predict pancreatic exocrine insufficiency in patients with chronic pancreatitis. Pancreas 2012;41(5):724–8.
28. Dominguez-Muñoz JE. Pancreatic exocrine insufficiency: diagnosis and treatment. J Gastroenterol Hepatol 2011;26(suppl 2):12–6.

29. Domínguez-Muñoz JE, Nieto L, Vilariño M, et al. Development and diagnostic accuracy of a breath test for pancreatic exocrine insufficiency in chronic pancreatitis. Pancreas 2016;45(2):241–7.

30. Domínguez-Muñoz JE, Iglesias-García J, Vilariño-Insua M, et al. ^{13}C-mixed triglyceride breath test to assess oral enzyme substitution therapy in patients with chronic pancreatitis. Clin Gastroenterol Hepatol 2007;5(4):484–8.

31. Domínguez-Muñoz JE, Hardt PD, Lerch MM, et al. Potential for screening for pancreatic exocrine insufficiency using the fecal elastase-1 test. Dig Dis Sci 2017;62(5):1119–30.

32. Boivin M, Lanspa SJ, Zinsmeister AR, et al. Are diets associated with different rates of human interdigestive and postprandial pancreatic enzyme secretion? Gastroenterology 1990;99(6):1763–71.

33. Holtmann G, Kelly DG, Sternby B, et al. Survival of human pancreatic enzymes during small bowel transit: effect of nutrients, bile acids, and enzymes. Am J Physiol 1997;273(2 Pt 1):G553–8.

34. Suzuki A, Mizumoto A, Sarr MG, et al. Bacterial lipase and high-fat diets in canine exocrine pancreatic insufficiency: a new therapy of steatorrhea? Gastroenterology 1997;112(6):2048–55.

35. Singh S, Midha S, Singh N, et al. Dietary counseling versus dietary supplements for malnutrition in chronic pancreatitis: a randomized controlled trial. Clin Gastroenterol Hepatol 2008;6(3):353–9.

36. Ladas SD, Giorgiotis K, Raptis SA. Complex carbohydrate malabsorption in exocrine pancreatic insufficiency. Gut 1993;34(7):984–7.

37. Caliari S, Benini L, Sembenini C, et al. Medium-chain triglyceride absorption in patients with pancreatic insufficiency. Scand J Gastroenterol 1996;31(1):90–4.

38. Dutta SK, Hlasko J. Dietary fiber in pancreatic disease: effect of high fiber diet on fat malabsorption in pancreatic insufficiency and in vitro study of the interaction of dietary fiber with pancreatic enzymes. Am J Clin Nutr 1985;41(3):517–25.

39. Lordan JT, Phillips M, Chun JY, et al. A safe, effective, and cheap method of achieving pancreatic rest in patients with chronic pancreatitis with refractory symptoms and malnutrition. Pancreas 2009;38(6):689–92.

40. Skipworth JR, Raptis DA, Wijesuriya S, et al. The use of nasojejunal nutrition in patients with chronic pancreatitis. JOP 2011;12(6):574–80.

41. Meier R, Ockenga J, Pertkiewicz M, et al. ESPEN guidelines on enteral nutrition: pancreas. Clin Nutr 2006;25(2):275–84.

42. Caliari S, Benini L, Bonfante F, et al. Pancreatic extracts are necessary for the absorption of elemental and polymeric enteral diets in severe pancreatic insufficiency. Scand J Gastroenterol 1993;28(8):749–52.

43. Ferrie S, Graham C, Hoyle M. Pancreatic enzyme supplementation for patients receiving enteral feeds. Nutr Clin Pract 2011;26(3):349–51.

44. Shlieout G, Koerner A, Maffert M, et al. Administration of CREON(R) pancrelipase pellets via gastrostomy tube is feasible with no loss of gastric resistance or lipase activity: an in vitro study. Clin Drug Investig 2011;31(7):e1–7.

45. Hauenschild A, Ewald N, Klauke T, et al. Effect of liquid pancreatic enzymes on the assimilation of fat in different liquid formula diets. JPEN J Parenter Enteral Nutr 2008;32(1):98–100.

46. Löhr JM, Dominguez-Munoz E, Rosendahl J, et al. United European Gastroenterology evidence-based guidelines for the diagnosis and therapy of chronic pancreatitis (HaPanEU). United European Gastroenterol J 2017;5(2):153–99.

47. de la Iglesia-García D, Huang W, Szatmary P, et al. NIHR Pancreas Biomedical Research Unit Patient Advisory Group. Efficacy of pancreatic enzyme

replacement therapy in chronic pancreatitis: systematic review and meta-analysis. Gut 2017;66(8):1354–5.

48. D'Haese JG, Ceyhan GO, Demir IE, et al. Pancreatic enzyme replacement therapy in patients with exocrine pancreatic insufficiency due to chronic pancreatitis: a 1-year disease management study on symptom control and quality of life. Pancreas 2014;43(6):834–41.

49. Domínguez-Muñoz JE, Iglesias-García J, Iglesias-Rey M, et al. Effect of the administration schedule on the therapeutic efficacy of oral pancreatic enzyme supplements in patients with exocrine pancreatic insufficiency: a randomized, three-way crossover study. Aliment Pharmacol Ther 2005;21(8):993–1000.

50. Capurso G, Signoretti M, Archibugi L, et al. Systematic review and meta-analysis: small intestinal bacterial overgrowth in chronic pancreatitis. United European Gastroenterol J 2016;4(5):697–705.

51. Bustillo I, Larson H, Saif MW. Small intestine bacterial overgrowth: an underdiagnosed cause of diarrhea in patients with pancreatic cancer. JOP 2009;10(5): 576–8.

52. Phillips ME. Pancreatic exocrine insufficiency following pancreatic resection. Pancreatology 2015;15(5):449–55.

The Role of Diet in the Treatment of Irritable Bowel Syndrome: A Systematic Review

Rajdeep Singh, MD[a], Ahmed Salem, MD[b], Julie Nanavati, MLS, MA[c], Gerard E. Mullin, MD[d],*

KEYWORDS

- Nutrition • Diet • Irritable bowel syndrome • FODMAPs • Gluten • Food sensitivities
- Fiber • Elimination diets

KEY POINTS

- Irritable bowel syndrome (IBS) is characterized by recurrent abdominal pain and altered stool frequency and form, which is diagnosed according to the updated Rome IV criteria.
- Food may induce symptoms that have a range of effects in the human body, including increases in luminal osmolarity, induction of gut motility, intestinal spasms immune activation, and other poorly understood processes.
- Elimination diets are helpful in improving IBS symptoms; however, it is impossible predict which subset(s) of patients will benefit from specific restriction regimens.
- A group of foods that include fructooligosaccharides, oligosaccharides, disaccharides, monosaccharides, and polyols (FODMAPs) represents a range of foods may provoke IBS.
- Restricting FODMAPS from the diet is associated with improved IBS symptoms and quality of life.

INTRODUCTION

Irritable bowel syndrome (IBS) is characterized by abdominal discomfort and alterations in bowel habits, including diarrhea (diarrhea-predominant IBS [IBS-D]), chronic constipation (constipation-predominant IBS), or a combination of both (IBS-mixed). A diverse range of digestive tract symptoms is associated with IBS, including constipation, diarrhea, pain, and/or discomfort, distension, and flatulence.

Disclosure: The authors have nothing to disclose.
[a] Department of Internal Medicine, Sinai Hospital of Baltimore, 2421 Cylburn Avenue, Baltimore, MD 21215, USA; [b] Gastroenterology Department, University of Rochester Medical Center, 101 Portsmouth Terrace, Rochester, NY 14642, USA; [c] The Johns Hopkins University School of Medicine, Welch Medical Library, 2024 East Monument Street, Baltimore, MD 21287, USA; [d] Division of Gastroenterology and Hepatology, Johns Hopkins University School of Medicine, 600 North Wolfe Street CARN 464B, Baltimore, MD 21287, USA
* Corresponding author.
E-mail address: gmullin1@jhmi.edu

Gastroenterol Clin N Am 47 (2018) 107–137
https://doi.org/10.1016/j.gtc.2017.10.003
0889-8553/18/© 2017 Elsevier Inc. All rights reserved.

There are 4 disease subtypes of disease in equal proportions: diarrhea, constipation, mixed, and undefined.[1] People with IBS may also experience bloating, intense abdominal pain, and a myriad of other intestinal and extraintestinal comorbidities (ie, anxiety, depression, fibromyalgia, chronic pelvic pain, chronic fatigue syndrome, temporomandibular joint dysfunction; **Fig. 1**).[2,3]

In the past, IBS was a diagnosis of exclusion, unless red flag symptoms were present, thereby indicating that another condition was present, such as celiac disease; others may have overlapping symptoms. The use of the Rome criteria has shifted

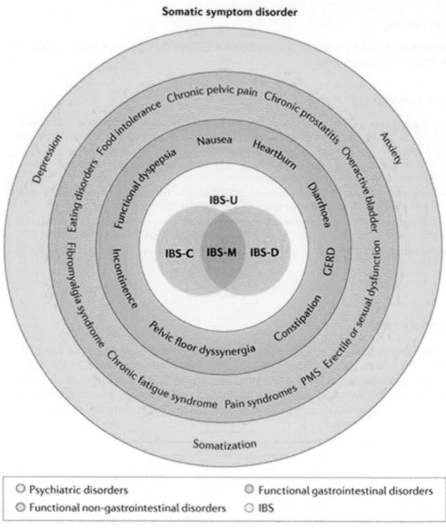

Fig. 1. A model of irritable bowel syndrome (IBS) and its associations with other clinical, intestinal, extraintestinal and psychiatric conditions. GERD, gastroesophageal reflux disease; IBS-C, IBS with constipation; IBS-D, IBS with diarrhea; IBS-M, mixed-type IBS; IBS-U, unsubtyped IBS; PMS, premenstrual syndrome. (*From* Enck P, Aziz Q, Barbara G, et al. Irritable bowel syndrome. Nat Rev Dis Primers 2016;2. https://doi.org/10.1038/nrdp.2016.14; with permission.)

the diagnosis of IBS away from a diagnosis of exclusion to one that is based on defined criteria. The Rome IV criteria were recently updated from Rome III (**Box 1**, **Fig. 2**)[4] and are used to diagnose IBS.

The revised Rome IV diagnostic criteria represent significant changes that are likely to impact disease prevalence by improving specificity. For instance, a survey of 5931 people in North America and the United Kingdom who used these updated criteria resulted in decreasing the prevalence of IBS to 5.7%.[5] The term "discomfort," as used in Rome III, has been replaced by "pain," and its frequency has increased from 3 days per month (Rome III) to at least 1 day per week. Abdominal pain no longer needs to be related to changes in stool frequency or form, and the relationship of abdominal pain to defecation is no longer restricted to "improvement," because it may be worsened by bowel movements; thus, the terminology used in Rome IV becomes abdominal pain "related to defecation."

The prevalence of IBS varies across the globe; however, the accepted prevalence in the United States and Europe is thought to be approximately 5% to 10%. A metaanalysis of 90 studies across 33 countries reported a pooled global prevalence of 11.2% (95% confidence interval [CI], 9.8–12.8).[6] Enck and colleagues[7] extended the study by Lovell and Ford,[6] and estimated the global prevalence to be 8.23%.

IBS can occur at any age but mainly presents in young adults and rarely manifests after the age of 50.[8] Most IBS experts agree that a pathophysiologic disruption of gut homeostasis and or psychological event is a trigger for the vast majority

---

Box 1
Rome IV criteria for IBS

According to Rome IV, a diagnosis of IBS can be made if recurrent abdominal pain (at least once weekly) is associated with 2 or more of the following:

- Related to defecation;
- Associated with a change in frequency of stool; or
- Associated with a change in form (appearance) of stool.

The patient needs to have none of the following warning signs:

- Are greater than 50 years of age at onset, no previous colon cancer screening, and with the presence of symptoms.
- Recent change in bowel habit.
- Evidence of overt GI bleeding (ie, melena or hematochezia).
- Nocturnal pain or passage of stools.
- Unintentional weight loss.
- Family history of colorectal cancer or inflammatory bowel disease.
- Palpable abdominal mass or lymphadenopathy.
- Evidence of iron deficiency anemia on blood testing.
- Positive test for fecal occult blood.

Abbreviations: GI, gastrointestinal; IBS, irritable bowel syndrome.
Data from Palsson OS, Whitehead WE, van Tilburg MA, et al. Rome IV diagnostic questionnaires and tables for investigators and clinicians. Gastroenterology 2016;150:6:1481–91.

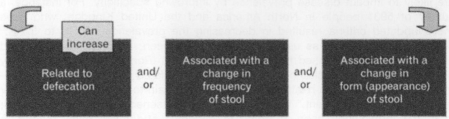

It is a nonspecific term, has different meanings in
different languages and is ambiguous to patients

Recurrent abdominal pain on average at least 1 d/wk in the last 3 mo, associated with
2 or more of the following[a]:

| Can increase — Related to defecation | and/ or | Associated with a change in frequency of stool | and/ or | Associated with a change in form (appearance) of stool |

[a]Criterion fulfilled for the last 3 mo with symptom onset at least 6 mo prior to diagnosis.

Fig. 2. Changes in diagnostic criteria for irritable bowel syndrome (IBS) from Rome III to
Rome IV. (*Data from* Drossman DA, Chang L, Kellow WJ, et al. Rome IV functional gastrointestinal disorders – disorders of gut-brain interaction. J Gastro 2016;150(6):1257–61; with
permission.)

of cases. IBS is more commonly identified in women than in men by 2:1 in Western
countries, and is associated with an adverse economic impact related to absen-
teeism from work and loss of productivity, with health care costs measured in
the billions of dollars annually.[9–11] IBS is well-known to have an adverse impact
on quality of life.

PATHOPHYSIOLOGY OF IRRITABLE BOWEL SYNDROME

The pathophysiology of IBS is complex and involves altered enteric neurotransmitters,
imbalances in the gut microbiota, neuroendocrine disruption, visceral hypersensitivity,
altered gut barrier function, disordered motility, a maladaptive stress response, and a
dysfunctional psychological component.[12–16] These mechanisms influence the
expression of the disease, but are not universally operative in all patients, and nor
are they pathognomic of IBS.

The pathophysiology of IBS involves the interaction of factors that collaborate to
produce chronic disease (**Fig. 3**). Psychological factors elicit neurotransmitters and
hypothalamic–pituitary axis hormones, which interfere with the balance of signaling
between the central and enteric nervous systems.[17] Early life experiences, such as
dysfunctional family influences, and traumatic life events, such as psychological
and physical abuse, have been linked to IBS disease susceptibility.[18] Impaired
coping mechanisms and comorbid psychiatric disorders, such as anxiety and
depression, may additionally influence sensitivity to pain, gut dysmotility, immune
function, and quality of life.[19] Further, genetics are known to play an antecedent
role in IBS, because the disease has a higher concordance in monozygotic twins
than dizygotic pairs.[20] A number of mechanisms have been explored for genetic
variation linkages to disease development.[21] To date, the best associations have
been linked to genetic variations in the serotonin transporter, the 5-hydroxytrypta-
mine transporter-linked polymorphic region (*5-HTTLPR*), and tumor necrosis factor
alpha superfamily member 15.[22] Vaiopoulou and colleagues[23] and Gazouli and colleagues[24] summarized the available molecular genetic data on IBS risk genes that
have since been replicated.

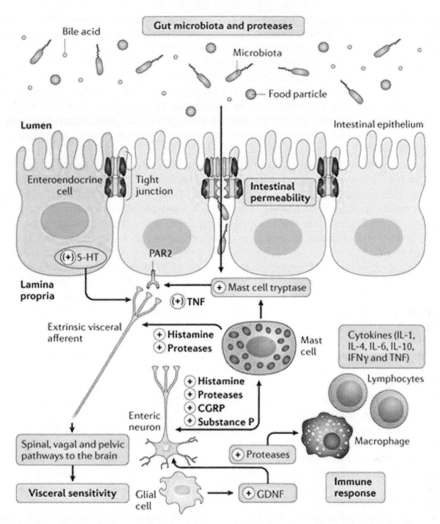

Fig. 3. Overview of the pathophysiology of irritable bowel syndrome (IBS). 5-HT, 5-hydroxytryptamine (also known as serotonin); CGRP, calcitonin gene-related peptide; GDNF, glial cell-derived neurotrophic factor; IFN, interferon; IL, interleukin; PAR2, proteinase-activated receptor 2; TNF, tumor necrosis factor. (*From* Enck P, Aziz Q, Barbara G, et al. Irritable bowel syndrome. Nat Rev Dis Primers 2016;2:16014; with permission.)

The contribution of the gut microbiota in disease pathogenesis is supported by the presence of small intestine bacterial overgrowth in the majority of patients with IBS.[25] Symptoms of small intestine bacterial overgrowth include bloating, constipation, diarrhea, and flatulence, all of which overlap with symptoms of IBS.[26,27] Approximately 25% of patients with IBS have a definable initiating event, which follows an enteric infection producing a disease subtype called postinfectious IBS, which tends to be diarrhea dominant.[28] Patients who are most at risk for acquiring IBS after an enteric infection are females, those with severe enteritis, those taking antibiotics during enteritis, and those with underlying psychiatric comorbidity.[29]

The intestinal mucosa of the postinfectious subset of patients with IBS has an increased density of lamina propria T cells, intraepithelial lymphocytes, mucosal mast cells, and serotonin-containing enteroendocrine cells, all of which promote a proinflammatory milieu via the resulting elaboration of inflammatory mediators.[30] Low-grade chronic inflammation, which is characterized by the increased production and secretion of mast cell mediators, is in juxtaposition to enteric nerves, contributes toward visceral hypersensitivity, and is noticeable in a number of IBS subtypes (ie, postinfectious IBS, IBS-D).[31,32] Studies have suggested an association of between mast cell mediators with worsened symptoms severity and psychosocial comorbidity.[31,32]

Food is a well-known provocateur in triggering IBS symptoms, having numerous putative mechanisms for symptom induction. Mechanisms by which food may influence IBS symptoms include fermentation of short chain carbohydrates by enteric bacteria, true food allergy, nonimmune food sensitivity, alterations in gut motility, luminal fluid shifts from poorly transported disaccharides and highly osmotic dietary substances, changes in gut hormones, and alterations in the gut microbiome.[1]

There are many known triggers for the flare-up of IBS symptoms, such as stress, infections, antibiotics, nonsteroidal antiinflammatory medications, and surgery. However, symptoms are most commonly provoked by foods.[13] When compared with the general population, individuals with IBS report a greater sensitivity to food and intolerance. According to the double-blind challenge methodologies, approximately two-thirds of patients with IBS have at least 1 food intolerance, and some have multiple intolerances.[33,34] Overall, IBS symptoms worsen in 60% of patients after the ingestion of food with 28% within 15 minutes after eating and 93% within 3 hours. A study from Sweden led by Bohn[35] reported that 84% of patients with IBS described a provocation of symptoms in response to one or more food items. Symptoms were related to the intake of foods rich in fermentable oligosaccharides, disaccharides, monosaccharides, and polyols (FODMAPs), but also included foods rich in biogenic amines and histamine-releasing foods. Risk factors for having more food items trigger IBS symptoms included a higher symptom severity score, female gender, and more somatic symptoms. Likewise, provocative foods, when restricted from the diet, have demonstrated improvements in symptomatology and quality of life.

A preliminary evaluation of the medical literature revealed that there have been thousands of articles written on the relationship of food to IBS. Thus, a systematic approach was chosen to most accurately analyze the influence of diet on symptoms, disease activity, and quality of life in patients with IBS.

METHODOLOGY FOR DATA ANALYSIS AND EXTRACTION
Search Methodology for Articles on Fructosaccharides, Oligosaccharides, Disaccharides, and Monosaccharides and Polyols and Irritable Bowel Syndrome

Applicable studies on FODMAPs and IBS were identified through a library literature search spanning this study's inception to August 16, 2017, using PubMed, Embase, the Cochrane Library, and Web of Science. The search strategy was developed by an informationist (JN) in collaboration with the co-authors of this study (GM, RS). There were no language restrictions or restrictions on publication types placed on the search. The PRISMA checklist[36] and the Cochrane review reporting guidelines (6.6.2.2)[37] (Appendix 1) were used to ensure reproducibility. Also, the references of studies cited by the selected articles were examined for further pertinent studies.

Selection Criteria for Systematic Analysis of Fructosaccharides, Oligosaccharides, Disaccharides, and Monosaccharides and Polyols and Irritable Bowel Syndrome

Based on the inclusion and exclusion criteria (see **Box 1**), 2 reviewers carefully reviewed the title and abstract of all studies. The study was selected for further analysis if there was an agreement between the 2 reviewers. A third reviewer studied whether there was any disagreement to determine whether the study qualified for inclusion. A full text review and data extraction were completed once the articles met the criteria.

Inclusion criteria were (1) patients with IBS, as diagnosed using any of the following criteria for IBS: Manning Criteria, Rome I, II, III, IV diagnostic criteria; (2) ages 18 or older; (3) organic disease excluded; and (4) randomized controlled clinical trials. Exclusion criteria were (1) patients having an organic disease, (2) studies with patients who have not had organic disease excluded, and (3) age less than 18 years.

Data Extraction of Low Fructosaccharides, Oligosaccharides, Disaccharides, and Monosaccharides and Polyols Studies

Regarding the role of FODMAPs for IBS, a total of 11 studies were included for eligibility (see Appendix 1). Two independent reviewers extracted data based on data quality, sufficiency, and relevance. A third reviewer resolved disagreements to reach a consensus. The following data were extracted: last name of the first author, publication year, authors' country of origin, patients' demographic information, sample size, food or dietary component under study, and primary endpoint. The risk of bias was assessed independently in duplicate using tools specific to each included study based on the inclusion and exclusion criteria for each question[37] (**Table 1**).

Primary and Secondary Dietary Factors in the Dietary Management of Irritable Bowel Syndrome

The PubMed, Embase, Cochrane, and Web of Science databases were used to search for pertinent articles for foods that were provocative and upon withdrawal, therapeutic for the IBS (see Appendix 1).

Primary dietary factors in the dietary management of irritable bowel syndrome
Foods rich in carbohydrates, as well as fatty foods, coffee, alcohol, and hot spices, were identified as being the most frequently reported to cause symptoms.[38]

Alcohol The consumption of alcohol may be related to changes in IBS symptomatology. The search on the aforementioned methodology yielded 246 potential papers on alcohol and IBS, with only 3 original articles meriting inclusion. Redding and colleagues found that there was an inconsistent relationship.[39] However, binge drinking (>4 drinks per day) had the strongest association of symptom provocation (diarrhea $P = 0.01$), whereas moderate to light drinking showed little to no IBS symptom induction. Simren and colleagues[40] conducted a case-controlled study on 330 IBS and 80 healthy controls and reported that the alcohol-induced symptoms were most commonly in the form of loose stools in 33% of IBS subjects. Further, Hayes and colleagues,[41] in a case-controlled study of 135 IBS and 111 health controls, reported that more patients with IBS reported alcohol intolerance (14.1 vs 2.7%; $P<0.01$).

Fat Our search methodology yielded 399 potential papers on the role of fat in IBS, with 5 original articles included in the analysis. The role of fat as a potential inducer of IBS

Table 1
Risk of bias assessment for studies on FODMAPs and IBS

Author, Year	Selection Bias	Performance Bias	Detection Bias	Attrition Bias	Reporting Bias	Bias in Design	Interpretation Bias
Bohn et al,[101] 2014	Low risk	High risk	High risk	Low risk	Low risk	High risk	High risk
Bohn et al,[102] 2015	Low risk	High risk	High risk	Low risk	Low risk	High risk	High risk
Eswaran et al,[103] 2016	Unknown	High risk	Low risk	High risk	Low risk	High risk	High risk
Halmos et al,[104] 2014	Low risk	High risk	High risk	Low risk	Low risk	High risk	High risk
McIntosh et al,[105] 2017	Low risk	High risk	High risk	High risk	High risk	High risk	High risk
Laatikainen et al,[106] 2016	High Risk	Low Risk	Unclear	Low Risk	Low Risk	Low Risk	Low Risk
Ong et al,[107] 2010	Low risk	High risk	High risk	Low risk	Low risk	High risk	High risk
Pedersen et al,[108] 2014	Low risk	High risk	High risk	High risk	High risk	High risk	Low risk
Peters et al,[109] 2016	Low risk	High risk	High risk	Low risk	Low risk	High risk	Low risk
Staudacher et al,[110] 2012	Low risk	High risk	High risk	Low risk	High risk	High risk	High risk
Staudacher et al,[111] 2017	Low risk	Low risk	Low risk	Low risk	Low risk	High risk	Low risk

Abbreviations: FODMAPS, fermentable oligo-, di-, mono-saccharides-and polyols; IBS, irritable bowel syndrome.

symptoms has been evaluated in several studies using a variety of means.[40–44] Interestingly, lipid infusion studies have shown impairments in gut motility leading to gas trapping, luminal distention, and bloating.[45] Significantly more patients with IBS than controls reported high-fat–induced symptoms in males (15% vs 4%; $P<0.04$) but not for females (24% vs 9%; $P<0.001$).[43] IBS subjects also reported more symptoms after fat ingestion than controls in case-controlled studies.[40–42] One randomized controlled trial with duodenal lipid infusion of 6.7 g over 2 hours in 15 IBS and 15 controls demonstrated increased intestinal symptoms in IBS subjects, which was caused by lipid infusion.[44]

Caffeine Most patients with IBS that we see in practice will tell you that eliminating caffeine is one of the most reliable means of improving symptomatology. Caffeinated products can increase colon motor activity, stimulate rectosigmoid activity, and produce a laxative effect, even in healthy individuals. This is particularly true for those with IBS-D. We only discovered 25 potential papers on this topic in applying our search methodology, with only 4 original articles meriting inclusion. Saito and colleagues[46] reported that patients with IBS do not drink more coffee and tea than patients without IBS in a population-based case control study. Surprisingly, our systematic evaluation disclosed a limited number of case-controlled studies.[39–41,43] Faresjo and colleagues[43] reported that females drinking coffee and tea reported more IBS symptoms than controls (21% vs 11%; $P = 0.004$). Hayes and colleagues[41] reported a greater number of patients with IBS than controls had a gastrointestinal intolerance to caffeine (11.9% vs 1.8%; $P<0.01$). In a study that included 330 patients with IBS, Simren and colleagues[40] found caffeine intolerance in 13% of tea drinkers and in 39% who consumed coffee. In contrast, Reding and colleagues[39] did not find an association between the light/moderate consumption of caffeine and exacerbation of IBS symptoms.

Spicy foods There are observational studies to support the contention that common spices, such as red chili used in cooking, may alter IBS symptoms. Pathophysiologic mechanisms, such as capsaicin (the active component in red chili), have been shown to hasten gut motility and may even cause a burning sensation in healthy subjects.[47] Capsaicin acts on the transient receptor potential vanilloid type-1, thus causing a sensation of burning and pain. In IBS, increases in the number of transient receptor potential vanilloid type-1 receptors have been found, thereby suggesting susceptibility to the painful effects of ingesting this spice.[48] We identified 140 articles related to this topic, with 5 original articles found to merit extraction. There are a number of studies showing that patients with IBS are more susceptible to spicy foods, in particular, red chili.[35,49,50] Faresjo and colleagues[43] reported that males with IBS were more susceptible than females with this condition or controls.

Chronic ingestion or rectal application of capsaicin may cause long-term desensitization in patients with IBS and occurs after an initial period of intense burning pain by inducing the release, followed by the depletion of substance P, a mediator of pain.[51] The only randomized controlled trial was a study from Thailand that compared the effects of either a spicy meal containing 2 g of chili versus a standard meal accompanied with 2 g of chili capsules versus a standard meal (control). 1patients with IBS reported significant abdominal pain, diarrhea, and rectal burning for up to 2 hours when ingesting the chili in a meal or in capsule form, but not after the standard meal.[52]

Milk and dairy products Lactose is a disaccharide that is enzymatically digested to monosaccharides, glucose, and galactose, by the intestinal brush border enzyme lactase. When it is not digested and absorbed in the small intestine, it is fermented by colonic bacteria to short chain fatty acids, hydrogen, methane, carbon dioxide, and other gases. The delivery of lactose to the intestinal lumen may exert an osmotic effect and result in more luminal water, thereby increasing the liquidity of intestinal contents and transit. Gastrointestinal symptoms that result from lactose malabsorption include abdominal cramping, bloating, flatulence, and diarrhea. Gastrointestinal symptoms after lactose ingestion are seen more frequently in IBS than controls.[53] More than one-third of patients with IBS have symptoms after the ingestion of lactose products.[34] Unfortunately, lactase supplementation does not improve symptoms in patients with IBS who ingest lactose products.[35] Our search methodology yielded 262 potential papers on this topic, and 5 original

Table 2
Studies of milk and dairy intolerance in IBS

Author, Year, Reference	Country	Design	Subjects	LHBT	Intervention	Primary Outcome
Bohmer & Tuynman,[79] 1996	Holland	DB non-RCT	70 IBS	Positive	Low lactose diet (<9 g/d) × 6 wk	Symptoms score return to baseline P<001
Bohmer & Tuynman,[80] 2001	Holland	Non-RCT	16 IBS	Positive	Low lactose diet × 5 y	Symptoms score return to baseline P<001
Bozzani et al,[81] 1986	Italy	Non-RCT	40 IBS	Positive	Low lactose diet (<9 g/d) × 4 mo	Symptoms improved (P>.05)
Parker et al,[82] 2001	UK	Non-RCT	33 IBS	Positive	Low lactose diet (<1 g/d) × 3 wk	No difference in symptoms (P>.05)
Vernia et al,[83] 1995	Italy	Non-RCT	110 IBS	Positive	Lactose-free diet for 3 mo	No difference in symptoms (P>.05)

Abbreviations: DB, double-blind; IBS, irritable bowel syndrome; LHBT, lactose hydrogen breath test; RCT, randomized controlled trial.

articles merited extraction. **Table 2** displays the results of lactose restriction to clinical response in IBS.

Secondary dietary factors in the dietary management of irritable bowel syndrome
Dietary fiber Fiber has a number of properties that can modify IBS symptoms. Fiber sources that are slowly, incompletely, or essentially not fermented in the large intestine provide bulk to the stool and therefore help to regulate bowel movements. These nonfermentable fibers, known as insoluble fibers, include wheat bran, corn bran, and defatted ground flaxseed. Oat bran is a 50/50 mixture of soluble and insoluble fiber. Fibers can modify gut transit, microbiome composition, stool viscosity, and vary regarding the degree of fermentability. The readily fermented fibers, such as β-glucan and inulin, can lead to rapid gas formation, whereas the poorly fermented (ie, wheat bran) and nonfermented fibers (ie, psyllium) often result in less flatulence.[54,55] A number of systematic reviews and metaanalyses have been performed on the role of dietary fiber for IBS.[56–59] However, the role of dietary fiber for IBS remains a matter of debate because there is a dearth of high-quality evidence and an abundance of contradictory trials. A Cochrane metaanalysis by Ruepert and colleagues[59] encompassing 12 included studies and 621 subjects failed to demonstrate any benefit for either soluble or insoluble fiber for IBS and was limited by high heterogeneity. A more recent systematic review by Moayyedi and colleagues[60] of 14 included randomized controlled trials involving 906 patients demonstrated efficacy for soluble fiber (relative risk, 0.83; 95% CI 0.73–0.94 with a number needed to treat of 7; 95% CI, 4–25), whereas there was no effect seen with bran (relative risk, 0.90; 95% CI, 0.79–1.03) and neither was there any provocation of symptoms. Our search resulted in 88 potential randomized clinical trials to review on dietary fiber and IBS, of which 17 original articles were included for the systematic analysis. **Table 3** displays the results of our systematic review of the literature of randomized controlled trials of dietary fiber for the treatment of IBS.

Table 3
Dietary fiber intake and IBS

Author, Year, Reference	Country	Design	Subjects	Intervention Time	Primary Outcome
Aller et al,[84] 2004	Spain	SB RCT	56 IBS	High-fiber vs low-fiber diet 3 mo	Pain and bloating improved both groups (P<.05), no difference
Arffmann et al,[85] 1985	Denmark	DB CO RCT	20 IBS-C or IBS-M	30 g wheat bran vs placebo 30 g colored breadcrumbs 6 wk washout not stated	No difference in abdominal symptoms (P<.05)
Bijkerk et al,[86] 2009	Holland	DB RCT 3 arm	275 IBS	4 g wheat bran vs 4 g psyllium vs placebo white rice	Symptom severity less for psyllium vs placebo (P = .03); no difference for symptoms between wheat bran and placebo
Cockerell et al,[87] 2012	UK	Open-label RCT	40 IBS	Whole linseeds 21 g/d vs ground linseeds 18 g/d vs controls 4 wk	No significant differences in overall symptoms; abdominal pain severity (P = .011) and days of pain (P = .042) improved for whole linseeds
Erdogan et al,[88] 2016	USA	DB RCT	72 IBS	Mixed fiber or psyllium, 5 g bid for 4 wk	Mean complete spontaneous bowel movement/week increased with both mixed fiber (P<.0001) and psyllium (P = .0002) without group difference
Fowlie et al,[89] 1992[a]	UK	Non-RCT	49 IBS-C	4.1 g of cereal and fruit fiber in 5 tablets vs placebo starch in 5 tablets 3 mo	No significant difference for symptoms between groups
Hebden et al,[90] 2002	UK	DB CO RCT	12 IBS	30 g of wheat bran vs placebo: 30 g of plain biscuits for 2 wk	Wheat bran increased pain and bloating compared with placebo (P<.02)
Jalihal & Kurian,[91] 1990	India	DB CO RCT	20 IBS	30 g of ispaghula husk vs placebo (polished white rice powder–roasted refined wheat powder 19:1) 4 wk then 7–10 d washout	Improvement in global symptoms and satisfaction with daily bowel movements (P<.001)

(continued on next page)

Table 3
(continued)

Author, Year, Reference	Country	Design	Subjects	Intervention Time	Primary Outcome
Kruis et al,[92] 1986	Germany	DB RCT	80 IBS	15 g of wheat bran vs placebo 16 wk	No significant difference for symptoms between groups
Longstreth et al,[93] 1981	USA	DB RCT	77 IBS	Ispaghula husk vs placebo 8 wk	Five symptom variables were significantly correlated ($P<.05$) with patient's subjective global assessment (R = 0.64)
Lucey et al,[94] 1987	UK	DB CO RCT	38 IBS	12 g of wheat bran vs placebo: 12 g of plain biscuits 16 wk	No significant difference for symptoms between groups; global symptoms improved for both groups ($P<.01$)
Manning et al,[95] 1977	UK	RCT	26 IBS	High (20 g) or low (not defined) wheat fibre content for 6 wk	High-wheat fiber regimen with significant improvement in symptoms; not with the low-fibre regimen
Prior and Whorell,[96] 1987	UK	DB RCT	80 IBS, 49% IBS-C	Ispaghula husk vs placebo 12 wk	Global assessment improved in 82% with ispaghula and 53% of the placebo group ($P<.02$)
Rees et al,[97] 2005	UK	SB RCT	28 IBS-C or IBS-M	10–20 g of wheat bran vs placebo: low-fiber crispbread 12 wk	No significant difference for symptoms between groups
Snook & Shepherd,[98] 1994	UK	DB CO RCT	80 IBS	40 g of wheat bran vs placebo: wheat and rice flour with 2-wk washout	No significant difference for symptoms between groups
Soltoft et al,[99] 1976	Denmark	RCT	59 IBS	Miller's bran biscuits vs wheat biscuits for 6 wk	No significant difference for symptoms between groups
Tarpila et al,[100] 2004	Finland	SB RCT	55 IBS-C	Ground linseeds ($\leq$24 g, 10.6 g) vs psyllium ($\leq$24 g, 13.5 g) 3 mo	In the flaxseed group, constipation and abdominal symptoms were decreased significantly ($P = .002$), whereas in the psyllium group the reduction was not statistically significant

Abbreviations: bid, twice a day; DB CO RCT, double-blind, cross-over randomized controlled trial; IBS, irritable bowel syndrome; IBS-C, constipation-predominant irritable bowel syndrome; IBS-M, irritable bowel syndrome-mixed; ND, no difference; SB RCT, single-blind randomized controlled trial.
[a] P value not reported: Fowlie et al.

Table 4
Foods with proven high FODMAPs content

Fruit: and Fruit Products	Vegetables and Vegetable Products	Milk Products	Grain and Starch-Based Foods	Legumes, Nuts and Seeds	Others
Apple	Artichoke globe	Cow's milk	Barley-, kamut, rye-, and wheat-based bread, crackers pasta, cereal, couscous, gnocchi, noodles, croissants, muffins, and crumpets	Cashews	Agave
Apricots	Artichoke, Jerusalem	Custard		Chickpeas	Fructose
Asian pears	Artichokes	Dairy desserts		Legumes (ie, red kidney beans, soy beans, Borlotti beans)	Fructo-oligosaccharides
Blackberries	Asparagus	Evaporated milk			Fruit juice concentrates
Boysenberry	Cauliflower	Goat's milk		Lentils	High-fructose corn syrup
Cherries	Garlic	Ice cream		Pistachios	Honey
Clingstone peach	Leek	Milk powder			Inulin
Custard apples	Mushroom	Sheep's milk			Isomalt[a]
Mango	Onion	Sweetened condensed milk			Malitol[a]
Nashi fruit	Shallot				Polydextrose[a]
Nectarines	Snow peas				Sorbitol[a]
Peaches	Spring onion (white part only)				
Pears	Sugar snap peas				
Plums					
Prunes					
Persimmon					
Tamarillo					
Watermelon					
White peaches					

Abbreviation: FODMAPs, fermentable oligo-, di-, and monosaccharides and polyols.
[a] Used as sweeteners in "diet" or "sugar-free" or "low-carbohydrate" desserts.
Data from Gibson PR, Shepherd SJ. Personal view: food for thought–western lifestyle and susceptibility to Crohn's disease. The FODMAP hypothesis. Aliment Pharmacol Ther 2005;21(12):1399–409.

Table 5
Foods with low and low or moderate FODMAPs content

Fruit and Fruit Products	Vegetables and Vegetable Products	Milk Products	Grain and Starch-Based Foods	Legumes, Nuts and Seeds	Others
Avocado[a]	Alfalfa	Ripened cheeses, for example, blue vein, brie, cheddar, Colby, Edam, feta, Gouda, mozzarella, parmesan, and Swiss	Buckwheat	Almonds[a]	Chewing gum, candy, mint sweetened with sucrose
Banana (unripened)	Bamboo Shoots		Corn	Chia seeds	Ginger spices
Blueberry	Bean sprouts		Gluten-free bread, cracker,[a] and cereal products	Hazelnuts[a]	Garlic-infused olive oil
Cantaloupe	Beans (green)	Butter	Linseed (flaxseed), poppy seeds, pumpkin seeds (pepita), sesame seeds, sunflower seeds, tahini[a]	Herbs
Carambola	Beetroot[a]	Cream	Millet		Maple syrup,
Cherries[a]	Bok Choy	Margarine	Oats		Sugar (sucrose), glucose,
Dragon fruit	Broccoli[a]	Oat milk	Oat bran		Stevia, any other artificial
Dried fruit[a]	Brussels sprouts[a]	Rice milk	Polenta		sweeteners not ending in
Durian	Butternut pumpkin[a]	Lactose-free ice cream	Quinoa		"-ol"
Grapefruit	Cabbage (savoy)[a]	Lactose-free yogurt	Rice		(eg, aspartame)
Grapes	Capsicum	Fromage frais[a]	Sweet biscuit[a]		Regular milk or milk powder as
Honeydew melon	Carrot	Yogurt[a] (cow, sheep, goat)	All grain- and flour-based products must be labeled gluten free		an ingredient in milk chocolate[a]
Kiwifruit	Celery[a]	Soft cheeses,[a] for example, cottage, ricotta, cream cheese, mascarpone, crème fraiche			
Lemon	Chives				
Lime	Choy sum				
Longon[a]	Cucumber				
Lychee[a]	Eggplant				
Mandarin	Endive				
Orange	Fennel bulb[a]				
Passionfruit	Green peas[a]				
Pawpaw	Lettuce				
Pineapple	Olives				
Pomegranate[a]	Parsnip				
Prickly pear	Potato				

Rambutan[a]	Pumpkin (Japanese)
Raspberry	Radish
Rhubarb	Rocket
Strawberry	Silverbeet
Tangelo	Spinach
	Spring onion (green part only)
	Squash
	Swede
	Sweet corn[a]
	Sweet potato[a]
	Tomato
	Turnip
	Zucchini

Abbreviation: FODMAPs, fermentable oligo-, di-, and monosaccharaides and polyols.

[a] Contain moderate amounts of FODMAPs per serving; a small intake is suitable on low FODMAP diet.

Data from Gibson PR, Shepherd SJ. Personal view: food for thought–western lifestyle and susceptibility to Crohn's disease. The FODMAP hypothesis. Aliment Pharmacol Ther 2005;21(12):1399–409.

Fermentable carbohydrates (fructosaccharides, oligosaccharides, disaccharides, and monosaccharides and polyols) FODMAPs are a group of short chain carbohydrates that share 3 common features: (1) they are poorly absorbed in the small intestine, (2) they are rapidly fermented by colonic bacteria, and (3) owing to their high osmotic activity, increase water delivery into the bowel.[61] A high FODMAP food is determined if the food exceeds any of the following amounts per serving for any FODMAP: less than 4 g of lactose, less than 0.3 g of mannitol, less than 0.3 g of sorbitol, less than 0.3 g of galacto-oligosaccharides, less than of 0.3 g fructans if cereal-based product (otherwise, <0.2 g of fructans for non–cereal-based products), and 0.2 g of excess fructose (ie, fructose in excess of glucose).[62] Implementation of the low FODMAP diet involves 2 phases.[61] The first phase or induction phase is the stringent restriction of all high-FODMAP foods to obtain symptom relief (**Table 4**). Patients are encouraged to consume foods that are low in FODMAPs (**Table 5**). The first phase is usually undertaken for 6 to 8 weeks. Then, in phase 2, which is the rechallenge phase, patients are encouraged to rechallenge FODMAPs by reintroducing foods that contain 1 type of FODMAP at a time over a period of 2 to 3 days, to determine individual tolerance of the type and amount of each FODMAP. This process individualizes the diet for the patient, encouraging a long-term maximum variety in the diet (avoiding unnecessary overrestriction), while still maintaining the symptom management achieved in the first phase. Details regarding the classification, mechanisms of action, and mode of absorption of FODMAPs are shown in **Fig. 4**. Our search methodology yielded 310 potential papers on this topic. Eleven original articles were included for analysis after review by the team (**Fig. 5**). The results of the dietary studies using FODMAPs restriction to treat IBS are shown in **Table 6**.[63]

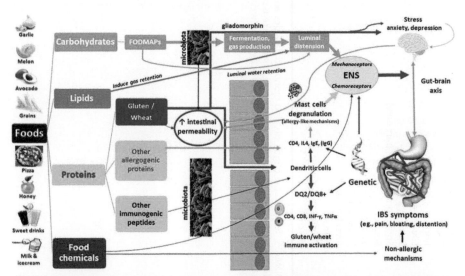

Fig. 4. Mechanisms of action of fructo, oligo-, di-, and monosaccharides and polyols (FODMAPS) in triggering irritable bowel syndrome (IBS) symptoms. ENS, enteric nervous system; IgE, immunoglobulin E; IgG, immunoglobulin G; IL4, interleukin-4; INF-γ, interferon-γ; TNF-α, tumor necrosis factor -α. (*Reproduced from* BMJ; with permission; and *From* De Giorgio R, Volta U, Gibson PR. Sensitivity to wheat, gluten and FODMAPS in IBS: facts or fiction? Gut 2016;65:169–78; with permission.)

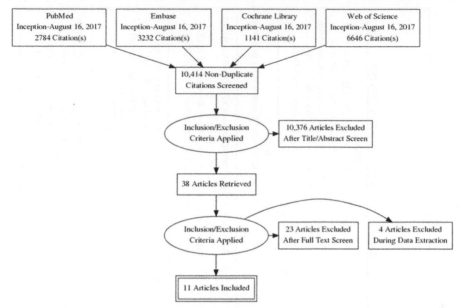

Fig. 5. Flow chart of studies on low fructo, oligo-, di-, and monosaccharides and polyols (FODMAPs) diet and irritable bowel syndrome (IBS).

Gluten One of the most controversial areas of dietetics is the potential contribution of wheat, because it is a gluten-containing grain and is among the top 8 food allergens owing to its high fructan content and because it is a part of the family of highly fermentable carbohydrates (FODMAPs). Wheat and related grain species, including barley and rye, are also a source of gluten, which induces an abnormal mucosal immune response in predisposed individuals. This susceptibility can range from mild gluten sensitivity (nonceliac gluten sensitivity) to autoimmunity, as seen in individuals with celiac disease. There are conflicting data in the literature about the relationship of celiac disease to IBS, with 2 metaanalyses by the same investigators showing an association.[64,65] However, a multicenter study comparing 492 patients with symptomatic nonconstipated patients with IBS with healthy individuals undergoing screening colonoscopy did not find a difference in the prevalence of celiac disease.[37] Interventional studies on gluten withdrawal suggest that there is a population of patients with IBS who may benefit from the gluten-free diet and that markers may help to predict responders. Our search methodology yielded 664 papers on the topic of gluten, wheat, or rye withdrawal for IBS, with 5 articles meriting extraction (**Table 7**).

Food allergies and food sensitivities Food sensitivities have been long postulated to play a provocative role in IBS.[34] The most common bonafide allergens known to provoke IBS are dairy products (40%–44%) and grains (40%–60%).[66] A number of elimination diet trials have shown benefits[67–75]; however, the most controversial is that of immunoglobulin (Ig)G4 antibody-based exclusion. Eliminating foods based on IgG4 antibody testing has shown to improve IBS symptoms and quality of life in a number of studies.[67–69,73,75] However, there are many criticisms of using IgG4 testing, which include a lack of validity, out-of-pocket expense, and limited availability.[76] The application of IgG4 testing leads to the restriction of multiple food

Table 6
Studies of randomized trials of low FODMAPs dietary intervention in IBS

First Author, Year, Reference	Country	Design	Sample Size	Intervention/Time	Definition of Response/Primary Outcome
Bohn et al,[101] 2014	Sweden	Parallel, Multicenter	82	LFD vs THD 4 wk No follow-up	>50% reduction in IBS-SSS. LFD reduced the IBS-SSS from 337 (287–382) (median, 231; 25th-75th percentile, 154–350; P = .001). THD reduced the symptom score from 312 (25th-75th percentile, 250–346) to 240 (25th-75th percentile, 171–296) (P<.001). No difference in reduction.
Bohn et al,[102] 2015	Sweden	Parallel, single center	75	LFD vs NICE diet guidelines 4 wk No follow-up	>50% reduction in IBS-SSS. Change in IBS-SSS LFD vs NICE was similar between groups (P = .62).
Eswaran et al,[103] 2016	USA	Parallel, single center	92	LFD vs NICE diet guidelines 4 wk No follow-up	Adequate relief of symptoms. >50% of last 2 wk of study. Fifty-two percent of the LFD vs 41% of the NICE group reported adequate relief of their IBS-D symptoms (P = .31).
Halmos et al,[104] 2014	Australia	Cross-over with washout ≥21 d, single center	30	LFD vs typical Australian diet 3 wk of each diet with ≥3-wk washout	10-mm difference on 100-mm VAS considered clinically significant. LFD had significant improvements in global symptoms, compared with control diet for IBS (all P<.001).
McIntosh et al,[105] 2017	UK	Parallel Single center	40	LFD vs HFD 3 wk No follow-up	Symptoms were assessed using the IBS-SSS. The IBS-SSS was reduced in the low FODMAP diet group (P<.001) but not the high FODMAP group.
Laatikainen et al,[106] 2016	UK	Cross-over design, single center 4 wk	87	LF rye bread vs HF rye bread	IBS-SSS and VAS were used to assess individual symptoms. Abdominal pain, wind, bloating improved on LF rye (P<.05) but IBS-SSS no different vs HF rye.

Study	Country	Design	N	Intervention	Results
Ong et al,[107] 2010	Australia	Cross-over with washout 7 d, single center	15	LFD vs HFD 2 d No follow-up	Composite scale of gastrointestinal symptoms based on a 3-point Likert scale. HFD has higher scale of symptoms (wind, abdominal pain, bloating; median, 6; range, 1–9) vs LFD (median, 2; range, 0–7; $P = .002$).
Pedersen et al,[108] 2014	Denmark	Parallel, single center	123 Web-based app	Dietary advice or probiotics: Intervention = LFD Control = probiotic (LGG)[a] or normal Danish Diet 6 wk No follow-up	>50% reduction in IBS-SSS. Reduction of IBS-SSS for LFD vs control at 6 wk (75; 95% CI, 24–126; $P<.01$) but not for LGG vs control (32; 95% CI, 18–80; $P = .2$).
Peters et al,[109] 2016	UK	Parallel, single center	74	Gut-directed hypnotherapy, LFD vs both 6 wk therapy 6 mo follow-up	>20-mm improvement on 100-mm VAS for GI symptoms. Improvements in overall symptoms were observed from baseline to week 6 for hypnotherapy (mean difference, −33 [95% CI, −41 to −25]; diet: mean difference, −30 [95% CI, −42 to −19]; combination: mean difference, −36 [95% CI, −45 to −27]. There were no differences across groups ($P = .67$).
Staudacher et al,[110] 2012	UK	Parallel, single center	41	LFD vs Australian habitual diet 4 wk No follow-up	Global symptoms rating scale not defined. Low FODMAP diet has significant improvements in global symptoms ($P = .006$).
Staudacher et al,[111] 2017	UK	Cross-over 2 × 2 factorial design, 2 centers	104	LFD or sham diet (placebo) vs probiotic VSL#3 or placebo. 4 wk Follow-up period unclear	Mean IBS-SSS scores were lower for patients on the LFD (173 ± 95) than sham (224 ± 89; $P = .001$). LFD had a trend toward adequate symptom relief (57%) vs the sham diet group (38%; $P = .051$).

Abbreviations: CI, confidence interval; FODMAP, fermentable oligosaccharides, disaccharides, monosaccharides and polyols; GI, gastrointestinal; HF, high FOD-MAP; IBS, irritable bowel syndrome; IBS-D, diarrhoea-predominant irritable bowel syndrome; IBS-SSS, IBS-Symptom Severity Score; LF, low FODMAP; LFD, low FOD-MAPs diet; LGG, *Lactobacillus rhamnosus* GG; NICE, National Institute for Health and Care Excellence; THD, traditional habitual diet; VAS, visual analog scale.

[a] *L rhamnosus* GG (1.2 9 10^{10} CFU in 2 capsules day^{-1}).

Table 7
Studies of wheat and gluten intolerance in IBS

Author, Year, Reference	Country	Design	Subjects	Intervention	Primary Outcome
Biesiekierski et al,[112] 2011	Australia	DB RCT	39 IBS with NCGS	2 slices bread, muffin daily either gluten free or 16 g/d of gluten plus GFD × 6 wk.	1 wk: VAS, overall symptoms, pain, bloating, tiredness, stool consistency dissatisfaction worse with gluten (P<.05) 6 wk: worse for tiredness, pain, and stool consistency (P<.05) dissatisfaction.
Biesiekierski et al,[113] 2013	Australia	DB RCT 3 arms, rechallenge; run-in: 2-wk GFD and low FODMAP	40 IBS with diagnosed NCGS	Feeding study. High gluten 16 g/d, low gluten 2 g/d + 14 g whey for 1 wk then 2 wk washout Rechallenge: gluten (16 g/d), whey 16 g/d or control (no additional protein) for 3 d	Overall symptom improvement for run-in (P = .001), symptom deterioration for intervention in all groups (P = .001). No change in symptoms for rechallenge vs baseline.
Carroccio et al,[114] 2012	Italy	DB PCT challenge: rechallenge study.	920 Rome II patients with IBS	Elimination diet followed by wheat challenge; subjects with positive provocation responses undergo cow's milk protein challenge	276 with wheat and cow's milk sensitivity, of these, 70 with wheat sensitivity alone; these patients had a higher prevalence of anemia, coexistent atopy, eosinophils in duodenal biopsies and basophil activation vs controls
Shahbazkhani et al,[115] 2015	Iran	DB RCT	148 patients with IBS Rome III criteria	All on a GFD for 6 wk then ingested powders gluten vs placebo	Overall symptoms worse in gluten group (74.3%) vs placebo (16.2%) (P<.001)
Wahnschaffe et al,[116] 2007	Germany	Nonrandomized evaluation of 6 mo of GFD	41 IBS-D Stratified according to CDAA and HLA-DQ2 status.	41 subjects on GFD then assessed for global IBS symptoms	IBS-D subjects with IgG-CDAA and HLA-DQ2 expression responded to GFD (P<.05) vs nonexpression
Vasquez-Rogue et al,[117] 2012	USA	DB RCT	45 IBS-D	Feeding Study. GCD vs GFD	GCD showed improved mean stool frequency (not form) compared with GFD (P = .04), and was greater in HLA-DQ2 or HLA-DQ-8 positive patients

Abbreviations: CDAA, celiac disease-associated antibodies; DB, double-blind; FODMAPs, fermentable oligo-, di-, monosaccharides and polyols; GCD, gluten containing diet; GFD, gluten free diet; IBS, irritable bowel syndrome; IBS-D, diarrhea-predominant irritable bowel syndrome; IgG, immunoglobulin G; NCGS, nonceliac gluten sensitivity; PCT, Placebo control trial; RCT, randomized controlled trial; VAS, visual analog scale.

groups that matches a generalized elimination dietary program.[76] Ligaarden and colleagues[77] conducted a large trial on IgG antibodies in IBS and the general population, which included 269 subjects with IBS and 277 control subjects. After correction for subject characteristics and diet, there were no differences with regard to food- and yeast-specific IgG and IgG4 antibodies between subjects with IBS and controls. Finally, allergy and immunology societies have recommended against the use of IgG4 testing as a diagnostic tool for food reactions.[78] Our search methodology yielded 239 potential papers on this topic, and 6 original articles merited extraction. **Table 8** provides the current evidence for IgG4-based food testing for the IBS.

Table 8
Results of studies of IgG4 antibodies elimination diets for IBS

Author, Year, Reference	Number of Subjects	Trial	Results
Atkinson et al,[73] 2004	150 IBS	TD vs sham diet 3 mo	TD lead to a 10% greater reduction in symptom score than sham diet ($P = .024$). The value increased to 26% in fully compliant patients ($P<.001$).
Drisko et al,[68] 2006	15 IBS Refractory to medical therapy	Elimination-rotational diet 6 mo	100% of the study subjects having serum IgG antibodies to food(s) and mold ($P<.005$). Stool frequency ($P<.05$), pain ($P<.05$), and IBS-QOL scores ($P<.0001$) improved with the elimination diet.
Guo et al,[118] 2012	77 IBS-D, 26 controls	Elimination diet based on specific IgG antibodies vs 14 common food antigens 12 wk	When compared with baseline, IBS-D patients experienced improved abdominal pain, stool form and frequency, distension, general feelings of distress and total symptom score. P values not provided.
Tan et al,[119] 2013	117 IBS 50 controls	Elimination diet based on specific IgG antibodies vs 14 common food antigens 12 wk	Food elimination diets could significantly improve disease severity score in patients with IBD-D or IBS-C, but had no influence in those with mixed type or nontyped disease.
Yang & Li,[67] 2007	55 IBS-D 32 IBS-C 18 controls	IgG-specific 8 wk elimination diet	IgG antibodies vs food(s) were 63.5% in patients with IBS-D and 43.8% in IBS-C. Elimination diet Improved IBS symptom relief. The P values were not specified.

Abbreviations: IBS, irritable bowel syndrome; IBS-C, constipation-predominant IBS, irritable bowel syndrome; IBS-D, diarrhea-predominant irritable bowel syndrome; IBS-QOL, Irritable Bowel Syndrome Quality of Life score; IgG, immunoglobulin G; TD, true diet.

SUMMARY

IBS is an enigmatic disorder that involves a number of pathophysiologic mechanisms that produce chronic gastrointestinal symptoms from a complex interplay of mediators, neural circuits, gut microbes, immune cells, and dietary triggers. There is increasing interest and evidence in support of nutrition as an emerging line of therapy that is often overlooked by many health care providers. The clinician should become aware of the influence of diet on the course of illness. A careful dietary history to

Table 9
Evidence for use of therapeutic diets in IBS

Therapy	Description	Level of Evidence	Quality of Evidence Strength of Recommendation
Targeted elimination diets	Remove suspected food groups then gradual reintroduction 1 food group at a time to confirm provocative foods to avoid. Suspect foods not limited to but include alcohol, caffeinated products, spicy foods, dairy, wheat, gluten, known food allergens, suspected food allergens.	IIB	3, moderate
Elimination diets based on IgG4 serum testing	Remove foods showing IgG4 antibody reactivity.	IIB	2, low
Generalized elimination diets	Remove top 8 allergenic food groups then reintroduce one at a time.	IV	1, low
FODMAPs elimination diet	Remove FODMAPs	IA	4, high
Fiber	Ispaghula	IA	3, moderate
Fiber	Wheat bran	IA	2, low

The Grading of Recommendations Assessment, Development and Evaluation (GRADE) analysis was used to assess the quality of evidence by 2 independent reviewers (GM, RS): very low = 1, low = 2, moderate = 3, high = 4.[120,121] A third reviewer was recruited (AS) to resolve disagreements about GRADE assessment and the strength of recommendations (high vs moderate vs low). We used the evidence-based Health Care Practice guidelines, as well as levels of evidence and grades of recommendations used by the National Guideline Clearinghouse.[122,123]

"IA, Evidence from meta-analysis of randomized controlled trials; IB evidence from at least one randomized controlled trial; IIA, evidence from at least one controlled study without randomization; IIB, Evidence from at least one other type of quasi-experimental study; III, Evidence from non-experimental descriptive studies, such as comparative studies, correlation studies, and case-control studies; IV, evidence from expert committee reports or opinions or clinical experience of respected authorities, or both."[122]

Quality of evidence was determined using GRADE methods based on the study design, in addition to study quality, consistency, and directness. Randomized trials provide high levels of initial quality. Adjustors that decrease quality include risk of bias, inconsistency, indirectness, imprecision, and publication bias, among others. Observational studies and expert consensus provide low levels of evidence. Quality adjustors help to increase quality, as well as large effect size, dose response, adjustment for all plausible residual confounders.[121]

Abbreviations: FODMAPS, fermentable oligo-, di-, mono-saccharides-and polyols; IBS, irritable bowel syndrome; IgG, immunoglobulin G.

discern whether food intolerances are provoking symptoms should be performed on every patient with IBS. The consumption of highly fermentable foods, such as the FODMAPs, food allergies, sensitivities, and intolerances, should be considered in every patient with this IBS who experiences a provocation of symptoms owing to the ingestion of certain foods. Thus, the strategic elimination of food items eliciting symptomatology along with lifestyle changes, such as stress management, should be considered for integration into the IBS management plan. Soluble viscous fibers can improve bowel regularity and seem to improve IBS symptoms. Future studies on the influence of food and food-based nutrients on IBS are warranted. Evidence for the use of therapeutic diets for the treatment of IBS is shown in **Table 9**.

REFERENCES

1. Eswaran S, Tack J, Chey WD. Food: the forgotten factor in the irritable bowel syndrome. Gastroenterol Clin North Am 2011;40(1):141–62.
2. Fond G, Loundou A, Hamdani N, et al. Anxiety and depression comorbidities in irritable bowel syndrome (IBS): a systematic review and meta-analysis. Eur Arch Psychiatry Clin Neurosci 2014;264(8):651–60.
3. Hausteiner-Wiehle C, Henningsen P. Irritable bowel syndrome: relations with functional, mental, and somatoform disorders. World J Gastroenterol 2014; 20(20):6024–30.
4. Schmulson MJ, Drossman DA. What Is New in Rome IV. J Neurogastroenterol Motil 2017;23(2):151–63.
5. Palsson OS, Whitehead WE, van Tilburg MA, et al. Rome IV Diagnostic Questionnaires and Tables for Investigators and Clinicians. Gastroenterology 2016; 150(6):1481–91.
6. Lovell RM, Ford AC. Global prevalence of and risk factors for irritable bowel syndrome: a meta-analysis. Clin Gastroenterol Hepatol 2012;10(7):712–21.e4.
7. Enck P, Aziz Q, Barbara G, et al. Irritable bowel syndrome. Nat Rev Dis Primers 2016;2:16014.
8. Choung RS, Locke GR 3rd. Epidemiology of IBS. Gastroenterol Clin North Am 2011;40(1):1–10.
9. Maxion-Bergemann S, Thielecke F, Abel F, et al. Costs of irritable bowel syndrome in the UK and US. Pharmacoeconomics 2006;24(1):21–37.
10. Monnikes H. Quality of life in patients with irritable bowel syndrome. J Clin Gastroenterol 2011;45(Suppl):S98–101.
11. Canavan C, West J, Card T. Review article: the economic impact of the irritable bowel syndrome. Aliment Pharmacol Ther 2014;40(9):1023–34.
12. Feng B, La JH, Schwartz ES, et al. Irritable bowel syndrome: methods, mechanisms, and pathophysiology. Neural and neuro-immune mechanisms of visceral hypersensitivity in irritable bowel syndrome. Am J Physiol Gastrointest Liver Physiol 2012;302(10):G1085–98.
13. Camilleri M, Lasch K, Zhou W. Irritable bowel syndrome: methods, mechanisms, and pathophysiology. The confluence of increased permeability, inflammation, and pain in irritable bowel syndrome. Am J Physiol Gastrointest Liver Physiol 2012;303(7):G775–85.
14. Zhou Q, Verne GN. New insights into visceral hypersensitivity–clinical implications in IBS. Nat Rev Gastroenterol Hepatol 2011;8(6):349–55.
15. O'Malley D, Quigley EM, Dinan TG, et al. Do interactions between stress and immune responses lead to symptom exacerbations in irritable bowel syndrome? Brain Behav Immun 2011;25(7):1333–41.

16. Hasler WL. Traditional thoughts on the pathophysiology of irritable bowel syndrome. Gastroenterol Clin North Am 2011;40(1):21–43.
17. Surdea-Blaga T, Baban A, Dumitrascu DL. Psychosocial determinants of irritable bowel syndrome. World J Gastroenterol 2012;18(7):616–26.
18. Prusator DK, Andrews A, Greenwood-Van Meerveld B. Neurobiology of early life stress and visceral pain: translational relevance from animal models to patient care. Neurogastroenterol Motil 2016;28(9):1290–305.
19. Drossman DA, Chang L, Bellamy N, et al. Severity in irritable bowel syndrome: a Rome Foundation Working Team report. Am J Gastroenterol 2011;106(10): 1749–59 [quiz: 60].
20. Makker J, Chilimuri S, Bella JN. Genetic epidemiology of irritable bowel syndrome. World J Gastroenterol 2015;21(40):11353–61.
21. Sasaki A, Sato N, Suzuki N, et al. Associations between Single-Nucleotide Polymorphisms in Corticotropin-Releasing Hormone-Related Genes and Irritable Bowel Syndrome. PLoS One 2016;11(2):e0149322.
22. Camilleri M, Katzka DA. Irritable bowel syndrome: methods, mechanisms, and pathophysiology. Genetic epidemiology and pharmacogenetics in irritable bowel syndrome. Am J Physiol Gastrointest Liver Physiol 2012;302(10): G1075–84.
23. Vaiopoulou A, Karamanolis G, Psaltopoulou T, et al. Molecular basis of the irritable bowel syndrome. World J Gastroenterol 2014;20(2):376–83.
24. Gazouli M, Wouters MM, Kapur-Pojskic L, et al. Lessons learned: resolving the enigma of genetic factors in irritable bowel syndrome. Nat Rev Gastroenterol Hepatol 2015;13:77–87.
25. Shah ED, Basseri RJ, Chong K, et al. Abnormal breath testing in IBS: a meta-analysis. Dig Dis Sci 2010;55(9):2441–9.
26. Lee HR, Pimentel M. Bacteria and irritable bowel syndrome: the evidence for small intestinal bacterial overgrowth. Curr Gastroenterol Rep 2006;8(4):305–11.
27. Chedid V, Dhalla S, Clarke JO, et al. Herbal therapy is equivalent to rifaximin for the treatment of small intestinal bacterial overgrowth. Glob Adv Health Med 2014;3(3):16–24.
28. Serghini M, Karoui S, Boubaker J, et al. Post-infectious irritable bowel syndrome. Tunis Med 2012;90(3):205–13 [in French].
29. Klem F, Wadhwa A, Prokop LJ, et al. Prevalence, risk factors, and outcomes of irritable bowel syndrome after infectious enteritis: a systematic review and meta-analysis. Gastroenterology 2017;152(5):1042–54.e1.
30. Barbara G, Cremon C, Pallotti F, et al. Postinfectious irritable bowel syndrome. J Pediatr Gastroenterol Nutr 2009;48(Suppl 2):S95–7.
31. Barbara G, Cremon C, Carini G, et al. The immune system in irritable bowel syndrome. J Neurogastroenterol Motil 2011;17(4):349–59.
32. Ford AC, Talley NJ. Mucosal inflammation as a potential etiological factor in irritable bowel syndrome: a systematic review. J Gastroenterol 2011;46(4):421–31.
33. Jones VA, McLaughlan P, Shorthouse M, et al. Food intolerance: a major factor in the pathogenesis of irritable bowel syndrome. Lancet 1982;2(8308):1115–7.
34. Mullin GE. Food allergy and irritable bowel syndrome. JAMA 1991;265(13): 1736.
35. Bohn L, Storsrud S, Tornblom H, et al. Self-reported food-related gastrointestinal symptoms in IBS are common and associated with more severe symptoms and reduced quality of life. Am J Gastroenterol 2013;108(5):634–41.
36. Hutton B, Salanti G, Caldwell DM, et al. The PRISMA extension statement for reporting of systematic reviews incorporating network meta-analyses of health

care interventions: checklist and explanations. Ann Intern Med 2015;162(11): 777–84.

37. Higgins JP, Altman DG, Gotzsche PC, et al. The Cochrane Collaboration's tool for assessing risk of bias in randomised trials. BMJ 2011;343:d5928.

38. Shepherd SJ, Parker FC, Muir JG, et al. Dietary triggers of abdominal symptoms in patients with irritable bowel syndrome: randomized placebo-controlled evidence. Clin Gastroenterol Hepatol 2008;6(7):765–71.

39. Reding KW, Cain KC, Jarrett ME, et al. Relationship between patterns of alcohol consumption and gastrointestinal symptoms among patients with irritable bowel syndrome. Am J Gastroenterol 2013;108(2):270–6.

40. Simren M, Mansson A, Langkilde AM, et al. Food-related gastrointestinal symptoms in the Irritable bowel syndrome. Digestion 2001;63(2):108–15.

41. Hayes P, Corish C, O'Mahony E, et al. A dietary survey of patients with irritable bowel syndrome. J Hum Nutr Diet 2014;27(Suppl 2):36–47.

42. Simren M, Agerforz P, Bjornsson ES, et al. Nutrient-dependent enhancement of rectal sensitivity in irritable bowel syndrome (IBS). Neurogastroenterol Motil 2007;19(1):20–9.

43. Faresjo A, Johansson S, Faresjo T, et al. Sex differences in dietary coping with gastrointestinal symptoms. Eur J Gastroenterol Hepatol 2010;22(3):327–33.

44. Serra J, Salvioli B, Azpiroz F, et al. Lipid-induced intestinal gas retention in irritable bowel syndrome. Gastroenterology 2002;123(3):700–6.

45. Caldarella MP, Milano A, Laterza F, et al. Visceral sensitivity and symptoms in patients with constipation- or diarrhea-predominant irritable bowel syndrome (IBS): effect of a low-fat intraduodenal infusion. Am J Gastroenterol 2005; 100(2):383–9.

46. Saito YA, Locke GR 3rd, Weaver AL, et al. Diet and functional gastrointestinal disorders: a population-based case-control study. Am J Gastroenterol 2005; 100(12):2743–8.

47. Gonlachanvit S, Fongkam P, Wittayalertpanya S, et al. Red chili induces rectal hypersensitivity in healthy humans: possible role of 5HT-3 receptors on capsaicin-sensitive visceral nociceptive pathways. Aliment Pharmacol Ther 2007;26(4):617–25.

48. Wouters MM, Balemans D, Van Wanrooy S, et al. Histamine receptor H1-mediated sensitization of TRPV1 mediates visceral hypersensitivity and symptoms in patients with irritable bowel syndrome. Gastroenterology 2016;150(4): 875–87.e9.

49. Agarwal MK, Bhatia SJ, Desai SA, et al. Effect of red chillies on small bowel and colonic transit and rectal sensitivity in men with irritable bowel syndrome. Indian J Gastroenterol 2002;21(5):179–82.

50. Bortolotti M, Porta S. Effect of red pepper on symptoms of irritable bowel syndrome: preliminary study. Dig Dis Sci 2011;56(11):3288–95.

51. Aniwan S, Gonlachanvit S. Effects of chili treatment on gastrointestinal and rectal sensation in diarrhea-predominant irritable bowel syndrome: a randomized, double-blinded, crossover study. J Neurogastroenterol Motil 2014;20(3): 400–6.

52. Gonlachanvit S, Mahayosnond A, Kullavanijaya P. Effects of chili on postprandial gastrointestinal symptoms in diarrhoea predominant irritable bowel syndrome: evidence for capsaicin-sensitive visceral nociception hypersensitivity. Neurogastroenterol Motil 2009;21(1):23–32.

53. Vesa TH, Seppo LM, Marteau PR, et al. Role of irritable bowel syndrome in subjective lactose intolerance. Am J Clin Nutr 1998;67(4):710–5.

54. McRorie JW Jr. Evidence-based approach to fiber supplements and clinically meaningful health benefits, part 2: what to look for and how to recommend an effective fiber therapy. Nutr Today 2015;50(2):90–7.

55. McRorie JW Jr. Evidence-based approach to fiber supplements and clinically meaningful health benefits, part 1: what to look for and how to recommend an effective fiber therapy. Nutr Today 2015;50(2):82–9.

56. Nagarajan N, Morden A, Bischof D, et al. The role of fiber supplementation in the treatment of irritable bowel syndrome: a systematic review and meta-analysis. Eur J Gastroenterol Hepatol 2015;27(9):1002–10.

57. Rao SS, Yu S, Fedewa A. Systematic review: dietary fibre and FODMAP-restricted diet in the management of constipation and irritable bowel syndrome. Aliment Pharmacol Ther 2015;41(12):1256–70.

58. Ford AC, Talley NJ, Spiegel BM, et al. Effect of fibre, antispasmodics, and peppermint oil in the treatment of irritable bowel syndrome: systematic review and meta-analysis. BMJ 2008;337:a2313.

59. Ruepert L, Quartero AO, de Wit NJ, et al. Bulking agents, antispasmodics and antidepressants for the treatment of irritable bowel syndrome. Cochrane Database Syst Rev 2011;(8):CD003460.

60. Moayyedi P, Quigley EM, Lacy BE, et al. The effect of fiber supplementation on irritable bowel syndrome: a systematic review and meta-analysis. Am J Gastroenterol 2014;109(9):1367–74.

61. Shepherd SJ, Lomer MC, Gibson PR. Short-chain carbohydrates and functional gastrointestinal disorders. Am J Gastroenterol 2013;108(5):707–17.

62. Gibson PR, Shepherd SJ. Personal view: food for thought–western lifestyle and susceptibility to Crohn's disease. The FODMAP hypothesis. Aliment Pharmacol Ther 2005;21(12):1399–409.

63. Barrett JS, Gibson PR. Fermentable oligosaccharides, disaccharides, monosaccharides and polyols (FODMAPs) and nonallergic food intolerance: FODMAPs or food chemicals? Therap Adv Gastroenterol 2012;5(4):261–8.

64. Ford AC, Chey WD, Talley NJ, et al. Yield of diagnostic tests for celiac disease in individuals with symptoms suggestive of irritable bowel syndrome: systematic review and meta-analysis. Arch Intern Med 2009;169(7):651–8.

65. Sainsbury A, Sanders DS, Ford AC. Prevalence of irritable bowel syndrome-type symptoms in patients with celiac disease: a meta-analysis. Clin Gastroenterol Hepatol 2013;11(4):359–65.e1.

66. Simonato B, De Lazzari F, Pasini G, et al. IgE binding to soluble and insoluble wheat flour proteins in atopic and non-atopic patients suffering from gastrointestinal symptoms after wheat ingestion. Clin Exp Allergy 2001;31(11):1771–8.

67. Yang CM, Li YQ. The therapeutic effects of eliminating allergic foods according to food-specific IgG antibodies in irritable bowel syndrome. Zhonghua Nei Ke Za Zhi 2007;46(8):641–3 [in Chinese].

68. Drisko J, Bischoff B, Hall M, et al. Treating irritable bowel syndrome with a food elimination diet followed by food challenge and probiotics. J Am Coll Nutr 2006; 25(6):514–22.

69. Zar S, Mincher L, Benson MJ, et al. Food-specific IgG4 antibody-guided exclusion diet improves symptoms and rectal compliance in irritable bowel syndrome. Scand J Gastroenterol 2005;40(7):800–7.

70. Hunter JO. Food elimination in IBS: the case for IgG testing remains doubtful. Gut 2005;54(8):1203 [author reply].

71. Zar S, Benson MJ, Kumar D. Food-specific serum IgG4 and IgE titers to common food antigens in irritable bowel syndrome. Am J Gastroenterol 2005; 100(7):1550–7.
72. Floch MH. Use of diet and probiotic therapy in the irritable bowel syndrome: analysis of the literature. J Clin Gastroenterol 2005;39(5 Suppl 3):S243–6.
73. Atkinson W, Sheldon TA, Shaath N, et al. Food elimination based on IgG antibodies in irritable bowel syndrome: a randomised controlled trial. Gut 2004; 53(10):1459–64.
74. Zar S, Kumar D, Kumar D. Role of food hypersensitivity in irritable bowel syndrome. Minerva Med 2002;93(5):403–12.
75. Aydinlar EI, Dikmen PY, Tiftikci A, et al. IgG-based elimination diet in migraine plus irritable bowel syndrome. Headache 2013;53(3):514–25.
76. Mullin GE, Swift KM, Lipski L, et al. Testing for food reactions: the good, the bad, and the ugly. Nutr Clin Pract 2010;25(2):192–8.
77. Ligaarden SC, Lydersen S, Farup PG. IgG and IgG4 antibodies in subjects with irritable bowel syndrome: a case control study in the general population. BMC Gastroenterol 2012;12:166.
78. Stapel SO, Asero R, Ballmer-Weber BK, et al. Testing for IgG4 against foods is not recommended as a diagnostic tool: EAACI Task Force Report. Allergy 2008; 63(7):793–6.
79. Bohmer CJ, Tuynman HA. The clinical relevance of lactose malabsorption in irritable bowel syndrome. Eur J Gastroenterol Hepatol 1996;8(10):1013–6.
80. Bohmer CJ, Tuynman HA. The effect of a lactose-restricted diet in patients with a positive lactose tolerance test, earlier diagnosed as irritable bowel syndrome: a 5-year follow-up study. Eur J Gastroenterol Hepatol 2001;13(8):941–4.
81. Bozzani A, Penagini R, Velio P, et al. Lactose malabsorption and intolerance in Italians. Clinical implications. Dig Dis Sci 1986;31(12):1313–6.
82. Parker TJ, Woolner JT, Prevost AT, et al. Irritable bowel syndrome: is the search for lactose intolerance justified? Eur J Gastroenterol Hepatol 2001;13(3):219–25.
83. Vernia P, Ricciardi MR, Frandina C, et al. Lactose malabsorption and irritable bowel syndrome. Effect of a long-term lactose-free diet. Ital J Gastroenterol 1995;27(3):117–21.
84. Aller R, de Luis DA, Izaola O, et al. Effects of a high-fiber diet on symptoms of irritable bowel syndrome: a randomized clinical trial. Nutrition 2004;20(9):735–7.
85. Arffmann S, Andersen JR, Hegnhoj J, et al. The effect of coarse wheat bran in the irritable bowel syndrome - a double-blind crossover study. Scand J Gastroenterol 1985;20(3):295–8.
86. Bijkerk CJ, de Wit NJ, Muris JW, et al. Soluble or insoluble fibre in irritable bowel syndrome in primary care? Randomised placebo controlled trial. BMJ 2009;339: b3154.
87. Cockerell KM, Watkins AS, Reeves LB, et al. Effects of linseeds on the symptoms of irritable bowel syndrome: a pilot randomised controlled trial. J Hum Nutr Diet 2012;25(5):435–43.
88. Erdogan A, Rao SSC, Thiruvaiyaru D, et al. Randomised clinical trial: mixed soluble/insoluble fibre vs. psyllium for chronic constipation. Aliment Pharmacol Ther 2016;44(1):35–44.
89. Fowlie S, Eastwood MA, Prescott R. Irritable bowel syndrome: assessment of psychological disturbance and its influence on the response to fibre supplementation. J Psychosom Res 1992;36(2):175–80.

90. Hebden JM, Blackshaw E, D'Amato M, et al. Abnormalities of GI transit in bloated irritable bowel syndrome: effect of bran on transit and symptoms. Am J Gastroenterol 2002;97(9):2315–20.

91. Jalihal A, Kurian G. Ispaghula therapy in irritable bowel syndrome: improvement in overall well-being is related to reduction in bowel dissatisfaction. J Gastroenterol Hepatol 1990;5(5):507–13.

92. Kruis W, Weinzierl M, Schussler P, et al. Comparison of the therapeutic effect of wheat bran, mebeverine and placebo in patients with the irritable bowel syndrome. Digestion 1986;34(3):196–201.

93. Longstreth GF, Fox DD, Youkeles L, et al. Psyllium therapy in the irritable bowel syndrome. A double-blind trial. Ann Intern Med 1981;95(1):53–6.

94. Lucey MR, Clark ML, Lowndes J, et al. Is bran efficacious in irritable bowel syndrome? A double blind placebo controlled crossover study. Gut 1987;28(2):221–5.

95. Manning AP, Heaton KW, Harvey RF. Wheat fibre and irritable bowel syndrome. A controlled trial. Lancet 1977;2(8035):417–8.

96. Prior A, Whorwell PJ. Double blind study of ispaghula in irritable bowel syndrome. Gut 1987;28(11):1510–3.

97. Rees G, Davies J, Thompson R, et al. Randomised-controlled trial of a fibre supplement on the symptoms of irritable bowel syndrome. J R Soc Promot Health 2005;125(1):30–4.

98. Snook J, Shepherd HA. Bran supplementation in the treatment of irritable bowel syndrome. Aliment Pharmacol Ther 1994;8(5):511–4.

99. Soltoft J, Krag B, Gudmand-Hoyer E, et al. A double-blind trial of the effect of wheat bran on symptoms of irritable bowel syndrome. Lancet 1976;1(7954):270–2.

100. Tarpila S, Tarpila A, Grohn P, et al. Efficacy of ground flaxseed on constipation in patients with irritable bowel syndrome. Curr Top Nutraceutical Res 2004;2:119–25.

101. Böhn L, Störsrud S, Liljebo T, et al. A multi-center, randomized, controlled, singleblind, comparative trial: low-FODMAP diet versus traditional dietary advice in IBS. United European Gastroenterol J 2014;2(1):A3.

102. Böhn L, Störsrud S, Liljebo TM, et al. A randomized, controlled trial comparing a diet low in fodmaps with traditional dietary advice in patients with IBS. Gastroenterology 2015;148(4):S654.

103. Eswaran SL, Chey WD, Han-Markey T, et al. A randomized controlled trial comparing the low FODMAP diet vs. modified NICE guidelines in US adults with IBS-D. Am J Gastroenterol 2016;111(12):1824–32.

104. Halmos EP, Power VA, Shepherd SJ, et al. A diet low in FODMAPs reduces symptoms of irritable bowel syndrome. Gastroenterology 2014;146(1):67–75.e5.

105. McIntosh K, Reed DE, Schneider T, et al. FODMAPs alter symptoms and the metabolome of patients with IBS: a randomised controlled trial. Gut 2017;66(7):1241–51.

106. Laatikainen R, Koskenpato J, Hongisto SM, et al. Randomised clinical trial: low-FODMAP rye bread vs. regular rye bread to relieve the symptoms of irritable bowel syndrome. Aliment Pharmacol Ther 2016;44(5):460–70.

107. Ong DK, Mitchell SB, Barrett JS, et al. Manipulation of dietary short chain carbohydrates alters the pattern of gas production and genesis of symptoms in irritable bowel syndrome. J Gastroenterol Hepatol 2010;25(8):1366–73.

108. Pedersen N, Vegh Z, Burisch J, et al. Ehealth monitoring in irritable bowel syndrome patients treated with low fermentable oligo-, di-, mono-saccharides and polyols diet. World J Gastroenterol 2014;20(21):6680–4.

109. Peters SL, Yao CK, Philpott H, et al. Randomised clinical trial: the efficacy of gut-directed hypnotherapy is similar to that of the low FODMAP diet for the treatment of irritable bowel syndrome. Aliment Pharmacol Ther 2016;44(5):447–59.

110. Staudacher HM, Lomer MC, Anderson JL, et al. Fermentable carbohydrate restriction reduces luminal bifidobacteria and gastrointestinal symptoms in patients with irritable bowel syndrome. J Nutr 2012;142(8):1510–8.

111. Staudacher HM, Lomer MCE, Farquharson FM, et al. Diet low in FODMAPs reduces symptoms in patients with irritable bowel syndrome and probiotic restores bifidobacterium species: a randomized controlled trial. Gastroenterology 2017;153(4):936–47.

112. Biesiekierski JR, Newnham ED, Irving PM, et al. Gluten causes gastrointestinal symptoms in subjects without celiac disease: a double-blind randomized placebo-controlled trial. Am J Gastroenterol 2011;106(3):508–14 [quiz: 15].

113. Biesiekierski JR, Peters SL, Newnham ED, et al. No effects of gluten in patients with self-reported non-celiac gluten sensitivity after dietary reduction of fermentable, poorly absorbed, short-chain carbohydrates. Gastroenterology 2013; 145(2):320–8.e1–3.

114. Carroccio A, Mansueto P, Iacono G, et al. Non-celiac wheat sensitivity diagnosed by double-blind placebo-controlled challenge: exploring a new clinical entity. Am J Gastroenterol 2012;107(12):1898–906 [quiz: 907].

115. Shahbazkhani B, Sadeghi A, Malekzadeh R, et al. Non-celiac gluten sensitivity has narrowed the spectrum of irritable bowel syndrome: a double-blind randomized placebo-controlled trial. Nutrients 2015;7(6):4542–54.

116. Wahnschaffe U, Schulzke JD, Zeitz M, et al. Predictors of clinical response to gluten-free diet in patients diagnosed with diarrhea-predominant irritable bowel syndrome. Clin Gastroenterol Hepatol 2007;5(7):844–50 [quiz: 769].

117. Vazquez-Roque MI, Camilleri M, Smyrk T, et al. Association of HLA-DQ gene with bowel transit, barrier function, and inflammation in irritable bowel syndrome with diarrhea. Am J Physiol Gastrointest Liver Physiol 2012;303(11):G1262–9.

118. Guo H, Jiang T, Wang J, et al. The value of eliminating foods according to food-specific immunoglobulin G antibodies in irritable bowel syndrome with diarrhoea. J Int Med Res 2012;40(1):204–10.

119. Tan QH, Li XH. Food-specific IgG antibody-directed restrictive diet treats irritable bowel syndrome. World Chinese Journal of Digestology 2013;21(34):3904–7.

120. McClave SA, DiBaise JK, Mullin GE, et al. ACG clinical guideline: nutrition therapy in the adult hospitalized patient. Am J Gastroenterol 2016;111(3):315–34 [quiz: 35].

121. Balshem H, Helfand M, Schunemann HJ, et al. GRADE guidelines: 3. rating the quality of evidence. J Clin Epidemiol 2011;64(4):401–6.

122. Cruz J, Germin F, Moore K, et al. Practice guideline development, grading, and assessment. Pharmacol Ther 2015;40(12):854–7.

123. Mearin F, Lacy B, Chang L, et al. The Rome IV Committees. Bowel disorders. In: Drossman DA, Kellow CL, William J, et al, editors. Rome IV functional gastrointestinal disorders – disorders of gut-brain interaction. Raleigh (NC): Gastroenterol 2016;150:1393–1407.

APPENDIX 1: SEARCH RESULTS OF DIET AND THE IRRITABLE BOWEL SYNDROME
Search Run August 16, 2017

PubMed (2784)

1. ("Diet"[mh:noexp] OR "Diet Therapy"[mh:noexp] OR diet[tiab] OR diets[tiab] OR dietary[tiab] OR "oligosaccharides"[mh] OR oligosaccharides[tiab] OR fructo oligosaccharide*[tiab] OR fructooligosaccharide*[tiab] OR galacto oligosaccharides[tiab] OR galactooligosaccharides[tiab] OR polyols[tiab] OR monosaccharide*[tiab] OR paleolithic[tiab] OR paleo[tiab] OR ketogenic[tiab] OR sucrose[tiab]

OR sorbitol[tiab] OR xylitol[tiab] OR "plantago seed"[tiab] OR "guar gum"[tiab] OR wheat[tiab] OR elimination[tiab] OR dairy[tiab] OR lactose[tiab] OR milk[tiab] OR sugar[tiab] OR sugars[tiab] OR fructose[tiab] OR exclusion diet*[tiab] OR gluten [tiab] OR "Diet, Gluten-Free"[mh] OR histamine[tiab] OR histamines[tiab] OR "low residue"[tiab] or "low-residue"[tiab] OR "dietary fiber"[mh] OR fiber[tiab] OR fiber[tiab] or bran[tiab] OR brans[tiab] OR metamucil[tiab] OR psyllium[tiab] OR "psyllium"[mh] OR "ispaghula"[tiab] OR "Diet, Western"[mh] OR western diet*[tiab] OR "Diet, Fat-Restricted"[mh] OR "low fat"[tiab] OR "fat restricted diet"[tiab] OR "low nickel"[tiab] OR "low-nickel"[tiab] OR "Healthy Diet"[mh] OR healthy diet*[tiab] OR habitual diet*[tiab] OR Australian diet*[tiab] OR ferment* [tiab] OR caffeine[tiab] OR alcohol[tiab] OR "Diet, Carbohydrate-Restricted"[mh] OR carbohydrate[tiab] OR carbo[tiab] OR "Diet, High-Fat"[mh] OR "high fat"[tiab] OR "high fats"[tiab] OR spices[tiab] OR spicy[tiab] OR spice[tiab] OR fodmap* [tiab] OR vegetarian*[tiab] OR "Carbonated Beverages"[Mesh] OR yogurt[tiab] OR yoghurt[tiab] OR whey[tiab] OR kefir[tiab] OR macrobiotic[tiab] OR keto-genic[tiab] OR "Prebiotics"[Mesh] OR prebiotic*[tiab] OR lifestyle*[tiab] OR starch*[tiab] OR igg4[tiab] OR "Allergens"[Mesh] OR allerg*[tiab] OR tea[tiab] OR coffee[tiab] OR fruit[tiab] OR fruits[tiab] OR vegetable*[tiab])

2. ("Irritable Bowel Syndrome"[mh] OR irritable bowel syndrome*[tiab] OR "Mucous Colitis"[tiab] OR "spastic colon"[tiab] OR irritable colon*[tiab] OR functional bowel*[tiab] OR colonic disease*[tiab] OR IBS[tiab] OR gastrointestinal syndrome*[tiab] OR fgid[tiab] OR functional gastrointestinal disorder*[tiab] OR Colon spasm*[tiab] OR Irritable colon syndrome*[tiab] OR "spastic colitis"[tiab] OR unstable colon*[tiab])

3. 1 AND 2.

Embase (3232)

1. 'diet'/de OR 'diet therapy'/exp OR diet:ti,ab OR diets:ti,ab OR dietary:ti,ab OR 'oligosaccharide'/exp OR 'oligosaccharides':ti,ab OR fructo oligosaccharide*:ti,ab OR fructooligosaccharide*:ti,ab OR 'galacto oligosaccharides':ti,ab OR galactooli-gosaccharides:ti,ab OR polyols:ti,ab OR monosaccharide*:ti,ab OR paleolithic:-ti,ab OR paleo:ti,ab OR ketogenic:ti,ab OR sucrose:ti,ab OR sorbitol:ti,ab OR xylitol:ti,ab OR 'plantago seed':ti,ab OR 'guar gum':ti,ab OR wheat:ti,ab OR elimi-nation:ti,ab OR dairy:ti,ab OR lactose:ti,ab OR milk:ti,ab OR sugar:ti,ab OR sugar-s:ti,ab OR fructose:ti,ab OR exclusion diet*:ti,ab OR gluten:ti,ab OR 'gluten free diet'/exp OR histamine:ti,ab OR histamines:ti,ab OR 'low residue':ti,ab OR 'low-residue':ti,ab OR 'dietary fiber'/exp OR fiber:ti,ab OR fiber:ti,ab OR bran:ti,ab OR brans:ti,ab OR metamucil:ti,ab OR psyllium:ti,ab OR 'ispagula'/exp OR ispaghula:-ti,ab OR 'Western diet'/exp OR 'western diet*':ti,ab OR 'low fat diet'/exp OR 'low fat':ti,ab OR 'fat restricted diet':ti,ab OR 'low nickel':ti,ab OR 'low-nickel':ti,ab OR 'healthy diet'/exp OR healthy diet*:ti,ab OR habitual diet*:ti,ab OR australian di-et*:ti,ab OR ferment*:ti,ab OR caffeine:ti,ab OR alcohol:ti,ab OR 'low carbohydrate diet'/exp OR carbohydrate:ti,ab OR carbo:ti,ab OR 'lipid diet'/exp OR 'high fat':-ti,ab OR 'high fats':ti,ab OR spices:ti,ab OR spicy:ti,ab OR spice:ti,ab OR fod-map*:ti,ab OR vegetarian*:ti,ab OR 'carbonated beverage'/exp OR yogurt:ti,ab OR yoghurt:ti,ab OR whey:ti,ab OR kefir:ti,ab OR macrobiotic:ti,ab OR ketogenic:-ti,ab OR prebiotic*:ti,ab OR lifestyle*:ti,ab OR starch*:ti,ab OR igg4:ti,ab OR 'allergen'/exp OR allerg*:ti,ab OR tea:ti,ab OR coffee:ti,ab OR fruit:ti,ab OR fruit-s:ti,ab OR vegetable*:ti,ab.

2. ('irritable colon'/exp OR 'irritable bowel syndrome*':ti,ab OR 'Mucous Colitis':ti,ab OR 'spastic colon*':ti,ab OR 'irritable colon*':ti,ab OR 'functional bowel*':ti,ab OR

'colonic disease*':ti,ab OR IBS:ti,ab OR 'gastrointestinal syndrome*':ti,ab OR fgid:-ti,ab OR 'functional gastrointestinal disorder*':ti,ab OR 'Colon spasm':ti,ab OR 'Irritable colon syndrome*':ti,ab OR 'spastic colitis':ti,ab OR 'unstable colon*':ti,ab)
3. 1 AND 2.

Web of Science (6646)–limited to journal articles.
1. Ts = (diet OR diets OR dietary OR oligosaccharides OR fructo oligosaccharide* OR fructooligosaccharide* OR galacto oligosaccharides OR galactooligosaccharides OR polyols OR monosaccharide* OR paleolithic OR paleo OR ketogenic OR sucrose OR sorbitol OR xylitol OR "plantago seed" OR "guar gum" OR wheat OR elimination OR dairy OR lactose OR milk OR sugar OR sugars OR fructose OR exclusion diet* OR gluten OR histamine OR histamines OR "low residue" or "low-residue" OR fiber OR fiber or bran OR brans OR metamucil OR psyllium OR "ispaghula" OR western diet* OR "low fat" OR "fat restricted diet" OR "low nickel" OR "low-nickel" OR healthy diet* OR habitual diet* OR Australian diet* OR ferment* OR caffeine OR alcohol OR carbohydrate OR carbo OR "high fat" OR "high fats" OR spices OR spicy OR spice OR fodmap* OR vegetarian* OR yogurt OR yoghurt OR whey OR kefir OR macrobiotic OR ketogenic OR prebiotic* OR lifestyle* OR starch* OR igg4 OR allerg* OR tea OR coffee OR fruit OR fruits OR vegetable*)
2. ts = ("Irritable Bowel Syndrome" OR "Mucous Colitis" OR "spastic colon" OR "irritable colon" OR "functional bowel" OR colonic disease* OR IBS OR gastrointestinal syndrome* OR fgid OR functional gastrointestinal disorder* OR Colon spasm* OR Irritable colon syndrome* OR "spastic colitis" OR "unstable colon")
3. 1 AND 2.

Cochrane (1141)
1. ("Diet"[mh:noexp] OR "Diet Therapy"[mh:noexp] OR "oligosaccharides"[mh] OR "Diet, Western"[mh] OR "psyllium"[mh] OR "Diet, Fat-Restricted"[mh] OR OR "Healthy Diet"[mh] OR "Diet, Carbohydrate-Restricted"[mh] OR "Diet, High-Fat"[mh] OR "Allergens"[Mesh] OR "Carbonated Beverages"[Mesh] OR "Prebiotics"[Mesh] OR diet OR "diets" OR "dietary" OR "oligosaccharides" OR fructo oligosaccharide* OR fructooligosaccharide* OR galacto oligosaccharides OR galactooligosaccharides OR polyols OR monosaccharide* OR paleolithic OR paleo OR ketogenic OR sucrose OR sorbitol OR xylitol OR "plantago seed" OR "guar gum" OR wheat OR elimination OR dairy OR lactose OR milk OR sugar OR sugars OR fructose OR exclusion diet* OR gluten OR "Diet, Gluten-Free"[mh] OR histamine OR histamines OR "low residue" or "low-residue" OR "dietary fiber"[mh] OR fiber OR fiber or bran OR brans OR metamucil OR psyllium OR "ispaghula" OR western diet* OR "low fat" OR "fat restricted diet" OR "low nickel" OR "low-nickel" OR healthy diet* OR habitual diet* OR Australian diet* OR ferment* OR caffeine OR alcohol OR carbohydrate OR carbo OR "high fat" OR "high fats" OR spices OR spicy OR spice OR fodmap* OR vegetarian* OR yogurt OR yoghurt OR whey OR kefir OR macrobiotic OR ketogenic OR prebiotic* OR lifestyle* OR starch* OR igg4 OR allerg* OR tea OR coffee OR fruit OR fruits OR vegetable*)
2. ("Irritable Bowel Syndrome"[mh] OR "Irritable Bowel Syndrome" OR "Mucous Colitis" OR "spastic colon" OR "irritable colon" OR "functional bowel" OR colonic disease* OR IBS OR gastrointestinal syndrome* OR fgid OR functional gastrointestinal disorder* OR Colon spasm* OR Irritable colon syndrome* OR "spastic colitis" OR "unstable colon")
3. 1 AND 2.

Nutritional Consideration in Celiac Disease and Nonceliac Gluten Sensitivity

Rishi D. Naik, MD, Douglas L. Seidner, MD,
Dawn Wiese Adams, MD, MS*

KEYWORDS

- Celiac • Nonceliac gluten sensitivity • Gluten • Nutritional deficiencies
- Gluten-free diet • Drug development

KEY POINTS

- Celiac disease is a chronic enteropathy of the small intestine, which leads to various gastrointestinal and extraintestinal symptoms and is associated with specific micronutrient deficiencies.
- A strict gluten-free diet is currently the only therapy for nonrefractory celiac disease and typically leads to healing of the small intestine and improved absorption of nutrients.
- Nonceliac gluten sensitivity typically does not damage the small intestine and, therefore, is marked by symptoms that improve with gluten cessation, rather than significant nutritional deficiencies.
- A gluten-free diet needs to be monitored because it can lead to nutritional deficiencies.
- Adherence to a strict gluten-free diet in patients without celiac disease nor non-celiac gluten sensitivity is not advised.

INTRODUCTION

Celiac disease (CeD) is an autoimmune disorder in which gluten and gluten-related prolamins initiate an inflammatory response when they reach the small bowel enterocyte. CeD, which can only occur in genetically predisposed individuals (HLA DQ2 or DQ8), is an underrecognized entity with many nutritional considerations. The estimated prevalence is 1% worldwide, though it is has classically been underdiagnosed due to its wide range of presenting symptoms and underrecognition.[1] The prevalence of CeD has increased fivefold in the last 50 years with various hypotheses including the

Disclosure: The authors have nothing to disclose.
Division of Gastroenterology, Hepatology, and Nutrition, Center for Nutrition, Vanderbilt University Medical Center, 1211 21st Avenue South, Suite 514, Nashville, TN 37232, USA
* Corresponding author. Division of Gastroenterology, Hepatology, and Nutrition, Vanderbilt University Medical Center, 1211 21st Avenue South, Suite 514, Nashville, TN 37232.
E-mail address: Dawn.W.Adams@vanderbilt.edu

Gastroenterol Clin N Am 47 (2018) 139–154
https://doi.org/10.1016/j.gtc.2017.09.006
0889-8553/18/© 2017 Elsevier Inc. All rights reserved.

hygiene hypothesis and possible infection by reovirus at an early age.[2,3] CeD has important long-term health concerns, such as the increase in osteoporosis, depression, non-Hodgkin lymphoma, and small intestinal adenocarcinoma. Nutrient deficiencies are common, such as vitamin B12, folate, B6, iron, vitamin D, magnesium, copper, and zinc. It is important to perform monitoring of these in patients with CeD.

Some patients without CeD report having a sensitivity to gluten, a condition called nonceliac gluten sensitivity (NCGS) or nonceliac wheat sensitivity (NCWS). Though a biological basis has yet to be determined, there may be an immune response, which is distinctly different from that seen in CeD.

This article briefly reviews the pathogenesis and symptoms of CeD and NCGS and, in more detail, discusses the nutritional complications seen in CeD before and during treatment, and the nutritional consequences of a long-term gluten-free diet (GFD).

GLUTEN

Gluten is derived from the Latin word for glue due to its viscoelastic properties. Gluten is the material that remains after washing away starch and water soluble components of wheat dough. Gluten mainly consists of a group of proteins called prolamins, primarily soluble gliadins and insoluble glutenins. The properties of gluten can best be demonstrated during dough mixing in which dough stiffness increases due to optimization of these protein interactions.[4] Because of this, gluten is a common additive in many food products that are naturally devoid of gluten to optimize texture and storage properties, and is a large component of the food industry.[5]

Gluten is naturally found in wheat, rye, and barley. However, a GFD must eliminate all sources of gluten, which includes any foods or products that have added gluten. This can include anything from salad dressing to cheese to medications. Pure oats are devoid of gluten but the processing of oats with gluten-containing grains has caused many people to eliminate oats as part of a GFD (see later discussion). Gluten itself has little nutritional value; however, foods naturally containing gluten are a common source of whole grains, fiber, vitamins, and minerals.

CELIAC DISEASE

CeD involves a complex interplay of genetics, immunologic factors, and gluten (**Fig. 1**). The basis for treatment of CeD is avoidance of gluten, therefore it excludes wheat, barley, and rye.[6] Gluten and other proline-rich proteins are poorly digested in the small intestine due to lack of prolyl endopeptidases, resulting in large gluten proteins. Moreover, gluten is rich in glutamine which can be deamidated by the enzyme tissue transglutaminase and converted to negatively charged glutamic acid residues.[7] Some of these peptides can bind to human HLA class II molecules DQ2 and DQ8, which activate CD4[+] T cells in the intestinal mucosa. This leads to a T-cell–mediated response to gluten in genetically susceptible individuals, resulting in a malabsorptive enteropathy.[8] The humoral immune system is directed against the exogenous antigen gluten and the autoantigen tissue transglutaminase. Disease is exhibited through a complex interplay of the mucosal and epithelial barriers via the disruptions and alterations of intestinal epithelial cells and tight junction defects.[8,9] Histologically, this leads to intraepithelial lymphocytosis, crypt hyperplasia, and villous atrophy, which are the hallmarks of biopsy diagnosis.[10] A strict GFD can lead to mucosal healing, resulting in improvement in histologic findings, malabsorption, and symptoms.

CeD can present with a wide array of symptoms. The classic presentation was a thin child with weight loss, poor growth, and diarrhea. Now patients are presenting with more atypical symptoms (**Table 1**).[11] Given the high frequency of many of these symptoms in

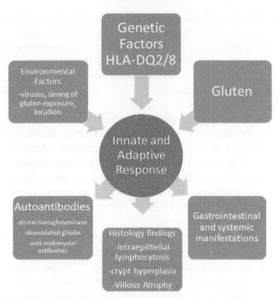

Fig. 1. Development of celiac disease.

the population, many individuals will be misdiagnosed with an average diagnosis time of 6 to 10 years from symptom onset. Diagnosis of CD is made by positive serology or a combination of serology and histology. Genetic testing is typically reserved to exclude CeD given its high negative predictive value but poor positive predictive value.

NONCELIAC GLUTEN SENSITIVITY

NCGS is a syndrome characterized by intestinal and extraintestinal symptoms related to the ingestion of gluten in patients who do not have CeD nor wheat allergy, but improve on a GFD.[12,13] Symptoms are vast and include abdominal pain, bloating, and irregular bowel movements, as well as fatigue, joint pain, migraines, and brain fog. Unlike CeD, which is due to an adaptive immune response characterized by the

Table 1 Symptoms of celiac disease	
Typical	**Atypical**
Diarrhea	Fatigue
Weight loss	Constipation
Bloating	Dyspepsia
Abdominal pain	Anemia
	vitamin deficiencies
	Osteoporosis
	Dermatitis herpetiformis
	Recurrent aphthous stomatitis
	Hepatitis
	Dental enamel hypoplasia
	Infertility
	Neuropathy
	Hyposplenism
	Delayed puberty

presence of gluten-reactive T cells and antibodies, the cause of NCGS is unknown. Some speculate that there is an innate immune response to dietary gluten; however, currently, there is no identified genetic predisposition or antibody formation, making NCGS a diagnosis based on clinical response to gluten in the absence of known serology and histology findings.[14] The current gold standard diagnostic test is a placebo-controlled crossover challenge.[15] This is used in clinical trials but is impractical in a current clinical setting.

It is important to distinguish gluten sensitivity from wheat sensitivity. Gluten is only a component of wheat. Wheat's other components, such as amylase-trypsin inhibitors, may be the inciting source of symptoms. Wheat contains fructans and, therefore, is part of a group of foods known as fermentable oligosaccharides, disaccharides, monosaccharides, and polyols (FODMAPs), which are known stimulants of GI symptoms in irritable bowel syndrome.[16,17] Because of this, some investigators have proposed the condition should be called NCWS rather than NCGS.[17]

Despite a lack of biomarkers or pathologic diagnosis, NCGS has been associated with increased mucosal immune activation via increased CD3-positive intraepithelial lymphocytes, increased interferon gamma response to gluten challenge, and signs of increased adaptive immune response with gluten.[18,19] In a study of ex vivo human duodenal biopsies, patients with NCGS and active CeD had increased intestinal permeability compared with patients with CeD in remission and controls.[20] Subsets of patients with NCGS have higher rates of anemia, weight loss, and osteoporosis, which brings up the question of whether some may have early CeD.[21] In addition, there is a higher rate of autoimmune disorders and atopic diseases in patients with NCGS as compared with patients with irritable bowel syndrome.[22] This condition is persistent and patients with NCGS or NCWS who initially respond to a GFD will continue to have negative response to wheat even years after initial exclusion.[23]

WHAT IS A GLUTEN-FREE DIET?

Ideally, in a GFD gluten is fully removed from the diet; however, gluten-free products are typically not fully devoid of gluten. Each country has different regulations on qualifications for gluten-free packaging. For instance, the US Food and Drug Administration reports a gluten-free product is either inherently gluten-free, does not contain an ingredient that is a gluten-containing grain, or derived from a gluten-containing grain that has been processed to remove gluten with less than 20 parts per million (ppm) of gluten. A similar cutoff of 20 ppm of gluten for gluten-free foods is seen in Spain, Italy, United Kingdom, and Canada. Some countries have more stringent criteria, such as Argentina (10 ppm) and Australia (3 ppm).[24] Several naturally gluten-free food groups include fruits, vegetables, meats, fish, dairy, beans, legumes, and nuts. Pure wheat grass and barley grass are gluten-free, but there is gluten in the seeds so there is a risk of contamination if not harvested correctly. There are many natural grains that are gluten-free, which include rice, corn, soy, quinoa, flax, chia, millet, yucca, nut flouts, and beans.

Common sources of gluten are shown in **Table 2**. The primary antigen prolamins found in wheat (gliadin), rye (secalin), and barley (hordein) are structurally different than the prolamines in oat (avenins) and are only a fraction of the total oat proteins.[25,26] There is controversy of the safety of oats with some investigators stating its harm, whereas others reported no toxicity, though most agree that pure oats are safe, but contamination with other cereals has to be avoided.[27,28] A large metaanalysis found no evidence that intake of oats with a GFD changes symptoms, histology, immunity, or serologies in patients with CeD.[29] This is an important acknowledgment because

Table 2		
Gluten-containing products and gluten-free grains		
Gluten Grains	**Hidden Sources of Gluten**	**Gluten-Free Grains**
• Wheat	• Oats harvested with wheat	• Corn
• Rye	• Sauces (marinades, soy sauce, salad dressing)	• Rice
• Barley	• Drug fillers	• Potato
	• Processed meats	• Amaranth
	• Shared food preparation (eg, toaster, deep fryer, pasta pot)	• Buckwheat
		• Millet
	• Church communion	• Sorghum
	• LIpstIcks or chopsticks	• Teff
		• Quinoa

oats may increase nutritional value of a GFD via improved amino acid, fiber, mineral, and vitamin balance with improved palatability.[30,31] Patients should be educated on how to select appropriate gluten-free oats to include in their diet.

NUTRITIONAL DEFICIENCIES OF CELIAC DISEASE AND THE GLUTEN-FREE DIET

The inflammation in CeD leads to malabsorption of important nutrients. The inflammation is improved with adherence to a GFD and should lead to improvement in nutrient absorption. However, a GFD itself has limitations in nutrient value (**Fig. 2**) and requires dietary counseling and monitoring to assure patients are meeting the recommended dietary intakes. The following are the important vitamins, minerals, and nutrients to be considered for CeD and those with NCGS on a GFD.

Iron

Iron is absorbed in the duodenum and upper part of the jejunum. CeD causes an enteropathy and iron deficiency is the most common nutrient deficiency in CeD.[32,33] At

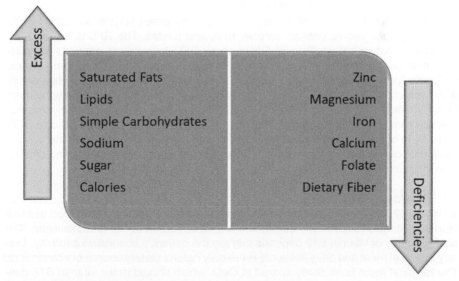

Fig. 2. Nutritional deficiencies and excess in gluten-free diet.

the time of diagnosis, 7% to 81% of patients may have iron deficiency anemia. It is estimated that 2% to 5% of patients presenting with iron deficiency anemia have CeD. Therefore, CeD should be excluded in all patients with iron deficiency of unclear cause.[34,35] The cause of iron deficiency is thought to be multifactorial, including a primary malabsorptive process and persistent inflammation.[36–38] With a strict GFD, iron stores typically improve. The duration of improvement depends largely on time to heal the intestinal mucosa, which typically occurs between 6 to 12 months.[39] Once intestinal healing is achieved, iron supplementation can be considered if there is persistent iron deficiency anemia. Oral iron supplementation can be difficult for patients due to difficult dosing and the common side effects of nausea and constipation. An intravenous route of iron should be selected if there are issues with compliance, intolerance, or ineffectiveness to oral iron.

Though iron stores typically improve after initiation of a GFD, this diet typically has lower amounts of iron, so patients should be counseled on eating foods rich in iron, including red meats, seafood, beans, leafy vegetables, and dried fruits. Iron stores should be checked periodically in patients with persistently active CeD.

Folate

Folate is a water-soluble vitamin not made by humans that is reliant on oral intake. Folate is absorbed in the proximal small intestine, mainly the duodenum and the proximal jejunum. Via enterocytes, folate is reduced and methylated, and eventually transported to the liver and then the systemic circulation. This process is disrupted with celiac enteropathy, leading to folate deficiency. Studies have shown correlation with increased villous atrophy and lower folate levels.[40–42] As in iron deficiency anemia, folate deficiency typically improves as the underlying enteropathy improves. Folate deficiency can present as a macrocytic anemia or pancytopenia, mouth ulcers, or various neuropsychiatric conditions. In addition, it is well known that folate deficiency is associated with neural tube defects in embryologic development and should be considered when patients with untreated CeD are considering pregnancy. It is important to check for vitamin B12 deficiency in folate deficient patients because repletion with folic acid in a vitamin B12 deficient patient can mask anemia while worsening neurologic manifestations of vitamin B12 deficiency.

Folate is found in variety of foods, including leafy green vegetables, citrus fruits, seeds and nuts, beans, breads, cereals, rice, and pastas. The GFD is typically low in folate. Biochemical profiling of GFDs show GFD have lower amounts of folate than their gluten counterparts, particularly in respect to breads and pastas. Hence, the underlying enteropathy has improved, but the oral nutritional intake has diminished, which has led to the proposal for routine folate measurements and supplementation if deficient.[43] Patients with CeD on a GFD commonly have below the estimated average requirement of folate and it has been shown that in controlled CeD on a GFD, up to 20% of patients will remain folate deficient.[44,45] One study showed the supplementation of folate and vitamin B12 for 6 months helped improve anxiety and depression in patients with CeD.[46]

Vitamin B12

Vitamin B12, also known as cobalamin, is released by gastric acid from food where it binds to intrinsic factor in the duodenum and is absorbed in the terminal ileum. The bioavailability of vitamin B12 depends fully on the patient's absorptive capacity. Dietary intake of meat and dairy products is the only natural dietary source of vitamin B12. The terminal ileum is relatively spared in CeD, which should make vitamin B12 deficiency less common. However, studies estimate a prevalence of 5% to 41% of vitamin

B12 deficiency in untreated CeD.[11,47,48] The mechanism of vitamin B12 deficiency in CeD is not completely understood but may be due to pancreatic insufficiency, decreased secretion of binding proteins, or concomitant pernicious anemia.[49] Vitamin B12 deficiency is typically corrected with a GFD but should be treated with vitamin B12 supplementation in the short term due to significant neurologic consequences of deficiency such as paresthesias, gait abnormalities, psychosis, and dementia.[50] In the same study that showed folate deficiency despite a GFD, vitamin B12 remained normal after a GFD.[44]

Vitamin D and Calcium

Vitamin D is produced mainly in the skin following sun exposure but can also be obtained via diet in which the prohormone of vitamin D is absorbed in the terminal ileum and released in the liver, converting vitamin D to 25-hydroxyvitamin D. This is converted to the active form of vitamin D by the kidneys, which regulates serum calcium levels by increasing intestinal calcium absorption and bone resorption.[51,52] Villous atrophy and fat malabsorption can lead to decreased absorption of vitamin D, leading to deficiency. Elimination of milk products in CeD with concomitant lactose intolerance will lead to poor vitamin D intake and contribute to vitamin D deficiency.

More than 90% of calcium is absorbed in the small intestine with highest rates in the duodenum. Because serum levels of calcium are tightly regulated, serum calcium is rarely low in patients with CeD and is not a good marker of calcium status. Calcium deficiency is thought to contribute to poor growth and fractures in children with CeD, and fractures and bone mineral density loss in adults with CeD.[53,54] The degree of calcium depletion may relate to disease severity. Patients with more severe disease, Marsh stage 3c, had lower serum calcium and higher parathyroid hormone levels compared with less severe CeD, suggesting overall lower total body calcium.[55]

Recognition of deficiencies in vitamin D and calcium are extremely important in CeD because up to 50% of patients with untreated CeD will have either osteopenia or osteoporosis.[56,57] Data are mixed, but several studies report vitamin D and calcium levels can normalize within 1 to 2 years of a strict GFD and, in some patients, reverse bone loss.[58–61] Despite this, adults and children on a GFD consume below the recommended intake of calcium and vitamin D.[53] Some of this may be due to continued avoidance of lactose-containing milk products even after intestinal healing has occurred, use of pH-raising medications for persistent dyspepsia, and lack of calcium and vitamin D fortification in gluten-free products. Assessment of calcium and vitamin D intake and needs should be determined by a trained dietitian because requirements vary by life-stage. Calcium and vitamin D should be supplemented in celiac patients with documented low serum levels, those with loss of bone mineral density, or those who cannot achieve adequate intake via diet.[62] Celiac patients with osteoporosis on a GFD have shown improvement in bone mineral density with the supplementation of vitamin D and calcium.[63,64]

Zinc

Zinc is an essential trace element that when deficient can lead to growth arrest and diminished protein synthesis. It is absorbed in the duodenum and jejunum, where it is taken up and bound by proteins for transport to the systemic circulation.[65,66] Zinc deficiency has been reported to be as high as 50% of patients with untreated CeD.[67–69] Several factors for zinc deficiency include primary villous atrophy, excessive zinc utilization due to enterocyte turnover, and chelation of zinc by fatty acids.[68] Deficiencies in zinc can be seen as impaired wound healing, dermatitis, hypogeusia, and poor growth.[70–72] With a strict GFD for 1 year, zinc deficiencies resolve and long-term supplementation is typically not needed.

Magnesium

Magnesium is a divalent intracellular cation that plays important roles in the metabolism of proteins, glucose, and fats. Its absorption and calibration are monitored by the small intestine and kidney.[73,74] In fact, 30% to 50% of magnesium is absorbed in the small intestine, which is partly dictated by Vitamin D, and is largely protein bound.[75,76] Approximately 20% of people with untreated CeD will have magnesium deficiencies. After adherence to a GFD, magnesium can still remain low due to the low magnesium contents of gluten-free cereal products. Continued monitoring and dietary education on intake of a magnesium-enriched GFD must be encouraged.[77,78]

Copper

Copper is an essential trace metal and plays key roles in the nervous system, catecholamine metabolism, and hematopoiesis.[79] Most copper absorption takes place in the proximal gastrointestinal tract where malabsorption leads to deficiency in CeD. Adequate copper supply is vital for hematopoiesis and development and maintenance of a healthy nervous system. Hypocupremia can present with hematological findings, such as anemia, neutropenia, and pancytopenia, as well as neurologic findings due to myeloneuropathy causing ataxia with gait unsteadiness and peripheral neuropathy.[80] With copper repletion, the hematological manifestations typically resolve, but the neurologic deficits can be irreversible.[81] Because of the important side effects of hypocupremia, screening for copper deficiency should be considered at time of diagnosis of CeD and when any associated deficiency symptoms are identified.

Pyridoxine (Vitamin B6)

Pyridoxine, also known as vitamin B6, is an essential nutrient in amino acid metabolism, hemoglobin synthesis, and gene expression. Pyridoxine is absorbed in the jejunum and ileum with high avidity, where celiac-induced enteropathy can lead to malabsorption.[82] Deficiencies of pyridoxine can lead to seborrheic dermatitis-like eruption, atrophic glossitis, angular cheilitis, neuropathy, somnolence, and a sideroblastic anemia.[83] Limited data are available on the pyridoxine content of a GFD with 1 study failing to show a statistical significant difference in serum level of pyridoxine in those on a GFD versus controls.[45] Initial screening for pyridoxine is advocated and subsequent monitoring if any symptoms develop or if multiple other B vitamin deficiencies are detected.

Other Nutritional Deficiencies in the Gluten-Free Diet

Macronutrients and energy intake is usually imbalanced both at the diagnosis of CeD but also with the adherence of a GFD. Despite adherence to a GFD as the treatment of CeD and NCGS, this diet typically leads to a consumption of an unbalanced diet. As opposed to the classic presentation of short stature and weight loss, overweight patients with CeD are becoming more prevalent with 1 study showing 40% of patients with CeD being overweight at diagnosis and 13% in the obese range.[84] Many gluten-free products are not enriched as their wheat-containing counterparts are, which can lead to low intake of common additives such as fiber, iron, folate, thiamine, riboflavin, and niacin.[85] The GFD is known to be low in fiber and many patients with CeD struggle to reach the recommended 25 to 30 g of daily fiber intake. This can lead to significant constipation, as well as removal of other health benefits of soluble and insoluble fiber. In 1 study of 18 children with CeD, those on a GFD were found to have increased intake of simple sugars, fats, and proteins, with higher energy intakes than controls.[86] The diet has also been shown to be higher in fat and protein content and lower in carbohydrates.[87,88] The results of how this diet affects body composition are mixed with some studies showing increased obesity in children.[88] Many processed gluten-free products have an increased glycemic index with increased fat and lower proteins compared with gluten-containing meals.[89,90] Moreover, gluten-free products have a high carbohydrate and lipid content with increased lipid intake (see **Fig. 2**).

BENEFITS OF GLUTEN-FREE DIET

The GFD is difficult for patients to maintain and adherence in patients with CeD is between 45% to 91%.[91] Strict compliance to a GFD in CeD typically leads to mucosal healing that, in addition to vast symptom improvement, is associated with decreased risk of cardiovascular disease and malignancy, two causes of mortality in CeD.[92–94] As previously mentioned, with continued compliance, there is improvement in iron stores and micronutrients with associated improvement in bone mineral density, body weight, body mass index, and fat mass. Patients typically take in fewer calories but have greater improvements in body composition.[7,59] In diabetic patients, nutritional parameters are improved on a GFD, though insulin requirement typically rises with no substantial change in diabetic control and should be monitored as disease heals.[95]

The GFD is not for everyone. There is concern in the lay public that gluten may promote inflammation, leading to obesity, neuropsychiatric problems, and cardiovascular disease even in patients without CeD or NCGS, causing an estimated 30% of the US population to report minimizing or avoiding gluten.[96–98] In a recent robust prospective cohort study examining 2,273,931 person-years, not only was there no increase in coronary heart disease with gluten intake, but avoidance of gluten reduced beneficial whole grain intake. Avoidance of gluten may worsen cardiovascular health; therefore, a GFD should not be advised in individuals without CeD or NCGS.[99]

DRUG DEVELOPMENT FOR CELIAC DISEASE

Many celiac patients desire a nondietary alternative to a strict GFD, which has innovated several new drug and vaccine therapies for CeD. The 3 main categories for current therapy are intraluminal therapies, immunotherapies, and immunosuppressants. Intraluminal therapies, include larazotide, latiglutenase, and BL-7010, which attempt to reduce gluten immunogenicity or prevent gluten uptake in intestinal epithelium.[100] Immunotherapies aim to restore immune tolerance. Examples of immunotherapies include Nexvax2 (see later discussion) and nanoparticle therapy designed to induce tolerance.[101] Finally, immunosuppressants, which include the IL-15 antagonist, target activation of the innate and adaptive immune system as treatment of refractory CeD.[102] Three important examples of celiac drug development follow.

Latiglutenase, also named IMGX-003 and formerly ALV-003, is a glutenase derived from a modified recombinant version of the proenzyme form of cysteine endoprotease derived from barley that has increasing interest for its potential benefit as an oral therapy for those with CeD. In a randomized study, subjects with biopsy-proven CeD were compared with controls for 6 weeks with a fixed gluten challenge of 2 g.[103] In the treatment arm, subjects given ALV003 showed no significant mucosal deterioration or change in CD3[+] intraepithelial lymphocytes compared with the placebo arm, which had mucosal injury.[103] Given the findings that AVL003 may attenuate gluten-induced small intestinal mucosal injury, a follow-up randomized control study was recently performed. Unfortunately, in this intention-to-treat population, this group failed to show a difference in morphologic change of small bowel mucosa, intraepithelial lymphocytes, or serologic markers of CeD.[104] Evaluation of these seemingly incongruent data has yielded several theories for these negative findings, which include the large trial-effect (all groups had significant improvement in histologic and symptom scores) and lack of defined amount of gluten intake.[104]

One crucial step in the pathogenesis of CeD is the interaction between gluten and gluten-reactive T cells in the lamina propria facilitated by paracellular permeability. Targeting this etiologic factor, larazotide acetate (also known as AT-1001) was developed as a tight junction regulator. Multiple clinical trials have shown safety, efficacy in protecting tight junction integrity and paracellular permeability, and symptom improvement when compared with placebo.[105,106] In an important multicenter, randomized, double-blind, placebo-controlled trial involving 342 subjects, larazotide acetate 0.5 mg reduced signs and symptoms in CeD on a GFD better than a GFD alone.[107]

Nexvax2 is an antigen-specific immunotherapy made up of 3 peptides that have immunodominant epitopes for gluten-specific CD4-positive T-cells. The goal of this therapy is to cause host CD4-positive T cells to become unresponsive to gluten antigenic stimulation.[108] Recent data from a combination of two randomized, double-blind, placebo-controlled, phase 1 studies have defined the maximal tolerated dose and have shown early signs of promise for immune responsiveness to Nexvav2 peptides without duodenal mucosal injury in the setting of a gluten challenge.[108]

These therapies offer promise for a burgeoning field for drug discovery and vaccine development for CeD to help with treatment of this chronic disease and its important nutritional consequences. However, all of the known and unknown adverse effects of these therapies must carefully be considered and balanced with the minimal risk of a strict GFD. Many of these therapies may be reserved for refractory CeD or prevention of cross-contamination and the GFD will remain the primary therapy for CeD.

SUMMARY

CeD is a common disease that leads to small intestinal enteropathy due to gluten toxicity. This enteropathy can lead to important nutritional deficiencies, specifically with iron, vitamin B12, folate, vitamin B6, vitamin D, calcium, copper, zinc, and magnesium. At the time of this publication, the only treatment of CeD is a strict GFD, which heals the small intestinal mucosa, leading to improvement in absorption of these important vitamins and minerals. A GFD has important limitations, including increased lipid and fat content, and reduced amounts of micronutrients. A GFD is also the treatment of patients with NCGS and poses similar after-diet need for nutritional monitoring and supplementation. Diets rich in fiber, folate, vitamin B12, magnesium, zinc, and vitamin D should be encouraged to help promote a wide array of health needs ranging from bone health to wound healing. Gluten should be avoided in patients with CeD and diagnosed NCGS, but there are important nutritional and mineral components of wheat that can have important health consequences. For this reason, a GFD in a patient without CeD nor NCGS should not be advised.

REVIEW CRITERIA

This review is based on extensive literature search of PubMed MEDLINE (National Library of Medicine). The PubMed search string contained the following terms: celiac, gluten, nonceliac gluten insensitivity, nutritional deficiencies, vitamin B12, folate, vitamin D, bone density, or iron deficiency; and drug development. The search string was limited to Title or Abstract; language or publication date did not serve as a search criterion. Articles were reviewed for the quality of evidence and whether they brought new understanding of the association of nutritional consideration in celiac and NCGS. Citations in these articles were reviewed similarly. All cited references were available in full-text.

REFERENCES

1. Rubio-Tapia A, Ludvigsson JF, Brantner TL, et al. The prevalence of celiac disease in the United States. Am J Gastroenterol 2012;107(10):1538–44 [quiz: 1537, 1545].
2. Rubio-Tapia A, Kyle RA, Kaplan EL, et al. Increased prevalence and mortality in undiagnosed celiac disease. Gastroenterology 2009;137(1):88–93.
3. Bouziat R, Hinterleitner R, Brown JJ, et al. Reovirus infection triggers inflammatory responses to dietary antigens and development of celiac disease. Science 2017;356(6333):44–50.
4. Shewry PR, Halford NG, Belton PS, et al. The structure and properties of gluten: an elastic protein from wheat grain. Philos Trans R Soc Lond B Biol Sci 2002; 357(1418):133–42.
5. Lamacchia C, Camarca A, Picascia S, et al. Cereal-based gluten-free food: how to reconcile nutritional and technological properties of wheat proteins with safety for celiac disease patients. Nutrients 2014;6(2):575–90.
6. Lebwohl B, Ludvigsson JF, Green PH. Celiac disease and non-celiac gluten sensitivity. BMJ 2015;351:h4347.
7. AGA Institute. AGA Institute Medical Position statement on the diagnosis and management of celiac disease. Gastroenterology 2006;131(6):1977–80.
8. Schumann M, Siegmund B, Schulzke JD, et al. Celiac disease: role of the epithelial barrier. Cell Mol Gastroenterol Hepatol 2017;3(2):150–62.
9. Clevers HC, Bevins CL. Paneth cells: maestros of the small intestinal crypts. Annu Rev Physiol 2013;75:289–311.
10. Ludvigsson JF, Leffler DA, Bai JC, et al. The Oslo definitions for coeliac disease and related terms. Gut 2013;62(1):43–52.
11. Schosler L, Christensen LA, Hvas CL. Symptoms and findings in adult-onset celiac disease in a historical Danish patient cohort. Scand J Gastroenterol 2016; 51(3):288–94.
12. Volta U, Bardella MT, Calabro A, et al, Study Group for Non-Celiac Gluten Sensitivity. An Italian prospective multicenter survey on patients suspected of having non-celiac gluten sensitivity. BMC Med 2014;12:85.
13. Fasano A, Sapone A, Zevallos V, et al. Nonceliac gluten sensitivity. Gastroenterology 2015;148(6):1195–204.
14. Escudero-Hernandez C, Pena AS, Bernardo D. Immunogenetic pathogenesis of celiac disease and non-celiac gluten sensitivity. Curr Gastroenterol Rep 2016; 18(7):36.
15. Volta U, Caio G, De Giorgio R, et al. Non-celiac gluten sensitivity: a work-in-progress entity in the spectrum of wheat-related disorders. Best Pract Res Clin Gastroenterol 2015;29(3):477–91.
16. Zanini B, Basche R, Ferraresi A, et al. Randomised clinical study: gluten challenge induces symptom recurrence in only a minority of patients who meet clinical criteria for non-coeliac gluten sensitivity. Aliment Pharmacol Ther 2015; 42(8):968–76.

17. Schuppan D, Pickert G, Ashfaq-Khan M, et al. Non-celiac wheat sensitivity: differential diagnosis, triggers and implications. Best Pract Res Clin Gastroenterol 2015;29(3):469–76.

18. Sapone A, Lammers KM, Casolaro V, et al. Divergence of gut permeability and mucosal immune gene expression in two gluten-associated conditions: celiac disease and gluten sensitivity. BMC Med 2011;9:23.

19. Brottveit M, Beitnes AC, Tollefsen S, et al. Mucosal cytokine response after short-term gluten challenge in celiac disease and non-celiac gluten sensitivity. Am J Gastroenterol 2013;108(5):842–50.

20. Hollon J, Puppa EL, Greenwald B, et al. Effect of gliadin on permeability of intestinal biopsy explants from celiac disease patients and patients with non-celiac gluten sensitivity. Nutrients 2015;7(3):1565–76.

21. Carroccio A, Soresi M, D'Alcamo A, et al. Risk of low bone mineral density and low body mass index in patients with non-celiac wheat-sensitivity: a prospective observation study. BMC Med 2014;12:230.

22. Carroccio A, D'Alcamo A, Cavataio F, et al. High proportions of people with non-celiac wheat sensitivity have autoimmune disease or antinuclear antibodies. Gastroenterology 2015;149(3):596–603.e1.

23. Carroccio A, D'Alcamo A, Iacono G, et al. Persistence of nonceliac wheat sensitivity, based on long-term follow-up. Gastroenterology 2017;153(1):56–8.e3.

24. Bascunan KA, Vespa MC, Araya M. Celiac disease: understanding the gluten-free diet. Eur J Nutr 2017;56(2):449–59.

25. Fric P, Gabrovska D, Nevoral J. Celiac disease, gluten-free diet, and oats. Nutr Rev 2011;69(2):107–15.

26. Rashid M, Butzner D, Burrows V, et al. Consumption of pure oats by individuals with celiac disease: a position statement by the Canadian Celiac Association. Can J Gastroenterol 2007;21(10):649–51.

27. Van De Kamer JH, Weijers HA, Dicke WK. Coeliac disease. IV. An investigation into the injurious constituents of wheat in connection with their action on patients with coeliac disease. Acta Paediatr 1953;42(3):223–31.

28. Baker PG, Read AE. Oats and barley toxicity in coeliac patients. Postgrad Med J 1976;52(607):264–8.

29. Pinto-Sanchez MI, Causada-Calo N, Bercik P, et al. Safety of adding oats to a gluten-free diet for patients with celiac disease: systematic review and meta-analysis of clinical and observational studies. Gastroenterology 2017;153(2):395–409.e3.

30. Comino I, Moreno Mde L, Sousa C. Role of oats in celiac disease. World J Gastroenterol 2015;21(41):11825–31.

31. Tapsas D, Falth-Magnusson K, Hogberg L, et al. Swedish children with celiac disease comply well with a gluten-free diet, and most include oats without reporting any adverse effects: a long-term follow-up study. Nutr Res 2014;34(5):436–41.

32. Murray JA. Celiac disease in patients with an affected member, type 1 diabetes, iron-deficiency, or osteoporosis? Gastroenterology 2005;128(4 Suppl 1):S52–6.

33. Farrell RJ, Kelly CP. Celiac sprue. N Engl J Med 2002;346(3):180–8.

34. Ransford RA, Hayes M, Palmer M, et al. A controlled, prospective screening study of celiac disease presenting as iron deficiency anemia. J Clin Gastroenterol 2002;35(3):228–33.

35. Lo W, Sano K, Lebwohl B, et al. Changing presentation of adult celiac disease. Dig Dis Sci 2003;48(2):395–8.

36. de Vizia B, Poggi V, Conenna R, et al. Iron absorption and iron deficiency in infants and children with gastrointestinal diseases. J Pediatr Gastroenterol Nutr 1992;14(1):21–6.
37. Oxford EC, Nguyen DD, Sauk J, et al. Impact of coexistent celiac disease on phenotype and natural history of inflammatory bowel diseases. Am J Gastroenterol 2013;108(7):1123–9.
38. Bergamaschi G, Markopoulos K, Albertini R, et al. Anemia of chronic disease and defective erythropoietin production in patients with celiac disease. Haematologica 2008;93(12):1785–91.
39. Bermejo F, Garcia-Lopez S. A guide to diagnosis of iron deficiency and iron deficiency anemia in digestive diseases. World J Gastroenterol 2009;15(37): 4638–43.
40. Dickey W, Ward M, Whittle CR, et al. Homocysteine and related B-vitamin status in coeliac disease: effects of gluten exclusion and histological recovery. Scand J Gastroenterol 2008;43(6):682–8.
41. Vilppula A, Kaukinen K, Luostarinen L, et al. Clinical benefit of gluten-free diet in screen-detected older celiac disease patients. BMC Gastroenterol 2011;11:136.
42. Saibeni S, Lecchi A, Meucci G, et al. Prevalence of hyperhomocysteinemia in adult gluten-sensitive enteropathy at diagnosis: role of B12, folate, and genetics. Clin Gastroenterol Hepatol 2005;3(6):574–80.
43. Thompson T. Folate, iron, and dietary fiber contents of the gluten-free diet. J Am Diet Assoc 2000;100(11):1389–96.
44. Hallert C, Grant C, Grehn S, et al. Evidence of poor vitamin status in coeliac patients on a gluten-free diet for 10 years. Aliment Pharmacol Ther 2002;16(7): 1333–9.
45. Valente FX, Campos Tdo N, Moraes LF, et al. B vitamins related to homocysteine metabolism in adults celiac disease patients: a cross-sectional study. Nutr J 2015;14:110.
46. Hallert C, Svensson M, Tholstrup J, et al. Clinical trial: B vitamins improve health in patients with coeliac disease living on a gluten-free diet. Aliment Pharmacol Ther 2009;29(8):811–6.
47. Bode S, Gudmand-Hoyer E. Symptoms and haematologic features in consecutive adult coeliac patients. Scand J Gastroenterol 1996;31(1):54–60.
48. Halfdanarson TR, Litzow MR, Murray JA. Hematologic manifestations of celiac disease. Blood 2007;109(2):412–21.
49. Dahele A, Ghosh S. Vitamin B12 deficiency in untreated celiac disease. Am J Gastroenterol 2001;96(3):745–50.
50. Stabler SP. Clinical practice. Vitamin B12 deficiency. N Engl J Med 2013;368(2): 149–60.
51. Battault S, Whiting SJ, Peltier SL, et al. Vitamin D metabolism, functions and needs: from science to health claims. Eur J Nutr 2013;52(2):429–41.
52. Barton SH, Kelly DG, Murray JA. Nutritional deficiencies in celiac disease. Gastroenterol Clin North Am 2007;36(1):93–108, vi.
53. Blazina S, Bratanic N, Campa AS, et al. Bone mineral density and importance of strict gluten-free diet in children and adolescents with celiac disease. Bone 2010;47(3):598–603.
54. Vasquez H, Mazure R, Gonzalez D, et al. Risk of fractures in celiac disease patients: a cross-sectional, case-control study. Am J Gastroenterol 2000;95(1): 183–9.

55. Posthumus L, Al-Toma A. Duodenal histopathology and laboratory deficiencies related to bone metabolism in coeliac disease. Eur J Gastroenterol Hepatol 2017;29(8):897–903.
56. Kemppainen T, Kroger H, Janatuinen E, et al. Osteoporosis in adult patients with celiac disease. Bone 1999;24(3):249–55.
57. Garcia-Manzanares A, Tenias JM, Lucendo AJ. Bone mineral density directly correlates with duodenal Marsh stage in newly diagnosed adult celiac patients. Scand J Gastroenterol 2012;47(8–9):927–36.
58. Mora S, Barera G, Beccio S, et al. A prospective, longitudinal study of the long-term effect of treatment on bone density in children with celiac disease. J Pediatr 2001;139(4):516–21.
59. Barera G, Mora S, Brambilla P, et al. Body composition in children with celiac disease and the effects of a gluten-free diet: a prospective case-control study. Am J Clin Nutr 2000;72(1):71–5.
60. Kavak US, Yuce A, Kocak N, et al. Bone mineral density in children with un-treated and treated celiac disease. J Pediatr Gastroenterol Nutr 2003;37(4): 434–6.
61. Keaveny AP, Freaney R, McKenna MJ, et al. Bone remodeling indices and sec-ondary hyperparathyroidism in celiac disease. Am J Gastroenterol 1996;91(6): 1226–31.
62. Krupa-Kozak U. Pathologic bone alterations in celiac disease: etiology, epidemi-ology, and treatment. Nutrition 2014;30(1):16–24.
63. Pistorius LR, Sweidan WH, Purdie DW, et al. Coeliac disease and bone mineral density in adult female patients. Gut 1995;37(5):639–42.
64. Walters JR, Banks LM, Butcher GP, et al. Detection of low bone mineral density by dual energy x ray absorptiometry in unsuspected suboptimally treated coeliac disease. Gut 1995;37(2):220–4.
65. Jeejeebhoy K. Zinc: an essential trace element for parenteral nutrition. Gastro-enterology 2009;137(5 Suppl):S7–12.
66. Tipton IH, Cook MJ. Trace elements in human tissue. II. Adult subjects from the United States. Health Phys 1963;9:103–45.
67. Crofton RW, Glover SC, Ewen SW, et al. Zinc absorption in celiac disease and dermatitis herpetiformis: a test of small intestinal function. Am J Clin Nutr 1983;38(5):706–12.
68. Solomons NW, Rosenberg IH, Sandstead HH. Zinc nutrition in celiac sprue. Am J Clin Nutr 1976;29(4):371–5.
69. Singhal N, Alam S, Sherwani R, et al. Serum zinc levels in celiac disease. Indian Pediatr 2008;45(4):319–21.
70. Hambidge KM, Hambidge C, Jacobs M, et al. Low levels of zinc in hair, anorexia, poor growth, and hypogeusia in children. Pediatr Res 1972;6(12): 868–74.
71. Hallbook T, Lanner E. Serum-zinc and healing of venous leg ulcers. Lancet 1972;2(7781):780–2.
72. Sandstead HH, Prasad AS, Schulert AR, et al. Human zinc deficiency, endocrine manifestations and response to treatment. Am J Clin Nutr 1967;20(5):422–42.
73. Rujner J, Socha J, Syczewska M, et al. Magnesium status in children and ado-lescents with coeliac disease without malabsorption symptoms. Clin Nutr 2004; 23(5):1074–9.
74. Musso CG. Magnesium metabolism in health and disease. Int Urol Nephrol 2009;41(2):357–62.

75. Kelepouris E, Agus ZS. Hypomagnesemia: renal magnesium handling. Semin Nephrol 1998;18(1):58–73.
76. Graham LA, Caesar JJ, Burgen AS. Gastrointestinal absorption and excretion of Mg 28 in man. Metabolism 1960;9:646–59.
77. Kupper C. Dietary guidelines and implementation for celiac disease. Gastroenterology 2005;128(4 Suppl 1):S121–7.
78. Shepherd SJ, Gibson PR. Nutritional inadequacies of the gluten-free diet in both recently-diagnosed and long-term patients with coeliac disease. J Hum Nutr Diet 2013;26(4):349–58.
79. Kumar N, Low PA. Myeloneuropathy and anemia due to copper malabsorption. J Neurol 2004;251(6):747–9.
80. Goodman BP, Mistry DH, Pasha SF, et al. Copper deficiency myeloneuropathy due to occult celiac disease. Neurologist 2009;15(6):355–6.
81. Halfdanarson TR, Kumar N, Hogan WJ, et al. Copper deficiency in celiac disease. J Clin Gastroenterol 2009;43(2):162–4.
82. Reinken L, Zieglauer H. Vitamin B-6 absorption in children with acute celiac disease and in control subjects. J Nutr 1978;108(10):1562–5.
83. Reinken L, Zieglauer H, Berger H. Vitamin B6 nutriture of children with acute celiac disease, celiac disease in remission, and of children with normal duodenal mucosa. Am J Clin Nutr 1976;29(7):750–3.
84. Dickey W, Kearney N. Overweight in celiac disease: prevalence, clinical characteristics, and effect of a gluten-free diet. Am J Gastroenterol 2006;101(10): 2356–9.
85. Thompson T. Thiamin, riboflavin, and niacin contents of the gluten-free diet: is there cause for concern? J Am Diet Assoc 1999;99(7):858–62.
86. Zuccotti G, Fabiano V, Dilillo D, et al. Intakes of nutrients in Italian children with celiac disease and the role of commercially available gluten-free products. J Hum Nutr Diet 2013;26(5):436–44.
87. Bardella MT, Fredella C, Prampolini L, et al. Body composition and dietary intakes in adult celiac disease patients consuming a strict gluten-free diet. Am J Clin Nutr 2000;72(4):937–9.
88. Mariani P, Viti MG, Montuori M, et al. The gluten-free diet: a nutritional risk factor for adolescents with celiac disease? J Pediatr Gastroenterol Nutr 1998;27(5): 519–23.
89. Penagini F, Dilillo D, Meneghin F, et al. Gluten-free diet in children: an approach to a nutritionally adequate and balanced diet. Nutrients 2013;5(11):4553–65.
90. Segura ME, Rosell CM. Chemical composition and starch digestibility of different gluten-free breads. Plant Foods Hum Nutr 2011;66(3):224–30.
91. Edwards George JB, Leffler DA, Dennis MD, et al. Psychological correlates of gluten-free diet adherence in adults with celiac disease. J Clin Gastroenterol 2009;43(4):301–6.
92. Ludvigsson JF, James S, Askling J, et al. Nationwide cohort study of risk of ischemic heart disease in patients with celiac disease. Circulation 2011; 123(5):483–90.
93. Holmes GK, Prior P, Lane MR, et al. Malignancy in coeliac disease–effect of a gluten free diet. Gut 1989;30(3):333–8.
94. Elfstrom P, Granath F, Ekstrom Smedby K, et al. Risk of lymphoproliferative malignancy in relation to small intestinal histopathology among patients with celiac disease. J Natl Cancer Inst 2011;103(5):436–44.

95. Scaramuzza AE, Mantegazza C, Bosetti A, et al. Type 1 diabetes and celiac disease: the effects of gluten free diet on metabolic control. World J Diabetes 2013; 4(4):130–4.

96. Soares FL, de Oliveira Matoso R, Teixeira LG, et al. Gluten-free diet reduces adiposity, inflammation and insulin resistance associated with the induction of PPAR-alpha and PPAR-gamma expression. J Nutr Biochem 2013;24(6): 1105–11.

97. Schiltz B, Minich DM, Lerman RH, et al. A science-based, clinically tested dietary approach for the metabolic syndrome. Metab Syndr Relat Disord 2009;7(3): 187–92.

98. Peters SL, Biesiekierski JR, Yelland GW, et al. Randomised clinical trial: gluten may cause depression in subjects with non-coeliac gluten sensitivity - an exploratory clinical study. Aliment Pharmacol Ther 2014;39(10):1104–12.

99. Lebwohl B, Cao Y, Zong G, et al. Long term gluten consumption in adults without celiac disease and risk of coronary heart disease: prospective cohort study. BMJ 2017;357:j1892.

100. McCarville JL, Nisemblat Y, Galipeau HJ, et al. BL-7010 demonstrates specific binding to gliadin and reduces gluten-associated pathology in a chronic mouse model of gliadin sensitivity. PLoS One 2014;9(11):e109972.

101. Attarwala H, Clausen V, Chaturvedi P, et al. Cosilencing intestinal transglutaminase-2 and interleukin-15 using gelatin-based nanoparticles in an in vitro model of celiac disease. Mol Pharm 2017;14(9):3036–44.

102. Abadie V, Jabri B. IL-15: a central regulator of celiac disease immunopathology. Immunol Rev 2014;260(1):221–34.

103. Lahdeaho ML, Kaukinen K, Laurila K, et al. Glutenase ALV003 attenuates gluten-induced mucosal injury in patients with celiac disease. Gastroenterology 2014; 146(7):1649–58.

104. Murray JA, Kelly CP, Green PH, et al. No difference between latiglutenase and placebo in reducing villous atrophy or improving symptoms in patients with symptomatic celiac disease. Gastroenterology 2017;152(4):787–98.e2.

105. Gopalakrishnan S, Durai M, Kitchens K, et al. Larazotide acetate regulates epithelial tight junctions in vitro and in vivo. Peptides 2012;35(1):86–94.

106. Gopalakrishnan S, Tripathi A, Tamiz AP, et al. Larazotide acetate promotes tight junction assembly in epithelial cells. Peptides 2012;35(1):95–101.

107. Leffler DA, Kelly CP, Green PH, et al. Larazotide acetate for persistent symptoms of celiac disease despite a gluten-free diet: a randomized controlled trial. Gastroenterology 2015;148(7):1311–9.e6.

108. Goel G, King T, Daveson AJ, et al. Epitope-specific immunotherapy targeting CD4-positive T cells in coeliac disease: two randomised, double-blind, placebo-controlled phase 1 studies. Lancet Gastroenterol Hepatol 2017;2(7): 479–93.

Nutritional Interventions in the Patient with Inflammatory Bowel Disease

Berkeley N. Limketkai, MD, PhD[a],*, Andrea Wolf, RD[b],
Alyssa M. Parian, MD[c]

KEYWORDS

- Diet • Prebiotics • Probiotics • Dietary supplements • Microbiome
- Clinical remission • Crohn's disease • Ulcerative colitis

KEY POINTS

- Foods that are consumed have effects on the intestinal microbiome and inflammation.
- There are sparse data on the effects of different diets on disease activity in inflammatory bowel disease.
- Nonetheless, there is emerging evidence to suggest that carbohydrate restriction may improve symptoms and inflammation.
- Curcumin may be effective for the maintenance of remission in ulcerative colitis.
- Probiotics (eg, VSL#3) may help induce remission in ulcerative colitis and prevent pouchitis.

INTRODUCTION

Inflammatory bowel disease (IBD), which primarily comprises Crohn disease (CD) and ulcerative colitis (UC), is a chronic relapsing and remitting inflammatory disorder of the gastrointestinal tract. The etiologic factors of IBD are currently unclear, although it is believed to stem from interactions between an individual's underlying genetic risk, the intestinal microbiome, and environmental factors. Because nutrients play a strong role in shaping the intestinal microbiome and may themselves modify the inflammatory response, the diet has emerged as a potential factor that influences IBD pathogenesis and activity.[1,2] Moreover, the increased risk of IBD among populations migrating to western countries[3,4] and the increasing incidence of IBD in regions that have

Disclosure Statement: The authors have nothing they wish to disclose.
[a] Division of Gastroenterology and Hepatology, Stanford University School of Medicine, 300 Pasteur Drive, Alway M211, Stanford, CA 94305, USA; [b] Department of Clinical Nutrition, Stanford Health Care, Stanford, 300 Pasteur Drive, Palo Alto, CA 94305, USA; [c] Division of Gastroenterology and Hepatology, Johns Hopkins University School of Medicine, 1800 Orleans Street, Baltimore, MD 21287, USA
* Corresponding author.
E-mail address: berkeley.limketkai@gmail.com

Gastroenterol Clin N Am 47 (2018) 155–177
https://doi.org/10.1016/j.gtc.2017.09.007
0889-8553/18/© 2017 Elsevier Inc. All rights reserved.

traditionally had a low incidence of IBD[5] have further led some investigators to suspect the westernization of diets to be an etiologic factor.

The principal premise of antiinflammatory diets used for the treatment of IBD relies on the reduction of proinflammatory food types and/or increase in food types thought to promote a favorable intestinal microbiota. For instance, the specific carbohydrate diet (SCD) and gluten-free diet recommend the elimination of certain carbohydrates and gluten, respectively, due to their suspected antigenic or proinflammatory effects. Diets that recommend a reduction in fat or meat intake relate to the knowledge that omega-6 fatty acids (found in red meats, fried fast foods, and pastries) are metabolic precursors of proinflammatory prostaglandins. On the other hand, other diets may recommend increased consumption of fish or omega-3 fatty acids because they are precursors of less inflammatory prostaglandins. Although the precise relationship between the intestinal microbial composition and inflammation is still unknown, the hypothesized relationship between the diet and the microbiome fuels recommendations to consume plant-based diets. This has also led to the investigation of probiotics and fecal microbiota transplantation as potential treatments for IBD. This article discusses the role of diverse diets and dietary supplements in the treatment of IBD.

ORAL DIETS
Specific Carbohydrate Diet

The SCD was initially conceived by Dr Sidney Haas, an American pediatrician, in the 1920s for the treatment of celiac disease.[6] The diet was later popularized in the 1980s by Canadian biochemist Elaine Gottschall in her book, *Breaking the Vicious Cycle*, after her 8-year-old daughter with UC was successfully treated with the SCD.[7] The SCD recommends the exclusion of complex carbohydrates in favor of monosaccharides that are purportedly easier for humans to digest and absorb. Consequently, fewer carbohydrates are available for bacterial fermentation, bacterial growth, and intestinal injury. The SCD is a rigid diet allowing unprocessed meats, poultry, eggs, fish, fruits, vegetables, all fats and oils, homemade fermented yogurts, and honey as a sweetener (**Table 1**).

A retrospective case series reported an improvement in clinical symptoms and laboratory indices in 7 children with active CD who were treated with the SCD for 5 to

Table 1 Permitted and prohibited foods in the specific carbohydrate diet	
Permitted Foods	**Prohibited Foods**
Unprocessed meats, poultry, eggs and fish	Preserved, packaged, deli meats
Most fresh fruits and vegetables (high amylose to amylopectin ratio)	Canned fruits or vegetables, starchy vegetables (eg, potatoes and yams)
All fats and oils including butter	
Aged cheeses >30 d	Soft cheeses (eg, cream, ricotta, mozzarella and cottage cheese)
Lactose free yogurt	Milk, store bought yogurts
Honey	Sugar, maple syrup, agave, artificial sweeteners
Legumes (lentils and most beans)	Grains (eg, wheat, rye, oats, rice, quinoa)
Nuts (almonds, pecans, peanuts, cashews, walnuts)	
Weak tea or coffee, water, club soda, scotch, gin, vodka, bourbon	Juice, soda, sweet wines, flavored liqueurs, beer

30 months.[8] In a prospective study of 9 children with active CD treated with the SCD, symptom scores and video capsule endoscopy findings significantly improved.[9] Seven subjects completed 52 weeks of the study and showed continued clinical improvement, whereas 2 subjects showed sustained mucosal healing.

Some evidence suggests that the liberalization of the SCD may be possible after induction of remission. One case report describes a 15-year-old boy with ileocolonic CD who weaned off pharmacotherapies after induction of remission with exclusive enteral nutrition (EEN), followed by maintenance of remission with the SCD.[10] After 6 months of a strict SCD, he added 1 non-SCD meal per week and continued to maintain remission for the subsequent 3 months of follow-up. Another case series of 11 children with CD found that after a mean of 7.7 months on the SCD, they were able to maintain clinical remission and adequate growth rates during the mean 4.2 months of follow-up despite adding a prohibited ingredient to their daily diet or a prohibited meal or snack periodically.[11] Evidence for the use of the SCD in adults is less robust. A survey of 50 adults with IBD (36 CD, 9 UC, 5 IBD undetermined) self-treated with the SCD reported a 66% clinical remission after a mean diet duration of 9.9 months.[12] Several subjects also reported the ability to stop corticosteroid therapy while on the SCD. An online survey was conducted on 417 IBD patients following the SCD to determine their perception of the diet.[13] After 12 months, most respondents perceived a clinical benefit with 42% self-reporting clinical remission with improvement in laboratory values.

The initial data of the SCD are promising but larger placebo-controlled studies are needed. The strict nature of the diet may decrease compliance and patient satisfaction as a long-term therapy, although liberalization of the diet after remission potentially seems to be possible.

Diet Low in Fermentable Carbohydrates

Fermentable oligosaccharides, disaccharides, monosaccharides, and polyols (FODMAPs) are short-chain carbohydrates that are poorly absorbed in the small intestine, leading to increased water secretion, bacterial fermentation, and the production of excess gas particles (ie, hydrogen, carbon dioxide, and methane).[14,15] These processes, in turn, lead to luminal distention, abdominal discomfort, dysbiosis, intestinal mucosal injury, and altered bowel habits. Although the putative mechanisms of effect for the low-FODMAP diet and SCD are similar, the former restricts simple carbohydrates and the latter favors simple carbohydrates.

A low-FODMAP diet involves the removal of high-FODMAP–containing foods from the diet for several weeks, followed by single reintroduction of foods with a food diary to identify individual triggers (**Table 2**). Research on FODMAP restriction has predominantly focused on the treatment of irritable bowel syndrome, although there are some data on its use in IBD.[16–20]

A randomized trial that serially exposed IBD subjects with functional gastrointestinal symptoms to a variety of FODMAPs and a glucose placebo found that fructans, but not galactooligosaccharides or sorbitol, aggravated their symptoms.[21] Several uncontrolled, retrospective studies have additionally shown the low-FODMAP diet to significantly improve gastrointestinal symptoms in IBD subjects.[22–25] One small crossover study of 8 subjects also found the low-FODMAP diet improved abdominal pain and diarrhea in IBD, but it did not affect fecal calprotectin levels.[26] Given that irritable bowel syndrome is present in greater than 30% of subjects with IBD,[27] these findings of benefit are not surprising. There are, nonetheless, some caveats. First, studies evaluating the effects of a low-FODMAP diet in the treatment of IBD have so far focused on improvement of symptoms and not on the control of inflammation, thus limiting the

Table 2
Foods containing low and high amounts of fermentable oligosaccharides, disaccharides, monosaccharides, and polyols

Food Group	Low-FODMAP Foods to Eat	High-FODMAP Foods to Avoid
Vegetables	Bamboo shoots, bok choy, carrots, celery, chives, eggplant, green beans, kale, leafy greens, parsnips, radish, red bell pepper, squash, sweet potato, tomatoes, white potato, zucchini	Artichokes, asparagus, beets, broccoli, Brussels sprouts, cabbage, cauliflower, fennel, garlic, leeks, mushrooms, onions, scallions
Fruits	Bananas (ripe), blueberries, cantaloupe, grapefruit, grapes, honeydew, kiwi, lemons, limes, oranges, papaya, passion fruit, pineapple, raspberries, rhubarb, strawberries * Avoid large amounts of any fruit	Apples, avocados, blackberries, dried fruits, fruit juice, stone fruits (apricots, cherries, mango, nectarines, peaches, plums, prunes), pears, persimmons, plums, watermelon
Dairy and dairy alternatives	Butter, lactose-free dairy products, hard or aged cheeses, almond milk, hemp milk, rice milk	Cow's milk, yogurt, ice cream, cottage cheese, ricotta cheese, soy milk (soy beans)
Grains	Wheat free grains or wheat free flours, gluten free products, quinoa, rice, millet, cornmeal, buckwheat, oatmeal (1/2 cup), popcorn, rice, tortillas chips	Wheat-containing foods (eg, bread, cereal, pasta), barley, rye, bran, couscous, granola, semolina, spelt
Nuts, seeds, and legumes	Small amount of most nuts or nut butters, sesame seeds, sunflower seeds, pumpkin seeds, firm tofu	Pistachios, cashews, almonds, beans, hummus, lentils, silken tofu, flaxseeds
Beverages	Espresso, coffee, green tea, peppermint tea, black tea	Drinks with high-fructose corn syrup, agave, fruit juices, instant coffee, chamomile tea, fennel tea, coconut water
Meat, protein	Eggs, beef, lamb, chicken, turkey, fish	Check ingredients for processed meats
Sweeteners	Granulated sugar, evaporated can juice, brown sugar, brown rice syrup, pure maple syrup, stevia, aspartame, saccharin sucralose	Agave, high fructose corn syrup, honey, inulin, isomalt, maltitol, mannitol, sorbitol, xylitol

ability to determine whether it would be helpful for the treatment of IBD. Second, a low-FODMAP diet can alter the microbiome toward dysbiosis with decreased butyrate-producing *Clostridium* cluster XIVa and *Akkermansia muciniphila*, and increased mucus-degrading *Ruminococcus torques*.[26,28] Third, as with all restrictive diets, there is a concern for undernutrition, especially in the IBD population already at risk for malnutrition. Patients who are recommended this diet should be followed closely with a nutritionist to ensure adequate nutrient intake.

Gluten-Free Diet

The gluten-free diet eliminates gliadin protein found in wheat, barley, rye, and other grains. This diet has traditionally been used for patients with celiac disease and, more recently, among individuals with nonceliac gluten sensitivity. Although individuals with nonceliac gluten sensitivity do not demonstrate abnormal genetic, serologic, or immunologic markers when consuming gluten, gluten restriction can lead to an improvement of gastrointestinal symptoms.[29] A putative mechanism for this effect involves the detrimental effect of gliadin on intestinal epithelial integrity.[30] Alternatively, the development of symptoms may instead stem from the nongliadin components that typically exist in gluten-containing foods, such as FODMAPs, amylase trypsin inhibitors, or wheat germ agglutinins.[31]

In an American cross-sectional study of 1647 subjects with IBD, 0.6% of subjects were diagnosed with celiac disease and 4.9% reported nonceliac gluten sensitivity.[32] Among the participants, 19.1% reported having tried a gluten-free diet and 8.2% had remained on the diet. Of those who had been on a gluten-free diet, 65.6% reported an improvement in at least 1 gastrointestinal symptom (ie, bloating, diarrhea, abdominal pain, nausea, and fatigue), 38.3% reported fewer or less severe flares, and 23.6% reported requiring fewer medications for their IBD. In a British cross-sectional study of 145 IBD subjects, 27.6% reported nonceliac gluten sensitivity.[33] Those with CD and nonceliac gluten sensitivity were more likely to have stricturing disease and greater disease activity. Those with UC and nonceliac gluten sensitivity had no difference in disease extent or severity of colitis. These studies suggest a potential benefit of the gluten-free diet for IBD; however, randomized trials are lacking and there are no studies to link gluten consumption with inflammatory activity in IBD.

Antiinflammatory Diet

An early concept of an antiinflammatory diet was The Zone Diet, which focused on balancing macronutrient ratios to improve cortisol and insulin levels. Other antiinflammatory diets that followed would focus on avoiding macronutrients with theoretic proinflammatory properties in favor of those with theoretic antiinflammatory properties. General principles include the increased consumption of fruits and vegetables, plant-based proteins, some lean animal protein, fatty fish, fiber, and certain herbs and spices.[34] Whole grains can be consumed in moderation. Olive oil could be used as a fat source. There should also be reduction in refined carbohydrates. The foods should focus on quality rather than quantity.

The antiinflammatory diet for IBD (IBD-AID) was derived from the SCD and follows the same assumptions that consumption of certain carbohydrates lead to dysbiosis, subsequent bowel injury, and increased intestinal permeability.[35] The 5 basic components of the IBD-AID are (1) restriction of carbohydrates (ie, lactose, refined or processed complex carbohydrates); (2) use of prebiotics and probiotics; (3) reduction of total and saturated fatty acids, hydrogenated oils, and increase of omega-3 fatty acids; (4) identification of missing nutrients and intolerances; and (5) reduction of food texture (ie, grinding, cooking) and intact fiber to improve absorption. In a case series published by the group that developed the IBD-AID, the diet was offered to 40 consecutive subjects with IBD. Of the 11 participants who met study eligibility criteria and had complete data, all were able to deescalate their drug therapy while on the diet. Among the 8 CD participants, the baseline Harvey-Bradshaw Index (HBI) score declined from a mean of 11 to 1.5. Among the 3 UC participants, the modified Truelove and Witts Severity Index declined from a mean of 7 to 0. However, with such a small sample size and in the absence of good controls, the data are insufficient to make any recommendations at this time.

Immunoglobulin-G4–Guided Exclusion Diet

A targeted exclusion diet has been investigated in subjects with IBD in a few studies based on serum immunoglobulin (Ig)-G4 antibody titers. In a British study of 40 subjects with active CD, serum IgG4 levels were measured for 14 common foods (egg white, egg yolk, potato, tomato, cheddar cheese, rice, beef, lamb pork, soy, peanuts, wheat, yeast, and chicken). The 4 most immunoreactive foods were excluded from the diet for 4 weeks. Of the 29 participants who completed the study, 90% reported an improvement in symptoms, such as a decline in mean daily bowel movements from 4 to 2, reduction in pain rating from 0.71 to 0.43, reduction in extraintestinal manifestations, and increase in general wellbeing scores. There was additionally a significant decrease in erythrocyte sedimentation rate from 23 to 17 mm per hour, although the C-reactive protein (CRP) and albumin levels did not significantly change. A follow-up randomized trial of the IgG-4 guided exclusion diet was performed by the same British group. The study enrolled 96 subjects with CD and tested IgG4 antibody titers against 16 different food types (milk, peanuts, soy, shrimp, egg, tomato, pork, beef, codfish, potato, wheat, yeast, cheddar cheese, chicken, lamb, and rice). Participants randomized to the IgG4-guided exclusion diet had 4 of the most immunoreactive food types excluded from their diet for 4 weeks, whereas those randomized to a sham diet had 4 of the least immunoreactive food types excluded from their diet.[36] Of the 76 participants who completed the trial, there was a modest yet statistically significant reduction in disease activity scores and Short Inflammatory Bowel Disease Questionnaire scores. There was otherwise no difference in CRP or fecal calprotectin levels. Although these studies show some benefit with the IgG4-guided exclusion diet in symptoms among CD subjects, there is not yet any evidence of benefit at reducing inflammation.

High-Fiber Diet

Dietary fibers are carbohydrate polymers not hydrolyzed by endogenous enzymes in the small intestine.[37] Intestinal bacteria ferment the otherwise indigestible fibers into short-chain fatty acids, which then lead to several downstream benefits, such as regulation of fluid and electrolyte absorption,[38] improved mucosal barrier function,[39] favorable alterations in the intestinal microbiota,[40] and antiinflammatory properties.[41] Given these potential benefits, there has been increasing interest in the role of dietary fiber in IBD. In an analysis of the Nurses' Health Study that included 170,776 women followed over 26 years, those at the highest quintile of energy-adjusted cumulative average dietary fiber intake (24 g/d), compared with those at the lowest quintile (12 g/d), had a 40% reduction in risk of CD but not UC.[42] The reduction in risk of CD was greatest for fibers derived from fruits. Although fiber may seem to have a protective effect against CD pathogenesis, the study was not designed to address its effect on those already diagnosed with IBD.

An early retrospective study published in 1979 evaluated 32 subjects with CD who were treated with a fiber-rich, unrefined carbohydrate diet for a mean of 52 months.[43] Those in the high-fiber diet group consumed an average of 33 g per day of fiber and 39 g per day of sugar; those in the control group, who received no dietary instruction, consumed an unreported amount of fiber and an average of 90 g per day of sugar. Compared with controls, the high-fiber diet group had fewer hospitalizations (11 vs 34; $P<.01$) and shorter total lengths of stay (111 vs 533 days; $P<.01$). No subjects developed any obstructive episodes; 1 participant on the high-fiber diet group required surgery compared with 5 controls. In a dietary survey of 1619 participants in the Crohn's and Colitis Foundation Partners Internet cohort (1130 CD; 489 UC or indeterminate colitis), CD subjects at the highest quartile of fiber consumption (median 23.7 g/d) had a 40% reduced odds of having a flare than those at the lowest quartile (median 10.4 g/d), although this trend was not detected for UC or indeterminate colitis subjects (median 24.5 g/d at highest quartile and 10.8 g/d at lowest quartile).[44] A potential confounder in this observation is disease severity. CD patients with more severe disease and complications (eg, intestinal stenosis) may not tolerate fiber as well and consequently consume less fiber. In a trial of 352 subjects with quiescent or mild CD, those randomized to a high-fiber, low-sugar diet consumed an average of 28 g per day, compared with those randomized to a low-fiber, unrestricted sugar diet who consumed an average of 18 g per day.[45] The study found no difference in hospitalizations or surgeries between the 2 groups. Currently, data on the effect of a high-fiber diet on inflammation are lacking.

Low-Residue Diet

Unlike the high-fiber diet, the low-residue diet focuses on reducing poorly digested nutrients (ie, fiber) to minimize stool output. This diet is often used in CD patients with stricturing disease and patients who undergo abdominal surgery. Similarly, an elemental diet includes predigested macronutrients to facilitate absorption and reduce downstream exposure of food antigens to the intestines. Some complex proteins are also thought to be allergenic for susceptible individuals. In a Japanese study of 60 subjects with quiescent CD provided a low-residue meal at 3 doses (0–799 kcal/d; 800–1599 kcal/d; or >1600 kcal/d), those at the highest dose level had significantly lower risk of relapse.[46] Those at the 2 highest doses also had lower risk of hospitalization. An Italian study of 70 subjects with nonstricturing CD randomly assigned a low-residue diet and a normal Italian diet over a mean of 29 months did not find any difference in symptoms, need for hospitalization, or need for surgery.[47] A randomized trial that compared a 6-mercaptopurine, elemental diet, and no therapy in 95 subjects with inactive CD found greater 24-month remission rates among those who received 6-mercaptopurine (60%) or continued an elemental diet (47%), compared with those on no maintenance treatment (27%).[48] Although the low-residue diet or elemental diets are occasionally used for CD patients with stricturing disease, there are currently insufficient data to make any recommendations for the treatment of IBD.

Semivegetarian Diet

A potential disadvantage of the low-residue diet is the lack of dietary fibers that have antiinflammatory properties and benefits for colonic function.[49] Contrary to the low-residue diet, the semivegetarian diet has a high amount of fiber. In a Japanese study of 22 subjects with quiescent CD who started a semivegetarian diet and were followed for 2 years, 16 subjects (74%) were able to maintain the semivegetarian diet throughout the study period.[50] Among those who remained on the diet, 15 (94%) maintained remission, compared with the 2 of 6 (33%) who did not remain on the diet.

Mediterranean Diet

The Mediterranean diet comprises the dietary patterns typical of countries along the Mediterranean Sea, such as southern France, Italy, and Greece. The diet generally involves a high consumption of plant-based foods (eg, fruits, vegetables) and olive oil; moderate consumption of dairy products, wine, fish, and poultry; and low consumption of red meat. The diet has been promoted primarily for its benefits on cardiovascular health, although meta-analyses reveal lower inflammatory markers among individuals who consume the diet.[51] There is nonetheless a dearth of studies of the Mediterranean diet for IBD. In a small study of 6 CD subjects on a Mediterranean-inspired diet, participants experienced normalization of the microbiota after 6 weeks but no change in CRP.[52] There are ongoing clinical trials evaluating the efficacy of the Mediterranean diet for IBD.

Paleolithic Diet

The Paleolithic diet, also referred to as Paleo, is a popular, yet controversial diet based on the evolutionary theory from a hunter-gatherer society. The premise of the Paleo diet is that the human digestive tract is not equipped to handle modern refined and processed foods, which can lead to chronic inflammation.[53] Wild game meats, high in polyunsaturated fatty acids and low in saturated fat, and fresh fruits and vegetables are the focus of the diet. The Paleo diet excludes foods such as cereal grains, meats from domesticated animals, refined sugars, and dairy products. Most studies involving the Paleo diet focus on its efficacy for weight loss and overall health.[54] There are no clinical data on the effect of the Paleo diet on the management and prevention of IBD. However, grain-based fibers that are typically excluded from the Paleo diet have demonstrated therapeutic benefits for patients with UC. Moreover, the restrictive nature of the Paleo diet creates the potential for nutrient deficiencies, especially in vitamin D.

DIETARY SUPPLEMENTS
Curcumin

Curcumin is the primary active constituent of the Asian spice turmeric. It has been effective in treating a variety of inflammatory conditions, including rheumatoid arthritis, uveitis, and IBD.[55] Several animal studies have reported that curcumin inhibits colonic inflammation in mice and rats, improving experimentally induced colitis and preventing the development of colorectal cancer.[56,57] Curcumin can prevent colon inflammation and carcinogenesis by several mechanisms. Notably, it has been observed to inhibit nuclear factor kappa beta (NF-κβ), which decreases inflammation and tumor growth.[58,59] It also blocks interferon-γ signaling in colonic epithelial cells to inhibit gene expression associated with IBD.[60]

Studies involving subjects with mild to moderate UC have shown mixed results, depending on the dosage of curcumin administered. A randomized, multicenter, double-blind, placebo-controlled trial treated 43 subjects with 3 g of oral curcumin per day, resulting in significantly fewer subjects experiencing a relapse than in the placebo group (4.6% vs 20.5%).[61] A study with a similar design reported that 3 g of curcumin daily in combination with mesalamine was effective in maintaining remission among subjects with UC.[62] A 2 g dose of curcumin in combination with mesalamine was also shown to reduce clinical and endoscopic activity among patients with UC.[63] However, another randomized, double-blind, placebo-controlled trial showed that oral curcumin at a lower dosage (450 mg daily) was ineffective at inducing remission. This 8-week trial of 16 subjects treated with curcumin and 25 subjects on placebo showed no significant difference in rates of clinical response, clinical remission, mucosal healing, or treatment failure.[64] The ability of curcumin to maintain remission among patients with UC and theoretically reduce the risk of carcinogenesis, coupled with few adverse effects, makes it a promising therapy for UC. Further dose defining research is needed to conclusively determine the optimal therapeutic use of curcumin for UC.

Omega-3

Omega-3 and omega-6 fatty acids are polyunsaturated fatty acids that are defined by the location of the carbon-carbon double bond along the carbon chain: the double bond is located 3 carbons from the end in omega-3 fatty acids and 6 carbons from the end in omega-6 fatty acids. Omega-3 fatty acids are believed to possess antiinflammatory properties and have been used to treat diverse medical ailments.

By contrast, omega-6 fatty acids may be proinflammatory when consumed in excess. The ideal ratio of omega-6 to omega-3 fatty acids is 4:1, whereas the ratio in Western diets is approximately 10:1.[65]

The prevalence of UC is reportedly lower among patients who consume a diet high in omega-3 fatty acids.[66] Studies have additionally found that omega-3 fatty acid supplementation leads to a decrease in inflammatory cytokines.[67,68] However, in 2 large related randomized, controlled trials of omega-3 fatty acid supplementation for the maintenance of remission in CD, the rate of relapse was similar between the omega-3 and placebo arms.[69] In a meta-analysis of these 2 studies and 4 others, there was a slight benefit of omega-3 fatty acids in the maintenance of remission in CD. The 4 other studies had substantial heterogeneity and a high risk of bias, making these results difficult to interpret.[70] In other studies, omega-3 fatty acids may be more effective when combined with mesalamine,[71] and used for colonic disease rather than ileal disease.[72]

The efficacy of omega-3 fatty acids for the induction and maintenance of UC has also been investigated in numerous studies. When compared with sulfasalazine (2 g daily), omega-3 fatty acids (5.4 g daily) was inferior in the treatment of mild to moderate UC.[73] One of the largest studies found a corticosteroid-sparing effect in active UC subjects but did not decrease the rate of relapse.[74] A Cochrane review from 2007 did not support the use of omega-3 fatty acids for the maintenance of remission in UC based on 3 included studies.[75] Omega-3 supplementation alone does not clearly confer benefit for the induction or maintenance of IBD in the current published studies. Further studies are needed to determine the efficacy of concomitant use of omega-3 fatty acids and standard medical therapy.

Glutamine

Glutamine is a small, nonessential, abundant amino acid that becomes conditionally essential under catabolic conditions. It is the main energy source for small intestinal enterocytes,[76,77] with the small bowel accounting for 30% of whole body glutamine utilization.[76,78] In addition, glutamine is a substrate for the synthesis of glutathione, the most abundant intracellular antioxidant.[79] Animal studies show rapid development of intestinal mucosal atrophy, increased gut permeability, and mucosal hypofunction when fed a glutamine-deficient diet.[80,81] In subjects on parental nutrition, glutamine supplementation improved gut permeability, prevented intestinal atrophy, and was vital for intestinal health.[82–84] The premise of glutamine use in IBD relates to a hypothesized reduction in intestinal permeability. In a small study of 14 CD subjects with altered intestinal permeability, oral glutamine (7 g 3 times a day) did not improve permeability, disease activity scores, CRP, or nutritional status compared with placebo.[85] A pediatric study of 18 children with CD found a glutamine-enriched diet, compared with a low-glutamine diet, did not improve clinical or laboratory parameters. In fact, improvement in mean disease activity score was significantly greater in children on the low-glutamine diet.[86] Despite the importance of glutamine in the small intestine, excessive glutamine in the colon leads to increased oxidative tissue injury and possible worsening colitis.[87] Therefore, glutamine is not currently recommended for the treatment of IBD.

Vitamin D

Vitamin D is a fat-soluble hormone that possesses immunomodulatory properties and is, therefore, hypothesized to help attenuate inflammation.[88] Murine studies had shown vitamin D-deficient mice to develop diarrhea, wasting disease, and death, which were absent in vitamin D-sufficient mice.[89] Exogenous vitamin D supplementation also improved colitis in IBD mouse models.[89,90] In humans, an analysis of the Nurses' Health Study found higher predicted vitamin D levels to be associated with a lower incidence of CD but not UC.[91] Cohort studies have also shown an inverse correlation between vitamin D levels and IBD activity,[92,93] although interpretation of these findings are challenged by reverse causation: Did low vitamin D worsen IBD or vice versa? A large retrospective study of 3217 subjects with IBD found that treatment to normalize vitamin D levels was associated with a lower risk of surgery in CD but not UC.[94] However, a benefit for vitamin D has not yet been demonstrated in randomized controlled trials. The largest trial to specifically evaluate the effects of vitamin D supplementation on CD activity randomized 94 subjects in remission to either 1200 IU vitamin D_3 or placebo.[95] The vitamin D group, compared with the placebo group, experienced a lower relapse rate (13% vs 29%), although the difference was not statistically significant. A metaanalysis of individual trials does not yet exist, but is registered and underway via the Cochrane Collaboration. For the moment, a benefit from vitamin D supplementation for IBD is unclear.

Prebiotics

Prebiotics are fermentable food ingredients that promote the growth of intestinal bacteria believed to confer health benefits. In a nonrandomized, open-label trial of subjects with quiescent UC on conventional therapy, 22 participants received 20 g per day of germinated barley foodstuff (GBF), which is a mixture of insoluble protein and dietary fiber, and 37 received nothing.[96] Over a 12-month follow-up period, those who received GBF supplementation had significantly lower clinical activity indices and relapse rates. A randomized, open-label trial of 46 subjects with UC found that 30 g per day of GBF for 2 months significantly reduces abdominal pain and cramping.[97] There was otherwise no significant difference in frequency of diarrhea, degree of visible blood in stool, nausea, vomiting, and anorexia. Baseline and follow-up CRP levels were similar between both groups.

A controlled study of 22 subjects with quiescent UC examined the effects of oat bran intake on butyrate levels.[98] Participants had 60 g of oat bran (equivalent to 20 g of dietary fiber) added to their daily diet for 12 weeks. Oat bran increased mean fecal butyrate concentrations by 36% at 4 weeks, although the fecal butyrate concentrations were not significantly different from baseline at 12 weeks. The oat bran group had no increase in gastrointestinal symptoms or relapse; instead, a subgroup of subjects who originally reported abdominal pain and reflux experienced significant improvement in symptoms. Another study of 39 subjects with quiescent UC divided participants into 2 groups. One group (24) increased its fiber intake through whole wheat bread, vegetables, and a supplement of 25 g of bran; the other group (15) continued on sulfasalazine without a change in diet.[99] Four subjects withdrew from the study due to intolerance to the diet. Over the 6-month follow-up, 75% of those in the high-fiber group experienced a relapse, compared with 20% in the sulfasalazine group. Fiber supplementation may help improve gastrointestinal symptoms but is currently not recommended as monotherapy for UC.

Probiotics

Probiotics are live microorganisms that, by definition, should confer a health benefit to the host. The mechanism of effect is believed to be mediated by introduction of beneficial bacteria to the intestinal microbiome.[100] Unfortunately, probiotics have so far been shown to be ineffective in inducing remission, maintaining remission,[101] and preventing postoperative recurrence of CD.[102,103] The data are nonetheless more promising in the treatment of UC. VSL#3, a multistrain probiotic, has been shown to induce remission in UC patients with mild to moderate disease activity.[104] Concomitant use of VSL#3 with standard therapy increases the rate of remission compared with standard therapy alone.[105–107] When compared to mesalamine, the probiotic *Escherichia coli Nissle 1917* was noninferior in maintaining remission in mild to moderate UC.[108,109] Another probiotic, *Lactobacillus GG*, was effective in prolonging the amount of time in remission in UC patients.[110] *Saccharomyces boulardii*, a probiotic strain of yeast, was found to improve clinical symptoms of UC when added to mesalamine therapy.[111]

The use of probiotics, specifically VSL#3, is most supported for the prevention of pouchitis in UC patients.[101,112] A randomized, placebo-controlled study of UC subjects with pouchitis showed an 85% decrease in relapse rates in subjects taking VSL#3.[113] Another study found VSL#3 was effective in the primary prevention of pouchitis in UC subjects.[114] A real-world experience published by the Cleveland Clinic reported that only 6 out of 31 subjects remained on VSL#3 therapy after 8 months. The rest had discontinued therapy due to disease recurrence or the development of adverse effects.[115] Overall, probiotics do not seem to have a role in the treatment of CD but may be efficacious in UC and pouchitis. Multiple studies have reported good safety data with use of probiotics; however, the cost, especially of VSL#3, could be prohibitive for many patients.

ENTERAL NUTRITION

EEN is the use of enteral nutrition (EN) formulae as the sole source of nutrition. Some hypothesized mechanisms include reduced exposure to antigens found in food, immunomodulatory properties, improvement of intestinal permeability, and alteration in the gut microbiota.[116–119] Several randomized trials have shown EEN to be as effective as corticosteroids for induction of remission in up to 85% of children with CD.[120] Although EN may also be effective for adults with active CD, a systematic review by the Cochrane Collaboration found it to be less effective than corticosteroids.[121] There was no difference in efficacy among elemental, semielemental, or polymeric EN formulations. The European Crohn's and Colitis Organisation (ECCO) recommends EEN use as a first-line choice for the induction of remission in pediatric CD.[122] Guidelines from the European Society for Clinical Nutrition and Metabolism (ESPEN) also consider it a first-line therapy in children with active CD and recommend its use as sole therapy in adults for whom corticosteroids may not be feasible.[123] However, the challenges for routine use in adults are long-term palatability and, alternatively, cosmetic considerations with nasogastric tube feeding.[124]

EEN also demonstrated potential efficacy in the closure of enterocutaneous fistulae. In a prospective study of 41 Chinese adults with stricturing or fistulizing CD who were administered EEN for 3 months, 81% achieved clinical remission and 75% experienced enterocutaneous fistula closure.[125] Another prospective study of 48 Chinese CD subjects with enterocutaneous fistulae who were administered a peptide-based EEN via nasogastric tube for 3 months showed a 63% closure rate.[126] However, the long-term effects, particularly after discontinuation of EEN, are unknown.

Given the challenges of EEN intake, the use of partial EN has been explored. The data for its efficacy in the induction of remission are inconsistent. A case series of 40 Israeli children and adolescents with active CD who received partial EN and a prescribed exclusion diet achieved a 68% remission rate after 6 weeks.[127] Another case series from the same investigators found partial EN to be effective for induction of remission after 6 weeks in 62% of 21 children who had previously failed biologic therapy.[128] There may have been 5 subjects who failed biologic therapy included in both retrospective reports. However, in a randomized trial

Table 3
Diets and treatment of inflammatory bowel disease

Diet	Premise	Components	Evidence of Efficacy
Specific carbohydrate diet	• Complex carbohydrates are less easily digested and absorbed, which facilitates bacterial fermentation, bacterial growth, and intestinal injury	• See Table 1	• Sparse data • Small studies show potential benefit for induction of remission in children • Few case reports show possibility for liberalization after remission has been achieved
Low-FODMAP diet	• Mono-chained and short-chained carbohydrates are poorly absorbed and facilitates bacterial fermentation, bacterial growth, and intestinal injury	• See Table 2	• Reasonable data to indicate benefit in reducing gastrointestinal symptoms, particularly with irritable bowel syndrome • Unknown effect on inflammation
Gluten-free diet	• Gliadin leads to increased intestinal permeability and immunologic activation	• Avoid gliadin protein found in wheat, barley, rye, and other grains	• Sparse data show potential benefit for nonspecific gastrointestinal symptoms • Unknown effect on inflammation
Antiinflammatory diet	• Consumption of certain carbohydrates leads to dysbiosis, bacterial overgrowth, mucosal injury, and altered intestinal permeability • Certain fatty acids are proinflammatory • Prebiotics and probiotics are beneficial for intestinal health	• Consumption of nutrients believed to be antiinflammatory (omega-3 fatty acids) • Avoidance of nutrients believed to be proinflammatory (eg, lactose, refined or processed complex carbohydrates, total and saturated fatty acids, hydrogenated oils) • Use of prebiotics and probiotics • Reduction of food texture (ie, grinding, cooking) and intact fiber to improve absorption	• Very sparse data
IgG4-guided exclusion diet	• Immune response to certain food antigens contribute to inflammation	• Systematic exclusion of food types that elicit an IgG4-mediated response	• Sparse data • Potential improvement of symptoms, although no current evidence of reduction in inflammation

Diet	Rationale	Foods	Evidence
High-fiber diet	• Fiber is fermented by intestinal bacteria into short-chain fatty acids, which possess antiinflammatory properties • Short-chain fatty acids also help regulate fluid and electrolyte absorption, improve mucosal barrier function, and promote microbial eubiosis	• Consumption of bran, whole grains, oats, lentils, beans, all fruits and vegetables, nuts, and seeds	• Sparse data show inconsistent effect on hospitalizations and surgeries • Very sparse data on its effects on inflammation • Fiber supplements may reduce symptoms, but results are inconsistent and fiber monotherapy is not recommended
Mediterranean diet	• The dietary patterns typical of the Mediterranean countries seem to confer good health and lower risk of chronic diseases	• High consumption of fruits, vegetables, and olive oil • Moderate consumption of wine, fish, poultry, and dairy products • Low consumption of red meat	• Weak evidence of lower inflammatory markers • Very sparse data on its efficacy in IBD
Low-residue and elemental diets	• Less food and stool passing to the lower segments of the gastrointestinal tract reduces the risk of obstruction among patients with strictures • Readily absorbed nutrients reduce downstream exposure of food antigens • Some complex proteins may also be allergenic	• Low-residue diet includes white breads with no nuts or seeds, well cooked vegetables without skin or seeds, canned fruits and vegetables, tender meats, smooth nut butters • Avoids bran, whole grains, fruit juice (prune juice), legumes, corn, raw fruits and vegetables, large amounts of dairy • Elemental diet contains predigested macronutrients and micronutrients	• Sparse data are inconsistent
Semivegetarian diet	• Dietary fibers possess antiinflammatory properties through its benefit on the intestinal microbiome and as short-chain fatty acids • Meats can be proinflammatory	• Plant-based diet with variable inclusion of eggs, dairy products, and occasional meats depending on the diet	• Sparse data show possible benefit for maintenance of remission
Paleolithic diet	• Diet of hunter-gatherers' are more natural for the human body	• Wild game meats, high in polyunsaturated fats and low in saturated fats • Fresh fruits and vegetables • Excludes grains, meats from domesticated animals, refined sugars, and dairy products	• No data

with 50 British children with active CD who were administered EEN or partial EN, EEN was superior than partial EN in achieving clinical remission (42% vs 15%; $P = .04$) after 4 weeks.[129] The efficacy of partial EN for the induction of remission is, therefore, still unknown.

For the maintenance of remission in CD, the long-term use of partial EN is more feasible than EEN. In study of 39 consecutive subjects with CD in clinical remission, 10 (48%) of the 21 who received an elemental diet supplement remained in remission after 12 months, compared with the 4 (22%) of the 18 who did not receive any supplementation ($P<.01$).[130] A follow-up trial of 33 subjects with inactive steroid-dependent CD revealed 12-month steroid-free remission rates of 42% in subjects on the elemental diet and 43% in those on the polymeric diet.[131] In a controlled trial of 51 subjects with inactive CD, the relapse rate was 35% in those on a half elemental diet and 64% in those on an unrestricted diet.[132] For subjects on infliximab maintenance therapy, a prospective study of 56 subjects with inactive CD did not find a difference in 56-week remission rates between those who received daytime EN or not (78% vs 67%; $P = .51$).[133] On the other hand, a meta-analysis of 4 trials (342 participants) evaluating infliximab therapy with and without EN have shown that the concurrent use of EN to be superior at maintenance of remission at 1 year (74.5% vs 49.2%; $P<.01$).[134] Similar to the use of partial EN for the induction of remission, there may be a benefit for the maintenance of remission, but more investigation is needed.

PARENTERAL NUTRITION

Parenteral nutrition (PN) involves the intravenous administration of a mixture of macronutrients (ie, carbohydrates, proteins, lipids), micronutrients (eg, vitamins, minerals), and electrolytes. The role of PN in the management IBD is typically limited to a few scenarios, such as malnutrition and stenotic disease. Because patients with active IBD often experience some degree of protein-calorie malnutrition secondary to the catabolic nature of inflammation and the detrimental effects of corticosteroids,[135] PN may serve as a source of nutrition when the patient cannot consume adequate oral or enteral intake to maintain fluid, electrolyte, and nutritional equilibrium. PN may also serve to provide nutrition in patients with CD strictures, although EEN and low-residue diets should be preferred options to consider.[136] PN has also use been used as a source of nutrition during bowel rest. The premise of bowel rest is to reduce antigenic stimuli to the inflamed segments of intestines, thus theoretically permitting mucosal healing. Moreover, it allows reduced drainage through enterocutaneous fistulae.[137] However, the benefit of bowel rest is currently unclear. In a prospective trial of 47 subjects with severe colitis treated with prednisolone and randomized to either receive an oral diet or undergo bowel rest with PN, there was no difference in clinical response, laboratory parameters, or need for surgery, or relapse rate between treatment arms.[138] An independent randomized trial of 51 subjects with CD, participants were provided either bowel rest with PN, EN via nasogastric tube, or partial PN with oral food.[139] There were no significant differences in induction or maintenance of remission. These studies highlight the unclear utility of bowel rest and PN for the treatment of IBD. The potential benefits of PN should also be balanced against the risks, such as bloodstream infections, PN-associated liver disease, and venous thromboses.

SUMMARY

Because diets play a strong role in shaping the intestinal microbiome and influencing intestinal inflammation, there is emerging evidence that nutritional interventions may

Table 4
Dietary supplements for the treatment of inflammatory bowel disease

Supplement	Evidence of Efficacy
Curcumin	• In a randomized trial of 43 UC subjects, 3 g of curcumin daily was superior to placebo in the maintenance of remission • In a randomized trial of 41 UC subjects, 450 mg daily was ineffective at inducing remission • May have benefit at reducing the risk of colon cancer
Omega-3	• Inconsistent data are present for the benefit of supplementation in the induction or maintenance of remission in IBD • Currently available data do not show clear evidence of benefit from supplementation with omega-3 fatty acids for IBD
Glutamine	• There are very sparse data, which currently do not show benefit from the use of glutamine for CD
Vitamin D	• A large retrospective cohort study has shown that normalization of vitamin D reduced the risk of surgery in CD but not UC • The largest randomized trial of 1200 IU vitamin D vs placebo found no difference in relapse rate in CD
Prebiotics	• Very sparse data for CD • Fiber supplementation may help improve gastrointestinal symptoms but is currently not recommended as monotherapy for UC
Probiotics	• Ineffective for inducing remission, maintaining remission, and preventing postoperative recurrence in CD • VSL#3, a multistrain probiotic, can help induce remission in mild-moderate UC • VSL#3 helps prevent pouchitis

help in the treatment of IBD. EN so far has the most robust supportive data and is also considered a first-line strategy in pediatric CD. However, the specific nutrient composition and diets are still ill-defined due to a dearth of research data. Although small studies show benefit of some diets in helping induce or maintain remission, the evidence is still weak or lacking (**Table 3**). These findings highlight the importance of additional and more robust investigation into dietary components and diets in the treatment of IBD. Dietary supplements, such as curcumin and probiotics, have relatively stronger evidence for use in UC (**Table 4**). The position of nutritional interventions as primary or adjunct therapies in the algorithm of the management of IBD is also still unclear. At present, the authors cannot endorse any particular diet, other than recommending a balanced plant-based diet that is high in fiber and low in refined sugars or processed foods. Given the general benefits of consuming a balanced healthy diet, even if it could not serve as primary monotherapy for IBD, there would be many advantages for improving the intestinal microbiome, gastrointestinal health, and health in general.

ACKNOWLEDGMENTS

We would like to thank Joanna Ye and Maryam Tajamal for their contributions.

REFERENCES

1. David LA, Maurice CF, Carmody RN, et al. Diet rapidly and reproducibly alters the human gut microbiome. Nature 2014;505(7484):559–63.
2. Chapman-Kiddell CA, Davies PS, Gillen L, et al. Role of diet in the development of inflammatory bowel disease. Inflamm Bowel Dis 2010;16(1):137–51.

3. Carr I, Mayberry JF. The effects of migration on ulcerative colitis: a three-year prospective study among Europeans and first- and second- generation South Asians in Leicester (1991-1994). Am J Gastroenterol 1999;94(10):2918–22.

4. Bar-Gil Shitrit A, Koslowsky B, Kori M, et al. Inflammatory bowel disease: an emergent disease among Ethiopian Jews migrating to Israel. Inflamm Bowel Dis 2015;21(3):631–5.

5. Molodecky NA, Soon IS, Rabi DM, et al. Increasing incidence and prevalence of the inflammatory bowel diseases with time, based on systematic review. Gastroenterology 2012;142(1):46–54.e42 [quiz: e30].

6. Haas SV, Haas MP. The treatment of celiac disease with the specific carbohydrate diet; report on 191 additional cases. Am J Gastroenterol 1955;23(4):344–60.

7. Gottschall E. Breaking the vicious cycle: intestinal health through diet. Canada: Baltimore: Kirkton Press, Limited; 1994.

8. Suskind DL, Wahbeh G, Gregory N, et al. Nutritional therapy in pediatric Crohn disease: the specific carbohydrate diet. J Pediatr Gastroenterol Nutr 2014; 58(1):87–91.

9. Cohen SA, Gold BD, Oliva S, et al. Clinical and mucosal improvement with specific carbohydrate diet in pediatric Crohn disease. J Pediatr Gastroenterol Nutr 2014;59(4):516–21.

10. Nakayuenyongsuk W, Christofferson M, Nguyen K, et al. Diet to the rescue: cessation of pharmacotherapy after initiation of exclusive enteral nutrition (EEN) followed by strict and liberalized specific carbohydrate diet (SCD) in Crohn's Disease. Dig Dis Sci 2017;62(10):2686–9.

11. Burgis JC, Nguyen K, Park KT, et al. Response to strict and liberalized specific carbohydrate diet in pediatric Crohn's disease. World J Gastroenterol 2016; 22(6):2111–7.

12. Kakodkar S, Farooqui AJ, Mikolaitis SL, et al. The specific carbohydrate diet for inflammatory bowel disease: a case series. J Acad Nutr Diet 2015;115(8):1226–32.

13. Suskind DL, Wahbeh G, Cohen SA, et al. Patients perceive clinical benefit with the specific carbohydrate diet for inflammatory bowel disease. Dig Dis Sci 2016; 61(11):3255–60.

14. Barrett JS, Gearry RB, Muir JG, et al. Dietary poorly absorbed, short-chain carbohydrates increase delivery of water and fermentable substrates to the proximal colon. Aliment Pharmacol Ther 2010;31(8):874–82.

15. Ong DK, Mitchell SB, Barrett JS, et al. Manipulation of dietary short chain carbohydrates alters the pattern of gas production and genesis of symptoms in irritable bowel syndrome. J Gastroenterol Hepatol 2010;25(8):1366–73.

16. Halmos EP, Power VA, Shepherd SJ, et al. A diet low in FODMAPs reduces symptoms of irritable bowel syndrome. Gastroenterology 2014;146(1):67–75.e5.

17. Staudacher HM, Whelan K, Irving PM, et al. Comparison of symptom response following advice for a diet low in fermentable carbohydrates (FODMAPs) versus standard dietary advice in patients with irritable bowel syndrome. J Hum Nutr Diet 2011;24(5):487–95.

18. Eswaran SL, Chey WD, Han-Markey T, et al. A randomized controlled trial comparing the low FODMAP diet vs. Modified NICE guidelines in US adults with IBS-D. Am J Gastroenterol 2016;111(12):1824–32.

19. Bohn L, Storsrud S, Liljebo T, et al. Diet low in FODMAPs reduces symptoms of irritable bowel syndrome as well as traditional dietary advice: a randomized controlled trial. Gastroenterology 2015;149(6):1399–407.e2.

20. Eswaran S, Chey WD, Jackson K, et al. A diet low in fermentable oligo-, di-, and mono-saccharides and polyols improves quality of life and reduces activity

impairment in patients with irritable bowel syndrome and diarrhea. Clin Gastro-enterol Hepatol 2017 [pii:S1542-3565(17)30791-7].

21. Cox SR, Prince AC, Myers CE, et al. Fermentable carbohydrates (FODMAPs) exacerbate functional gastrointestinal symptoms in patients with inflammatory bowel disease: a randomised, double-blind, placebo-controlled, cross-over, re-challenge trial. J Crohns Colitis 2017. [Epub ahead of print].

22. Gearry RB, Irving PM, Barrett JS, et al. Reduction of dietary poorly absorbed short-chain carbohydrates (FODMAPs) improves abdominal symptoms in pa-tients with inflammatory bowel disease-a pilot study. J Crohns Colitis 2009; 3(1):8–14.

23. Prince AC, Myers CE, Joyce T, et al. Fermentable carbohydrate restriction (Low FODMAP Diet) in clinical practice improves functional gastrointestinal symptoms in patients with inflammatory bowel disease. Inflamm Bowel Dis 2016;22(5):1129–36.

24. Maagaard L, Ankersen DV, Vegh Z, et al. Follow-up of patients with functional bowel symptoms treated with a low FODMAP diet. World J Gastroenterol 2016;22(15):4009–19.

25. Croagh C, Shepherd SJ, Berryman M, et al. Pilot study on the effect of reducing dietary FODMAP intake on bowel function in patients without a colon. Inflamm Bowel Dis 2007;13(12):1522–8.

26. Halmos EP, Christophersen CT, Bird AR, et al. Consistent prebiotic effect on gut microbiota with altered FODMAP intake in patients with Crohn's disease: a rand-omised, controlled cross-over trial of well-defined diets. Clin Transl Gastroen-terol 2016;7:e164.

27. Halpin SJ, Ford AC. Prevalence of symptoms meeting criteria for irritable bowel syndrome in inflammatory bowel disease: systematic review and meta-analysis. Am J Gastroenterol 2012;107(10):1474–82.

28. Halmos EP, Christophersen CT, Bird AR, et al. Diets that differ in their FODMAP content alter the colonic luminal microenvironment. Gut 2015;64(1):93–100.

29. Elli L, Tomba C, Branchi F, et al. Evidence for the presence of non-celiac gluten sensitivity in patients with functional gastrointestinal symptoms: results from a multicenter randomized double-blind placebo-controlled Gluten challenge. Nutrients 2016;8(2):84.

30. Heyman M, Abed J, Lebreton C, et al. Intestinal permeability in coeliac disease: insight into mechanisms and relevance to pathogenesis. Gut 2012;61(9): 1355–64.

31. Aziz I, Dwivedi K, Sanders DS. From coeliac disease to noncoeliac gluten sensi-tivity; should everyone be gluten free? Curr Opin Gastroenterol 2016;32(2): 120–7.

32. Herfarth HH, Martin CF, Sandler RS, et al. Prevalence of a gluten-free diet and improvement of clinical symptoms in patients with inflammatory bowel diseases. Inflamm Bowel Dis 2014;20(7):1194–7.

33. Aziz I, Branchi F, Pearson K, et al. A study evaluating the bidirectional relation-ship between inflammatory bowel disease and self-reported non-celiac gluten sensitivity. Inflamm Bowel Dis 2015;21(4):847–53.

34. Ricker MA, Haas WC. Anti-inflammatory diet in clinical practice: a review. Nutr Clin Pract 2017;32(3):318–25.

35. Olendzki BC, Silverstein TD, Persuitte GM, et al. An anti-inflammatory diet as treatment for inflammatory bowel disease: a case series report. Nutr J 2014; 13:5.

36. Gunasekeera V, Mendall MA, Chan D, et al. Treatment of Crohn's Disease with an IgG4-guided exclusion diet: a randomized controlled trial. Dig Dis Sci 2016;61(4):1148–57.

37. Jones JM. CODEX-aligned dietary fiber definitions help to bridge the 'fiber gap'. Nutr J 2014;13:34.

38. Bowling TE, Raimundo AH, Grimble GK, et al. Reversal by short-chain fatty acids of colonic fluid secretion induced by enteral feeding. Lancet 1993; 342(8882):1266–8.

39. Spaeth G, Gottwald T, Specian RD, et al. Secretory immunoglobulin A, intestinal mucin, and mucosal permeability in nutritionally induced bacterial translocation in rats. Ann Surg 1994;220(6):798–808.

40. Kleessen B, Hartmann L, Blaut M. Oligofructose and long-chain inulin: influence on the gut microbial ecology of rats associated with a human faecal flora. Br J Nutr 2001;86(2):291–300.

41. Inan MS, Rasoulpour RJ, Yin L, et al. The luminal short-chain fatty acid butyrate modulates NF-kappaB activity in a human colonic epithelial cell line. Gastroenterology 2000;118(4):724–34.

42. Ananthakrishnan AN, Khalili H, Konijeti GG, et al. A prospective study of long-term intake of dietary fiber and risk of Crohn's disease and ulcerative colitis. Gastroenterology 2013;145(5):970–7.

43. Heaton KW, Thornton JR, Emmett PM. Treatment of Crohn's disease with an unrefined-carbohydrate, fibre-rich diet. Br Med J 1979;2(6193):764–6.

44. Brotherton CS, Martin CA, Long MD, et al. Avoidance of fiber is associated with greater risk of Crohn's disease flare in a 6-month period. Clin Gastroenterol Hepatol 2016;14(8):1130–6.

45. Ritchie JK, Wadsworth J, Lennard-Jones JE, et al. Controlled multicentre therapeutic trial of an unrefined carbohydrate, fibre rich diet in Crohn's disease. Br Med J (Clin Res Ed) 1987;295(6597):517–20.

46. Koga H, Iida M, Aoyagi K, et al. Long-term efficacy of low residue diet for the maintenance of remission in patients with Crohn's disease. Nihon Shokakibyo Gakkai Zasshi 1993;90(11):2882–8 [in Japanese].

47. Levenstein S, Prantera C, Luzi C, et al. Low residue or normal diet in Crohn's disease: a prospective controlled study in Italian patients. Gut 1985;26(10):989–93.

48. Hanai H, Iida T, Takeuchi K, et al. Nutritional therapy versus 6-mercaptopurine as maintenance therapy in patients with Crohn's disease. Dig Liver Dis 2012; 44(8):649–54.

49. Hamer HM, Jonkers D, Venema K, et al. Review article: the role of butyrate on colonic function. Aliment Pharmacol Ther 2008;27(2):104–19.

50. Chiba M, Abe T, Tsuda H, et al. Lifestyle-related disease in Crohn's disease: relapse prevention by a semi-vegetarian diet. World J Gastroenterol 2010; 16(20):2484–95.

51. Dinu M, Pagliai G, Casini A, et al. Mediterranean diet and multiple health outcomes: an umbrella review of meta-analyses of observational studies and randomised trials. Eur J Clin Nutr 2017. [Epub ahead of print].

52. Marlow G, Ellett S, Ferguson IR, et al. Transcriptomics to study the effect of a Mediterranean-inspired diet on inflammation in Crohn's disease patients. Hum Genomics 2013;7:24.

53. Whalen KA, McCullough ML, Flanders WD, et al. Paleolithic and mediterranean diet pattern scores are inversely associated with biomarkers of inflammation and oxidative balance in adults. J Nutr 2016;146(6):1217–26.

54. Pitt CE. Cutting through the Paleo hype: the evidence for the Palaeolithic diet. Aust Fam Physician 2016;45(1):35–8.
55. Jurenka JS. Anti-inflammatory properties of curcumin, a major constituent of Curcuma longa: a review of preclinical and clinical research. Altern Med Rev 2009;14(2):141–53.
56. Sugimoto K, Hanai H, Tozawa K, et al. Curcumin prevents and ameliorates trinitrobenzene sulfonic acid-induced colitis in mice. Gastroenterology 2002;123(6): 1912–22.
57. Deguchi Y, Andoh A, Inatomi O, et al. Curcumin prevents the development of dextran sulfate Sodium (DSS)-induced experimental colitis. Dig Dis Sci 2007; 52(11):2993–8.
58. Jobin C, Bradham CA, Russo MP, et al. Curcumin blocks cytokine-mediated NF-kappa B activation and proinflammatory gene expression by inhibiting inhibitory factor I-kappa B kinase activity. J Immunol 1999;163(6):3474–83.
59. Tong W, Wang Q, Sun D, et al. Curcumin suppresses colon cancer cell invasion via AMPK-induced inhibition of NF-kappaB, uPA activator and MMP9. Oncol Lett 2016;12(5):4139–46.
60. Midura-Kiela MT, Radhakrishnan VM, Larmonier CB, et al. Curcumin inhibits interferon-gamma signaling in colonic epithelial cells. Am J Physiol Gastrointest Liver Physiol 2012;302(1):G85–96.
61. Hanai H, Iida T, Takeuchi K, et al. Curcumin maintenance therapy for ulcerative colitis: randomized, multicenter, double-blind, placebo-controlled trial. Clin Gastroenterol Hepatol 2006;4(12):1502–6.
62. Lang A, Salomon N, Wu JC, et al. Curcumin in combination with mesalamine induces remission in patients with mild-to-moderate ulcerative colitis in a randomized controlled trial. Clin Gastroenterol Hepatol 2015;13(8):1444–9.e1.
63. Kumar S, Ahuja V, Sankar MJ, et al. Curcumin for maintenance of remission in ulcerative colitis. Cochrane Database Syst Rev 2012;(10):CD008424.
64. Kedia S, Bhatia V, Thareja S, et al. Low dose oral curcumin is not effective in induction of remission in mild to moderate ulcerative colitis: results from a randomized double blind placebo controlled trial. World J Gastrointest Pharmacol Ther 2017;8(2):147–54.
65. Simopoulos AP. The importance of the ratio of omega-6/omega-3 essential fatty acids. Biomed Pharmacother 2002;56(8):365–79.
66. John S, Luben R, Shrestha SS, et al. Dietary n-3 polyunsaturated fatty acids and the aetiology of ulcerative colitis: a UK prospective cohort study. Eur J Gastroenterol Hepatol 2010;22(5):602–6.
67. Gallai V, Sarchielli P, Trequattrini A, et al. Cytokine secretion and eicosanoid production in the peripheral blood mononuclear cells of MS patients undergoing dietary supplementation with n-3 polyunsaturated fatty acids. J Neuroimmunol 1995;56(2):143–53.
68. Fisher M, Levine PH, Weiner BH, et al. Dietary n-3 fatty acid supplementation reduces superoxide production and chemiluminescence in a monocyte-enriched preparation of leukocytes. Am J Clin Nutr 1990;51(5):804–8.
69. Feagan BG, Sandborn WJ, Mittmann U, et al. Omega-3 free fatty acids for the maintenance of remission in Crohn disease: the EPIC randomized controlled trials. JAMA 2008;299(14):1690–7.
70. Vasudevan A, Yu Y, Banerjee S, et al. Omega-3 fatty acid is a potential preventive agent for recurrent colon cancer. Cancer Prev Res (Phila) 2014;7(11): 1138–48.

71. Romano C, Cucchiara S, Barabino A, et al. Usefulness of omega-3 fatty acid supplementation in addition to mesalazine in maintaining remission in pediatric Crohn's disease: a double-blind, randomized, placebo-controlled study. World J Gastroenterol 2005;11(45):7118–21.

72. Lorenz-Meyer H, Bauer P, Nicolay C, et al. Omega-3 fatty acids and low carbohydrate diet for maintenance of remission in Crohn's disease. A randomized controlled multicenter trial. Study Group Members (German Crohn's Disease Study Group). Scand J Gastroenterol 1996;31(8):778–85.

73. Dichi I, Frenhane P, Dichi JB, et al. Comparison of omega-3 fatty acids and sulfasalazine in ulcerative colitis. Nutrition 2000;16(2):87–90.

74. Hawthorne AB, Daneshmend TK, Hawkey CJ, et al. Treatment of ulcerative colitis with fish oil supplementation: a prospective 12 month randomised controlled trial. Gut 1992;33(7):922–8.

75. Turner D, Steinhart AH, Griffiths AM. Omega 3 fatty acids (fish oil) for maintenance of remission in ulcerative colitis. Cochrane Database Syst Rev 2007;(3):CD006443.

76. Windmueller HG, Spaeth AE. Respiratory fuels and nitrogen metabolism in vivo in small intestine of fed rats. Quantitative importance of glutamine, glutamate, and aspartate. J Biol Chem 1980;255(1):107–12.

77. Windmueller HG. Glutamine utilization by the small intestine. Adv Enzymol Relat Areas Mol Biol 1982;53:201–37.

78. Labow BI, Souba WW. Glutamine. World J Surg 2000;24(12):1503–13.

79. Roth E, Oehler R, Manhart N, et al. Regulative potential of glutamine–relation to glutathione metabolism. Nutrition 2002;18(3):217–21.

80. Li J, Langkamp-Henken B, Suzuki K, et al. Glutamine prevents parenteral nutrition-induced increases in intestinal permeability. JPEN J Parenter Enteral Nutr 1994;18(4):303–7.

81. Horvath K, Jami M, Hill ID, et al. Isocaloric glutamine-free diet and the morphology and function of rat small intestine. JPEN J Parenter Enteral Nutr 1996;20(2):128–34.

82. Platell C, McCauley R, McCulloch R, et al. The influence of parenteral glutamine and branched-chain amino acids on total parenteral nutrition-induced atrophy of the gut. JPEN J Parenter Enteral Nutr 1993;17(4):348–54.

83. Platell C, McCauley R, McCulloch R, et al. Influence of glutamine and branched chain amino acids on the jejunal atrophy associated with parenteral nutrition. J Gastroenterol Hepatol 1991;6(4):345–9.

84. Tremel H, Kienle B, Weilemann LS, et al. Glutamine dipeptide-supplemented parenteral nutrition maintains intestinal function in the critically ill. Gastroenterology 1994;107(6):1595–601.

85. Den Hond E, Hiele M, Peeters M, et al. Effect of long-term oral glutamine supplements on small intestinal permeability in patients with Crohn's disease. JPEN J Parenter Enteral Nutr 1999;23(1):7–11.

86. Akobeng AK, Miller V, Stanton J, et al. Double-blind randomized controlled trial of glutamine-enriched polymeric diet in the treatment of active Crohn's disease. J Pediatr Gastroenterol Nutr 2000;30(1):78–84.

87. Sido B, Seel C, Hochlehnert A, et al. Low intestinal glutamine level and low glutaminase activity in Crohn's disease: a rational for glutamine supplementation? Dig Dis Sci 2006;51(12):2170–9.

88. Limketkai BN, Mullin GE, Limsui D, et al. Role of vitamin D in inflammatory bowel disease. Nutr Clin Pract 2017;32(3):337–45.

89. Cantorna MT, Munsick C, Bemiss C, et al. 1,25-Dihydroxycholecalciferol prevents and ameliorates symptoms of experimental murine inflammatory bowel disease. J Nutr 2000;130(11):2648–52.
90. Daniel C, Radeke HH, Sartory NA, et al. The new low calcemic vitamin D analog 22-ene-25-oxa-vitamin D prominently ameliorates T helper cell type 1-mediated colitis in mice. J Pharmacol Exp Ther 2006;319(2):622–31.
91. Ananthakrishnan AN, Khalili H, Higuchi LM, et al. Higher predicted vitamin D status is associated with reduced risk of Crohn's disease. Gastroenterology 2012;142(3):482–9.
92. Ulitsky A, Ananthakrishnan AN, Naik A, et al. Vitamin D deficiency in patients with inflammatory bowel disease: association with disease activity and quality of life. JPEN J Parenter Enteral Nutr 2011;35(3):308–16.
93. Blanck S, Aberra F. Vitamin d deficiency is associated with ulcerative colitis disease activity. Dig Dis Sci 2013;58(6):1698–702.
94. Ananthakrishnan AN, Cagan A, Gainer VS, et al. Normalization of plasma 25-hydroxy vitamin D is associated with reduced risk of surgery in Crohn's disease. Inflamm Bowel Dis 2013;19(9):1921–7.
95. Jorgensen SP, Agnholt J, Glerup H, et al. Clinical trial: vitamin D3 treatment in Crohn's disease - a randomized double-blind placebo-controlled study. Aliment Pharmacol Ther 2010;32(3):377–83.
96. Hanai H, Kanauchi O, Mitsuyama K, et al. Germinated barley foodstuff prolongs remission in patients with ulcerative colitis. Int J Mol Med 2004;13(5):643–7.
97. Faghfoori Z, Shakerhosseini R, Navai L, et al. Effects of an oral supplementation of germinated barley foodstuff on serum CRP level and clinical signs in patients with ulcerative colitis. Health Promot Perspect 2014;4(1):116–21.
98. Hallert C, Bjorck I, Nyman M, et al. Increasing fecal butyrate in ulcerative colitis patients by diet: controlled pilot study. Inflamm Bowel Dis 2003;9(2):116–21.
99. Davies PS, Rhodes J. Maintenance of remission in ulcerative colitis with sulphasalazine or a high-fibre diet: a clinical trial. Br Med J 1978;1(6126):1524–5.
100. Hill C, Guarner F, Reid G, et al. Expert consensus document. The International Scientific Association for Probiotics and Prebiotics consensus statement on the scope and appropriate use of the term probiotic. Nat Rev Gastroenterol Hepatol 2014;11(8):506–14.
101. Shen J, Zuo ZX, Mao AP. Effect of probiotics on inducing remission and maintaining therapy in ulcerative colitis, Crohn's disease, and pouchitis: meta-analysis of randomized controlled trials. Inflamm Bowel Dis 2014;20(1):21–35.
102. Prantera C, Scribano ML, Falasco G, et al. Ineffectiveness of probiotics in preventing recurrence after curative resection for Crohn's disease: a randomised controlled trial with lactobacillus GG. Gut 2002;51(3):405–9.
103. Rahimi R, Nikfar S, Rahimi F, et al. A meta-analysis on the efficacy of probiotics for maintenance of remission and prevention of clinical and endoscopic relapse in Crohn's disease. Dig Dis Sci 2008;53(9):2524–31.
104. Sood A, Midha V, Makharia GK, et al. The probiotic preparation, VSL#3 induces remission in patients with mild-to-moderately active ulcerative colitis. Clin Gastroenterol Hepatol 2009;7(11):1202–9, 1209.e1.
105. Tursi A, Brandimarte G, Giorgetti GM, et al. Low-dose balsalazide plus a high-potency probiotic preparation is more effective than balsalazide alone or mesalazine in the treatment of acute mild-to-moderate ulcerative colitis. Med Sci Monit 2004;10(11):PI126–31.

106. Bibiloni R, Fedorak RN, Tannock GW, et al. VSL#3 probiotic-mixture induces remission in patients with active ulcerative colitis. Am J Gastroenterol 2005; 100(7):1539–46.
107. Huynh HQ, deBruyn J, Guan L, et al. Probiotic preparation VSL#3 induces remission in children with mild to moderate acute ulcerative colitis: a pilot study. Inflamm Bowel Dis 2009;15(5):760–8.
108. Kruis W, Schutz E, Fric P, et al. Double-blind comparison of an oral Escherichia coli preparation and mesalazine in maintaining remission of ulcerative colitis. Aliment Pharmacol Ther 1997;11(5):853–8.
109. Kruis W, Fric P, Pokrotnieks J, et al. Maintaining remission of ulcerative colitis with the probiotic Escherichia coli Nissle 1917 is as effective as with standard mesalazine. Gut 2004;53(11):1617–23.
110. Zocco MA, dal Verme LZ, Cremonini F, et al. Efficacy of lactobacillus GG in maintaining remission of ulcerative colitis. Aliment Pharmacol Ther 2006; 23(11):1567–74.
111. Guslandi M, Giollo P, Testoni PA. A pilot trial of Saccharomyces boulardii in ulcerative colitis. Eur J Gastroenterol Hepatol 2003;15(6):697–8.
112. Mimura T, Rizzello F, Helwig U, et al. Once daily high dose probiotic therapy (VSL#3) for maintaining remission in recurrent or refractory pouchitis. Gut 2004;53(1):108–14.
113. Gionchetti P, Rizzello F, Venturi A, et al. Oral bacteriotherapy as maintenance treatment in patients with chronic pouchitis: a double-blind, placebo-controlled trial. Gastroenterology 2000;119(2):305–9.
114. Gionchetti P, Rizzello F, Helwig U, et al. Prophylaxis of pouchitis onset with probiotic therapy: a double-blind, placebo-controlled trial. Gastroenterology 2003; 124(5):1202–9.
115. Shen B, Brzezinski A, Fazio VW, et al. Maintenance therapy with a probiotic in antibiotic-dependent pouchitis: experience in clinical practice. Aliment Pharmacol Ther 2005;22(8):721–8.
116. Feng Y, Li Y, Mei S, et al. Exclusive enteral nutrition ameliorates mesenteric adipose tissue alterations in patients with active Crohn's disease. Clin Nutr 2014; 33(5):850–8.
117. Teahon K, Smethurst P, Pearson M, et al. The effect of elemental diet on intestinal permeability and inflammation in Crohn's disease. Gastroenterology 1991; 101(1):84–9.
118. Leach ST, Mitchell HM, Eng WR, et al. Sustained modulation of intestinal bacteria by exclusive enteral nutrition used to treat children with Crohn's disease. Aliment Pharmacol Ther 2008;28(6):724–33.
119. Levine A, Wine E. Effects of enteral nutrition on Crohn's disease: clues to the impact of diet on disease pathogenesis. Inflamm Bowel Dis 2013;19(6):1322–9.
120. Heuschkel RB, Menache CC, Megerian JT, et al. Enteral nutrition and corticosteroids in the treatment of acute Crohn's disease in children. J Pediatr Gastroenterol Nutr 2000;31(1):8–15.
121. Zachos M, Tondeur M, Griffiths AM. Enteral nutritional therapy for induction of remission in Crohn's disease. Cochrane Database Syst Rev 2007;(1):CD000542.
122. Ruemmele FM, Veres G, Kolho KL, et al. Consensus guidelines of ECCO/ESPGHAN on the medical management of pediatric Crohn's disease. J Crohns Colitis 2014;8(10):1179–207.
123. Lochs H, Dejong C, Hammarqvist F, et al. ESPEN guidelines on enteral nutrition: gastroenterology. Clin Nutr 2006;25(2):260–74.

124. Wall CL, Day AS, Gearry RB. Use of exclusive enteral nutrition in adults with Crohn's disease: a review. World J Gastroenterol 2013;19(43):7652–60.
125. Yang Q, Gao X, Chen H, et al. Efficacy of exclusive enteral nutrition in complicated Crohn's disease. Scand J Gastroenterol 2017;52(9):995–1001.
126. Yan D, Ren J, Wang G, et al. Predictors of response to enteral nutrition in abdominal enterocutaneous fistula patients with Crohn's disease. Eur J Clin Nutr 2014;68(8):959–63.
127. Sigall-Boneh R, Pfeffer-Gik T, Segal I, et al. Partial enteral nutrition with a Crohn's disease exclusion diet is effective for induction of remission in children and young adults with Crohn's disease. Inflamm Bowel Dis 2014;20(8):1353–60.
128. Sigall Boneh R, Sarbagili-Shabat C, Yanai H, et al. Dietary therapy with the Crohn's disease exclusion diet is a successful strategy for induction of remission in children and adults failing biological therapy. J Crohns Colitis 2017;11(10): 1205–12.
129. Johnson T, Macdonald S, Hill SM, et al. Treatment of active Crohn's disease in children using partial enteral nutrition with liquid formula: a randomised controlled trial. Gut 2006;55(3):356–61.
130. Verma S, Kirkwood B, Brown S, et al. Oral nutritional supplementation is effective in the maintenance of remission in Crohn's disease. Dig Liver Dis 2000;32(9): 769–74.
131. Verma S, Holdsworth CD, Giaffer MH. Does adjuvant nutritional support diminish steroid dependency in Crohn disease? Scand J Gastroenterol 2001;36(4): 383–8.
132. Takagi S, Utsunomiya K, Kuriyama S, et al. Effectiveness of an 'half elemental diet' as maintenance therapy for Crohn's disease: a randomized-controlled trial. Aliment Pharmacol Ther 2006;24(9):1333–40.
133. Yamamoto T, Nakahigashi M, Umegae S, et al. Prospective clinical trial: enteral nutrition during maintenance infliximab in Crohn's disease. J Gastroenterol 2010;45(1):24–9.
134. Nguyen DL, Palmer LB, Nguyen ET, et al. Specialized enteral nutrition therapy in Crohn's disease patients on maintenance infliximab therapy: a meta-analysis. Therap Adv Gastroenterol 2015;8(4):168–75.
135. O'Keefe SJ, Ogden J, Rund J, et al. Steroids and bowel rest versus elemental diet in the treatment of patients with Crohn's disease: the effects on protein metabolism and immune function. JPEN J Parenter Enteral Nutr 1989;13(5): 455–60.
136. Hu D, Ren J, Wang G, et al. Exclusive enteral nutritional therapy can relieve inflammatory bowel stricture in Crohn's disease. J Clin Gastroenterol 2014;48(9): 790–5.
137. Polk TM, Schwab CW. Metabolic and nutritional support of the enterocutaneous fistula patient: a three-phase approach. World J Surg 2012;36(3):524–33.
138. McIntyre PB, Powell-Tuck J, Wood SR, et al. Controlled trial of bowel rest in the treatment of severe acute colitis. Gut 1986;27(5):481–5.
139. Greenberg GR, Fleming CR, Jeejeebhoy KN, et al. Controlled trial of bowel rest and nutritional support in the management of Crohn's disease. Gut 1988;29(10): 1309–15.

The Role of Prebiotics and Probiotics in Gastrointestinal Disease

Martin H. Floch, MD, MACG, AGAF

KEYWORDS

- Probiotics • Prebiotics • Dietary fiber • Symbiotics • FMT

KEY POINTS

- Prebiotics and probiotics are important to the gastrointestinal tract.
- Many dietary fiber substances are prebiotics.
- Probiotics are live organisms that when administered in adequate amounts confer health benefits to the host and improve the intestinal microbial balance.

INTRODUCTION

With the advent of the scientific realization that the microbiota of the gastrointestinal tract was more than the cells that exist in the body, the full importance of prebiotics and probiotics has come forth.[1] This importance has been stressed and is available in new textbook entitled, "The Microbiota in Gastrointestinal Pathophysiology: Implication for Human Health, Prebiotics, Probiotics and Dysbiosis."[2] There is enough evidence now published in the literature so that the scientific world now believes that prebiotics and probiotics are important in gastrointestinal disease.[1,2] At Yale University, 4 workshops were held and were attended by prominent scientists in the field to make recommendations on the use of probiotics in health.[3–6] Since the last workshop, much literature has appeared on probiotics and prebiotic experience in gastrointestinal disease around the world. This article reviews the gastrointestinal diseases and attempts to add the recent literature to this information.

In **Table 1**, the latest recommendations published from the Yale workshop from 2015 in human diseases are listed.[6]

Probiotics

Definitions of probiotics and prebiotics are important. There is much debate about them, but it is best to keep in mind the original definitions. Probiotics are defined by

Disclosure: M.H. Floch has nothing to disclose.
Section of Digestive Diseases, Yale University School of Medicine, 333 Cedar Street, 1089 LMP, New Haven, CT 06850, USA
E-mail address: martin.floch@yale.edu

Gastroenterol Clin N Am 47 (2018) 179–191
https://doi.org/10.1016/j.gtc.2017.09.011

Table 1
Recommendations for probiotic use: update 2015

Clinical Condition	Effectiveness	Specific Strain of Organism & Strain References	Analysis References
Diarrhea			
Infectious childhood—treatment	A	LGG, *S boulardii*, *L reuteri* SD2112	27–30
Prevention of infection	B	*S boulardii*, LGG	27,28,30
Prevention of AAD	A	*S boulardii*, LGG, combination of *Lactobacillus casei* DN114 G01, *L bulgaricus*, snf *S thermophilus*	31–33
Prevention of recurrent CDAD	B/C	*S boulardii*, LGG, FMT	34–37
Prevention of CDAD	B/C	LGG, *S boulardii*	34,37
IBD			
Pouchitis			
Preventing and maintaining remission	A	VSL#3	38–40
Induce remission	C	VSL#3	41
Ulcerative colitis			
Inducing remission	B	*E coli* Nissle, VSL#3	42–44
Maintenance	A	*E coli* Nissle, VSL#3	43–45
Crohn	C	*E coli* Nissle, *S boulardii*, LGG	46–48
IBS			
	B	*B infantis* 35624, VSL#3	49–53,a
	C	*B animalis*	54
		L plantarum 299V	55
Necrotizing enterocolitis			
	B	*Lactobacillus acidophilus* NCDO1748, *B bifidium* NCDO1453	56,57
Immune response			
	A	*L rhamnosus* GG, *L acidophilus* LAFT1, *L plantarum*, *Bifidobacterium lactis*, *Lactobacillus johnsonii*	58,59
Allergy			
Atopic eczema associated with cow's milk allergy			
Treatment	A	L G, *B lactis*	59
Prevention	A	LGG, *B lactis*	59
Radiation enteritis			
	C	VSL#3, *L acidophilus*	60,61
Vaginosis and vaginitis			
	C	*L acidophilus*, *L rhamnosus* GR-1, *L reuteri* RC14	62–64

(continued on next page)

Table 1
(continued)

Clinical Condition	Effectiveness	Specific Strain of Organism & Strain References	Analysis References
Liver disease			
Hepatic encephalopathy	A	VSL#3	8–12
Nonalcoholic fatty liver disease	C	VSL#3, combinations of *L plantarum, Lactobacillus delbrueckii, L bulgaricus, L acidophilus, L rhamnosus, B bifidium, S thermophilus, B longum*	8,9,13,15,16
Nonalcoholic fatty liver disease in children	C	VSL#3, LGG	17
Alcoholic liver disease	C	VSL#3, LGG, *L acidophilus, L bulgaricus, Bifidobacterium bifidium, B longum* w/ oligosaccharides	8–17

[a] Ref.[53] was made available after the workshop meeting on April 8, 2011 but believed to be significant enough to qualify this probiotic to be in a B category.
Data from Floch MH, Walker WA, Sanders ME, et al. Recommendations for probiotic use-2015 update; proceedings and consensus opinion. J Clin Gastroenterol 2015;49:S69–73.

the Food Agricultural Organization and the World Health Organization Expert Consultation on Evaluation of Health and Nutritional Properties of Probiotics. The definition is "Live microorganisms which, when administered in adequate amounts, confer a health benefit on the host."[7] Fuller's[8] original definition also included that they improved intestinal microbial balance. Although there is debate on definitions of probiotics, it is best to keep in mind the original ones that state probiotics are live organisms that when administered in adequate amounts confer health benefits to the host and improve the intestinal microbial balance. It is important to note that there are strains of probiotics. A specific strain might cause a very specific response, such as toll-like receptors. The specific strain of a probiotic might have different responses, although the same generic name. Therefore, in any of the discussions on probiotics, one must keep in mind that the specific strain must be identified if used to obtain a specific response.

Prebiotics

The original definition of prebiotics was presented by Gibson and Roberfroid[9] in 1995 and has persisted: "Non-digestible dietary ingredients that beneficially affect the host by selectively stimulating the growth and/or activity of one of a limited number of bacteria in the colon, thus improve host health." This definition includes substances that are natural as well as those produced chemically. This original definition by Gibson and Roberfroid is still accepted. Therefore, many dietary fiber substances are included under this definition.

Dietary fiber is defined in many places in the literature, but it depends on the chemical analysis used and the substances that result from that analysis. The classic definition put forth by Trowell and colleagues[10] can be summarized as "plant non-starch, polysaccharides that are not digested by human enzymes." This is a simple but good definition and includes cell wall substances, such as cellulose, semicelluloses, pectin, lignin, as well as intracellular polysaccharides such as gums and mucilages.[10,11]

Spiller[11] has defined these carefully, but it is important to remember that they are merely plant polysaccharides and are poorly digested by human enzymes. The term resistant starch is often used, but it refers, again, to starch and it is not digested by human enzymes that reach the colon.[11]

Probiotics are generally regarded as safe. Boyle and colleagues[12] published a review article in 2006 whereby they proposed risk factors for probiotic substances. Minor risk factors were central venous catheters, impaired intestinal epithelial barriers, administration of probiotic by jejunotomy, concomitant administration of broad spectrum antibiotics, to which a probiotic may be resistant, probiotics with properties of high mucosal adherence of known pathogenicity, and cardiac value disease (*Lactobacillus rhamnosus* or *Bacillus subtilis*). They also reviewed all of the cases of fungal sepsis in humans. There were 16 such reports containing 24 cases. In all of those, the organism identified was *Saccharomyces boulardii*. Many of these were controversial reports. That is the extent of the entire negative literature. The medical world and the Food and Drug Administration consider probiotics extremely safe, especially when considering the amount that is used in the world. The major concern is that probiotics adhere to the intestinal mucosa and could break through the barrier to be absorbed and create a sepsis situation. This should be considered when treating a high-risk patient, especially one that is immunocompromised.[13]

Irritable Bowel Syndrome

Irritable bowel syndrome (IBS) remains a worldwide problem.[14,15] With the advent of prebiotic and probiotic therapies, there is hope that this syndrome can be controlled.[16,17] It is important to define which part of IBS is being discussed when considering therapies. IBS is classified as follows. One of the major symptoms in IBS is constipation (IBS-c); the second is abdominal pain (IBS-ab pain), and the third is diarrhea (IBS-d). A mixture of these can be called the Mixed Syndrome. It is difficult to analyze the literature with outcome results specific to either constipation, diarrhea, abdominal pain, or a mixture. However, there are many studies that have attempted to focus their protocol on one of those symptoms.[18–20] In a review of the studies that specifically focus on IBS, Mearin and colleagues[18] reveal that probiotics may benefit selective groups of patients.

A study using *B lactis* DN-173 010 in 312 constipated patients demonstrated acceleration of transient, improvement in abdominal distention, and severity of symptoms after 4 to 6 weeks of treatment.[21] In another trial, there also was improvement in the constipation group over placebo.[22] In another large trial, it was much more difficult to isolate the constipation patients from within the group.[23]

Two important articles were published from the group in Ireland, and both showed that *Bacillus infantis* 35624 strain was extremely effective.[24,25] Both of these articles impressed the clinical community, and this probiotic has been used widely to treat IBS.[24,25] However, again, only this strain of *B infantis* has been shown to be effective.

Several studies have identified diarrhea as the main symptom, and those show a definite improvement of multiple probiotics over placebo.[26–28] The identification of abdominal pain and mixed symptoms has been easier to identify as outcomes in studies, and here the author has shown many studies that have improved symptoms. However, it must be kept in mind that the same strain of probiotic should be used that was used in the reference.[26–32] Studies using either *Lactobacillus plantarum*[29] or *Bacillus coagulans*[32] were effective but in single large studies. Therefore, one can conclude that there are many probiotic controlled studies that have shown effectiveness in either constipation, diarrhea, or mixed variety, but the correct strain must be used and may require several studies.

The Danone Laboratory in France reports on identification of intestinal microbiota from patients with severe IBS. With their colleagues in Sweden, they reported on severe IBS subjects as compared with healthy controls and found definite intestinal microbiota profiles associated with the severity of IBS symptoms.[33] It certainly is early in the studies to be reported on the microbiota, but there is no question that this will be important as more research evolves.

Inflammatory Bowel Disorders

Ulcerative colitis

Probiotics are somewhat effective in both reducing and maintaining remission in classic ulcerative colitis. *Escherichia coli* Nissle 1917 was demonstrated by Rembacken and colleagues[34] in a small study in 1999 as effective. More recently, VSL#3 (now Visbiome) has clearly been used in many studies to both induce remission and maintain remission.[35] Studies first reported by Biblioni and colleagues in 2005[36] and in larger studies by Miele and his group[37] and Sood and his group,[38] as well as Tursi and his group,[39] all demonstrated that VSL#3 is an effective probiotic. It is extremely important that the correct VSL be used. Recently, VSL manufacturers have changed, and the formulation used in the successful studies is now called Visbiome.[40] Numerous other probiotics have been used in smaller studies but none with the amount of effectiveness of *E coli* Nissle or VSL#3.[40] Similarly, symbiotics have been tried in smaller studies and have shown some mild effectiveness, but much more work is needed to meet the results shown with *E coli* Nissle and VSL.[40] Fecal microbial transplant (FMT) has been tried in ulcerative colitis, but no study has yet shown that it is definitely effective.[40]

Interesting observations, such as that of Machiels and colleagues,[41] were recorded by the latest identification methods, that *Roseburia hominis* and *Faecalibacterium prusnitzii* define the dysbiosis that is present in ulcerative colitis. Certainly more information will be forthcoming as research evolves, because a change in the flora and dysbiosis has been reported by latest identification methods.[40]

Crohn disease

Although Crohn disease is clearly classified among inflammatory bowel disorders (IBD), there have been no long-term effective studies with either prebiotics or probiotics, although there have been many attempts to do so.[35,41–43]

Pouchitis

The surgical treatment of patients with familial adenomatous polyposis is restorative colectomy with ileal pouch–anal anastomosis (IPAA).[44–46] Also, it is a treatment for patients with refractive ulcerative colitis or those that have dysplasia in severe ulcerative colitis. Inflammation of the ileal reservoir or "pouch" is called pouchitis and develops only in patients that undergo the surgical procedures. The incidence of pouchitis occurs in 24% to 60% of cases with a tendency to reoccur in about 60%. Approximately 30% will develop chronic pouchitis, which in turn, may lead to excision of the pouch in 10%.[44–46] The cause of pouchitis is still poorly understood. However, bacteriologic studies have revealed a dysbiosis with increased levels of *Clostridium perfringens* and a decrease in anaerobes, *Bifidobacteria* and *Lactobacilli*.[47,48] Probiotics have proven to be popular in the treatment of pouchitis. In a double-blind study with placebo control, VSL was shown to be effective with only 10% recurring, whereas 40% recurred in controls.[49] In another randomized study, it was shown that at 3, 6, and 12 months there was significant reduction of pouchitis.[50] From all of the literature, it appears that the most effective probiotic agent is VLS#3.[51,52] Furthermore, it has been shown to be effective in small doses, high doses, at the onset, and in recurrence.

In the older literature, nonpathogenic *E coli* was reported effective in one study[53] but not repeated. Tomasz and colleagues[54] reported that long-term use of *Lactobacillus* and *Bifidobacteria* in a randomized study had a positive effect on recurrent pouchitis. Further changes can be expected with more research in IPAA.

Acute Infectious Diarrhea

In most cases, especially in children, the onset of diarrhea is due to an episode of infectious gastroenteritis. It is generally defined as a decrease in the consistency of stool to loose or liquid and an increase in the frequency of evacuations, which are more than 3 in 24 hours.[55] Johnston and his group[56] showed that there was great variation in the data collection in acute diarrhea. The choice of treatment varies,[55–59] but Guandalini[58] and an expert panel reviewed the recent data up to 2015, and it was thought that *Lactobacillus* GG (LGG) is the best treatment for acute gastroenteritis diarrhea and that it saves at least 1 day of sickness.

The question of treatment, therefore, varies with the use of a probiotic, but it also raises the question of prevention in healthy adults and children. Most prevention studies have been performed with probiotic strains related to milk-based feedings. These initial studies demonstrated a definite reduction in the incidence of severity of acute disease.[59–61] However, studies question the data.[58–62] *Lactobacillus reuteri* DSM 17938 has been shown to be effective in a careful study, but there were few others to follow this even though the investigators claim it was cost-saving.[63]

Nevertheless, the American Academy of Pediatrics considered probiotics beneficial for use in special circumstances, such as in long-term health care facilities.[64]

Hospital-acquired Diarrhea

Hospital-acquired diarrheas are common, and rotavirus is probably the most common cause.[65,66] There have been some attempts to prevent hospital-acquired diarrhea, and the only reported successful one is with *LGG*.[67] Supplementation with *Bifidobacteria* to hospitalized infants has prevented the incidence of diarrhea and hospital-acquired diseases. The beneficial effect of *Bifidobacteria breve* strain occult has been recorded in immunocompromised children on chemotherapy[68] to cure infections and increased anaerobes.[68] Of all of the available literature, there seems to be 2 references that can be used for the use of probiotics in children with infections.[55,69]

Antibiotic-associated Diarrhea and Clostridium difficile–associated Diarrhea

A great number of random controlled trials have been performed, and there are many meta-analyses conducted on the efficacy of probiotics in preventing antibiotic-associated diarrhea (AAD) and *Clostridium difficile*–associated diarrhea (CDAD). These studies have been performed in adults and children.[70–72] Analysis shows that the risk of CDAD is reduced by 64%. It included 23 random controlled trials with 4213 patients studied in both adults and children. The analyses reveal that either *LGG* or *S boulardii* is effective.[70–72]

Fecal Microbial Transplant

Severe or refractive CDAD has been successfully treated by fecal microbial transplant (FMT), which is described in detail.[73] Early reports from Europe[74,75] and later confirming reports in the United States[76] lead to wide acceptance that FMT can be curative of refractory *C difficile* diarrhea. There are now guidelines for the treatment of refractory *C difficile* diarrhea[77] and long-term studies documenting its long-term effectiveness.[78] Although there were high hopes that FMT would be helpful in other diseases such as

IBD, it is not been proven effective yet for the treatment of ulcerative colitis or Crohn disease.[79,80]

Since the guidelines have been written,[77] there has been important technique advances. There is now evidence that FMT can be performed with fresh frozen volunteer specimens.[81–83] This technique is early in its development, but should be proven very helpful when the frozen specimens are appropriately marketed.

Although it is disappointing that FMT has not proven to help in IBD, one can expect future research will show areas in which it can be effective.

Liver Disease

There is no question that prebiotics and probiotics are extremely helpful in the treatment of hepatic encephalopathy. Now nonalcoholic fatty liver disease (NAFLD) can be added to the list of uses in liver disease.

Studies of the microbiota reveal definite dysbiosis in subjects with chronic liver disease.[84,85] Bacterial overgrowth, bacterial translocation, and dysmotility are other mechanisms that have been observed in cirrhosis.[86,87]

However, the most commonly used and effective treatment of hepatic encephalopathy has been the prebiotic lactulose.[88] The limiting factor in its use is the production of diarrhea.[89,90] It also is effective as a symbiotic in use with probiotics. The simplest use of probiotics in patients with liver disease has been the use of yogurt for the treatment of mild hepatic encephalopathy.[89] With the yogurt study, which contained *Lactobacillus bogaritus* and *Thiptocaccus thermophilus*, the subjects on the yogurt did not develop any symptoms. In another study where symbiotics (a prebiotic and a probiotic) were used, the symbiotic was subsequently effective compared with other forms of therapy.[90] In numerous studies, lactulose combined with a probiotic has been most effective in decreasing neuropsychiatric symptoms of encephalopathy.[91] The limiting factor of lactulose use is the development of diarrhea and abdominal cramps.[91,92] In a random controlled trial, the use of VSL#3 over an extended period was effective therapy for hepatic encephalopathy. The patients on VSL#3 and probiotic-treated patients developed fewer symptoms.[93] From the references cited, it is clear that the clinician must choose the therapy wanted: either a simple prebiotic if tolerated or a symbiotic. There are many therapeutic choices available in treating mild to severe hepatic encephalopathy, and it is the clinician's choice depending on the clinical situation.[91–93]

It also is apparent that symbiotics or probiotics can be helpful to prevent infectious complications in patients after liver transplantation. This has been shown in a prospective randomized study.[94] In a meta-analysis, it was confirmed.[95] Therefore, it would seem that probiotics should be used in all liver transplant patients.[94,95]

During the past decade, it has become clear that probiotics are effective in treating NAFLD, first in pediatric reports and more recently in adults. The biochemical studies have shown that it is related to choline deficiency.[96] There are now numerous studies that have shown a variety of probiotics are effective in controlling the course of NAFLD. In the studies reported, all combinations of probiotics have been effective, including VSL#3, *Lactobacillus bulgaris*, and *Streptococcus thermophilus*, a combination of *L plantarum*, *Bifidobacteria longum*, and *L rhamnonus*. The clinician has to pick his or her choice and follow the references carefully. This is an excellent good turn in the use of probiotics, and it should be used by clinicians treating NAFLD.[97–100]

The author has listed the main uses of probiotics, probiotics, and symbiotics, which are supported by meta-analysis in gastrointestinal disease, but there are many uses with less literature support that are certainly going to come forth, such as their use in obesity,[101] rare autoimmune disease,[102] and bee-sting desensitization,[103] to balance the microbiota[104] and effect stress.[105]

REFERENCES

1. Turnbaugh PJ, Ley RE, Hamady M, et al. The human microbiome project. Nature 2007;449:804–10.
2. Floch MH, Ringel Y, Walker WA. The microbiota in gastrointestinal pathophysiology: implications for human health, prebiotics, probiotics, and dysbiosis. Cambridge (MA): Elsevier Inc; 2017.
3. Floch MH, Madsen KK, Jenkins DJA, et al. Recommendations for probiotic use. J Clin Gastroenterol 2006;40:275–8.
4. Floch MH, Walker WA, Guandalini S, et al. Recommendations for probiotic use-2008. J Clin Gastroenterol 2008;42:S104–8.
5. Floch MH, Walker WA, Madsen K, et al. Recommendations for probiotic use-2011 update. J Clin Gastroenterol 2011;45:S168–71.
6. Floch MH, Walker WA, Sanders ME, et al. Recommendations for probiotic use-2015 update: proceedings and consensus opinion. J Clin Gastroenterol 2015; 49:S69–73.
7. Report of joint FAO/WHO expert consultation on evaluation of health and nutritional properties of probiotics in food including powder milk with live lactic acid bacteria, October 2001.
8. Fuller R. Probiotics in man and animals. J Appl Bacteriol 1989;66:365–78.
9. Gibson CR, Roberfroid MB. Dietary modulation of the human colonic microflora: introducing the concept of prebiotics. J Nutr 1995;125:401.
10. Trowell H, Burkitt D, Heaton K. Dietary fibre, fibre-depleted foods and disease. London: Academic Press; 1985.
11. Spiller GA. CRC handbook of dietary fiber in human nutrition. 2nd edition. Boca Raton (FL): CRC Press; 1992. p. 15–8.
12. Boyle RJ, Robins-Browne RM, Tang MLK. Probiotic use in clinical practice: what are the risks? Am J Clin Nutr 2006;83:1256–64.
13. Donohue D. Safety of probiotic organisms. In: Lee YK, Salminen S, editors. Handbook of probiotics and prebiotics. 2nd edition. Hoboken (NJ): John Wiley & Sons, Inc; 2009. p. 75–95.
14. Peery AF, Crockett SD, Barritt AS, et al. Burden of gastrointestinal, liver, and pancreatic diseases in the United States. Gastroenterology 2015;149(7): 1731–41.e3.
15. Chang JY, Locke GR III, McNally MA, et al. Impact of functional gastrointestinal disorders on survival in the community. Am J Gastroenterol 2010;105(4):822–32.
16. Ford AC, Quigley EMM, Lacy BE, et al. Efficacy of prebiotics, probiotics, and synbiotics in irritable bowel syndrome and chronic idiopathic constipation: systemic review and meta-analysis. Am J Gastroenterol 2014;109:1547–61.
17. Patel R, DuPont HL. New approaches for bacteriotherapy: prebiotics, new-generation probiotics, and synbiotics. Clin Infect Dis 2015;60:S108–21.
18. Mearin F, Lacy BE, Chang L, et al. Bowel disorders. Gastroenterology 2016;150: 1393–407.e5.
19. Kim HJ, Vazquez Roque MI, Camilleri M, et al. A randomized controlled trial of a probiotic combination VSL#3 and placebo in irritable bowel syndrome with bloating. Neurogastroenterol Motil 2005;17:687–96.
20. Enck P. A probiotic fermented milk may help manage mild gastrointestinal discomfort in healthy female adults. (Gut Microbiota Research & Practice Website). 2017. Available at: http://www.gutmicrobiotaforhealth.com/en/probiotic-fermented-milk-may-help-manage-mild-gastrointestinal-discomfort-healthy-female-adults/. Accessed March 18, 2017.

21. Agrawal A, Houghton LA, Morris J, et al. Clinical trial: the effects of a fermented milk production containing Bifidobacterium lactis DN-173 010 on abdominal distension and gastrointestinal transit in irritable bowel syndrome with constipation. Aliment Pharmacol Ther 2009;29:104–14.
22. Guyonnet D, Chassany O, Ducrotte P, et al. Effect of a fermented milk containing Bifidobacterium animalis DN-173 010 on the health-related quality of life and symptoms in irritable bowel syndrome in adults in primary care: a multicentre, randomized, double-blind, controlled trial. Aliment Pharmacol Ther 2007; 26(3):475–86.
23. Roberts LM, McCahon D, Holder R, et al. A randomised controlled trial of a probiotic 'functional food' in the management of irritable bowel syndrome. BMC Gastroenterol 2013;13:45.
24. Whorwell PJ, Altringer L, Morel J, et al. Efficacy of an encapsulated probiotic Bifidobacterium infantis 35624 in women with irritable bowel syndrome. Am J Gastroenterol 2006;101:1581–90.
25. Quigley EMM. Irritable bowel syndrome. In: Floch MH, Kim AS, editors. Probiotics: a clinical guide. Thorofare (NJ): SLACK Inc; 1999. p. 273–82.
26. Zeng J, Li YQ, Zuo XL, et al. Clinical trial: effect of active lactic acid bacteria on mucosal barrier function in patients with diarrhea-predominant irritable bowel syndrome. Aliment Pharmacol Ther 2008;28:994–1002.
27. Michail S, Kenche H. Gut microbiota is not modified by randomized, double-blind, placebo-controlled trial of VSL#3 in diarrhea-predominant irritable bowel syndrome. Probiotics Antimicrob Proteins 2011;3:1–7.
28. Kim HJ, Camilleri M, McKinzie S, et al. A randomized controlled trial of a probiotic, VLS#3, on gut transit and symptoms in diarrhoea-predominant irritable bowel syndrome. Aliment Pharmacol Ther 2003;17:895–904.
29. Ducrotte P, Sawant P, Jayanthi V. Clinical trials: Lactobacillus plantarum 299v (DSM 9843) improves symptoms of irritable bowel syndrome. World J Gastroenterol 2012;18:4012–8.
30. Kim HJ, Vazquez Roque MI, Camilleri M, et al. A randomized controlled trial of a probiotic combination VSL#3 and placebo in irritable bowel syndrome with bloating. Neurogastroenterol Motil 2005;22:387–94.
31. Kajander K, Hatakka K, Poussa T, et al. A probiotic mixture alleviates symptoms in irritable bowel syndrome patients: a controlled 6-month intervention. Aliment Pharmacol Ther 2005;22:387–94.
32. Kalman DS, Schwartz HI, Alvarez P, et al. A prospective, randomized, double-blind, placebo-controlled parallel-group dual site trial to evaluate the effects of a Bacillus coagulans-based product on functional intestinal gas symptoms. BMC Gastroenterol 2009;9:85.
33. Tap J, Derrien M, Tomblom H, et al. Identification of an intestinal microbiota signature associated with severity of irritable bowel syndrome. Gastroenterology 2017;152:111–23.
34. Rembacken BJ, Snelling AM, Hawkey PM, et al. Non-pathogenic Escherichia coli versus mesalazine for the treatment of ulcerative colitis: a randomized trial. Lancet 1999;354:635–9.
35. Orel R, Trop TK. Intestinal microbiota, probiotics, and prebiotics in inflammatory bowel disease. World J Gastroenterol 2014;20:11505–24.
36. Biblioni R, Fedorak RN, Tannock GW, et al. VSL#3 probiotic-mixture induces remission in patients with active ulcerative colitis. Am J Gastroenterol 2005; 100:1539–46.

37. Miele E, Pascarell F, Giannetti E, et al. Effect of a probiotic preparation (VSL#3) on induction and maintenance of remission in children with ulcerative colitis. Am J Gastroenterol 2009;104:437–43.

38. Sood A, Midha V, Makharia GK, et al. The probiotic preparation VSL#3 induces remission in patients with mild to moderately active ulcerative colitis. Clin Gastroenterol Hepatol 2009;7:1202–9.

39. Tursi A, Brandimarte G, Papa A, et al. Treatment of relapsing mild to moderately active ulcerative colitis with probiotic VSL#3 as adjunctive to a standard pharmaceutical treatment: a double-blind, randomized, placebo-controlled study. Am J Gastroenterol 2010;105:2218–27.

40. Chibbar R, Alahmadi A, Dieleman LA. Treatment of inflammatory bowel disease in ulcerative colitis. In: Floch MH, Ringel Y, Walker WA, editors. The microbiota in gastrointestinal pathophysiology; implications for human health, prebiotics, probiotics, and dysbiosis. Cambridge (MA): Elsevier Inc; 2017. p. 343–54.

41. Machiels K, Joossens M, Sabino J, et al. A decrease of the butyrate-producing species Roseburia hominis and Faecalibacterium prusnitzii defines dysbiosis in patients with ulcerative colitis. Gut 2014;63:1275–83.

42. Rahimi R, Nikfar S, Rahimi F, et al. A meta-analysis on the efficacy of probiotics for maintenance of remission and prevention of clinical and endoscopic relapse in Crohn's disease. Dig Dis Sci 2008;53:2524–31.

43. van Loo ES, Dijkstra G, Ploeg RJ, et al. Prevention of postoperative recurrent of Crohn's disease. J Crohns Colitis 2012;6:637–46.

44. Sandborn WJ. Pouchitis following ileal pouch-anal anastomosis: definition, pathogenesis and treatment. Gastroenterology 1994;107:1856–60.

45. Fazio VW, Ziv Y, Church JM, et al. Ileal pouch-anal anastomoses complications and function in 1005 patients. Ann Surg 1995;222:120–7.

46. Pardi DS, Sandborn WJ. Management of pouchitis. Aliment Pharmacol Ther 2006;23:1087–96.

47. Iwaya A, Iiai T, Okamoto H, et al. Change in the bacterial flora of pouchitis. Hepatogastroenterology 2006;53:55–9.

48. Komanduri S, Gillevet PM, Sikaroodi M, et al. Dysbiosis in pouchitis, evidence of unique microfloral patterns in pouch inflammation. Clin Gastroenterol Hepatol 2007;5:353–60.

49. Gionchetti P, Rizzello F, Morselli C, et al. High-dose probiotics for the treatment of active pouchitis. Dis Colon Rectum 2007;50:2075–84.

50. Gionchetti P, Rizzello F, Venturi A, et al. Oral bacteriotherapy as maintenance treatment in patients with chronic pouchitis; a double-blind, placebo-controlled trial. Gastroenterology 2000;119:305–9.

51. Mimura T, Rizzello F, Helwig U, et al. Once daily high dose probiotic therapy (VSL #3) for maintaining remission in recurrent refractory pouchitis. Gut 2004; 53:108–14.

52. Shen J, Zuo ZX, Mao AP. Effect of probiotics on inducing remission and maintaining therapy in ulcerative colitis, Crohn's disease and pouchitis: meta-analysis of randomized controlled trial. Inflamm Bowel Dis 2014;20:21–35.

53. Kuzela L, Kascak M, Vavrecka A. Induction and maintenance of remission with nonpathogenic Escherichia coli in patients with pouchitis. Am J Gastroenterol 2001;96:3218–9.

54. Tomasz B, Zoran S, Jaroslaw W, et al. Long-term use of probiotics Lactobacillus and Bifidobacterium has a prophylactic effect on the occurrence and severity of pouchitis: a randomized prospective study. Biomed Res Int 2014;2014:208064.

55. Guarino A, Ashkenazi S, Gendrel D, et al. European Society for Pediatric Gastro-enterology, Hepatology, and Nutrition/European Society for Pediatric Infectious Diseases Evidence-based Guidelines for management of acute gastroenteritis in children in Europe: update. J Pediatr Gastroenterol Nutr 2014;59:132–52.
56. Johnston BC, Shamseer L, de Costa BR, et al. Measurement issues in trials of pediatric acute-diarrheal diseases: a systemic review. Pediatrics 2010;126: e222–31.
57. Isolauri E, Juntunen M, Rautanen T, et al. A human Lactobacillus strain (Lactobacillus casei sp strain GG) promotes recovery from acute diarrhea in children. Pediatrics 1991;88:90–7.
58. Guandalini S. Probiotics for prevention and treatment of diarrhea. J Clin Gastroenterol 2011;45:S149–53.
59. Saavedra JM, Tschernia A. Human studies with probiotics and prebiotics: clinical implications. Br J Nutr 2002;87:S241–6.
60. Saran S, Gopalan S, Krishna TP. Use of fermented foods to combat stunting and failure to thrive. Nutrition 2002;18:393–6.
61. Karas J, Ashkenazi S, Guarino A, et al. A core outcome set for clinical trials in acute diarrhea. Arch Dis Child 2015;100:359–63.
62. Szajewska H, Setty M, Mrukowicz J, et al. Probiotics in gastrointestinal diseases in children: hard and not-so-hard evidence of efficacy. J Pediatr Gastroenterol Nutr 2006;42:454–75.
63. Gutierrez-Castrellon P, Lopez-Velazquez G, Diaz-Garcia L, et al. Diarrhea in preschool children and Lactobacillus reuteri: a randomized controlled trial. Pediatrics 2014;133:e904–9.
64. Thomas DW, Greer FR. American Academy of Pediatrics Committee on Nutrition, American Academy of pediatrics section on gastroenterology, hepatology, and nutrition. Probiotics and prebiotics in pediatrics. Pediatrics 2010;126: 1217–31.
65. Wittenberg DP. Management guidelines for acute infective diarrhea/gastroenteritis in infants. S Afr Med J 2012;102:104–7.
66. Chen W-Z, Ren L-H, Shi R-H. Enteric microbiota leads to new therapeutic strategies for ulcerative colitis. World J Gastroenterol 2014;20:15657–63.
67. European Food Safety Authority Panel on Dietetic Products, Nutrition and Allergies. Scientific opinion on the substantiation of health claims related to non-characterised microorganisms pursuant to Article 13(1) of Regulation (EC) No 1924/20061. EFSA J 2009;7:1247.
68. Wada M, Nagata S, Saito M, et al. Effects of the enteral administration of Bifidobacterium breve on patients undergoing chemotherapy for pediatric malignancies. Support Care Cancer 2010;18:751–9.
69. Szajewska H, Guarino A, Hojsak I, et al. Use of probiotics for management of acute gastroenteritis: a position paper by the ESPGHAN Working Group for probiotics and prebiotics. J Pediatr Gastroenterol Nutr 2014;58:531–9.
70. Goldenberg JZ, Ma SS, Saxton JD, et al. Probiotics for the prevention of Clostridium difficile-associated diarrhea in adults and children. Cochrane Database Syst Rev 2013;5:CD006096.
71. Szajewska H, Canani RB, Guarino A, et al. Probiotics for the prevention of antibiotic-associated diarrhea in children. J Pediatr Gastroenterol Nutr 2015; 62:495–506.
72. Pattani R, Palda VA, Hwang SW, et al. Probiotics for the prevention of antibiotic-associated diarrhea and Clostridium difficile infection among hospitalized patients: systemic review and meta-analysis. Open Med 2015;7:e56–67.

73. Fine S, Kelly CR. FMT in Clostridium difficile and other potential uses. In: Floch MH, Ringel Y, Walker WA, editors. The microbiota in gastrointestinal pathophysiology: implications for human health, prebiotics, probiotics, and dysbiosis. Cambridge (MA): Elsevier Inc; 2017. p. 315–26.

74. Eiseman B, Silen W, Bascom GS, et al. Fecal enema as an adjunct in the treatment of pseudomembranous enterocolitis. Surgery 1958;44:854–9.

75. Schwan A, Sjolin S, Trottestam U, et al. Relapsing Clostridium difficile enterocolitis cured by rectal infusion of homologous faeces. Lancet 1983;2:845.

76. Bartlett JG, Chang TW, Gurwith M, et al. Antibiotic-associated pseudomembranous colitis due to toxin-producing clostridia. N Engl J Med 1978;298:531–4.

77. Surawicz CM, Brandt LJ, Binion DG, et al. Guidelines for diagnosis, treatment, and prevention of Clostridium difficile infections. Am J Gastroenterol 2013; 108:478–98 [quiz: 499].

78. Brandt LJ, Aroniadis OC, Mellow M, et al. Long-term follow-up of colonoscopic fecal microbiota transplant for recurrent Clostridium difficile infection. Am J Gastroenterol 2012;107:1079–87.

79. Rossen NG, Fuentes S, van der Spek MJ, et al. Findings from a randomized controlled trial of fecal transplantation for patients with ulcerative colitis. Gastroenterology 2015;149:110–8.e4.

80. Colman RJ, Rubin DT. Fecal microbiota transplantation as therapy for inflammatory bowel disease: a systemic review and meta-analysis. J Crohns Colitis 2014; 8:1569–81.

81. Hamilton MJ, Weingarden AR, Sadowsky MJ, et al. Standardized frozen preparation for transplantation of fecal microbiota for recurrent Clostridium difficile infection. Am J Gastroenterol 2012;107:761–7.

82. Lee CH, Steiner T, Petrof EO, et al. Frozen vs. fresh fecal microbiota transplantation and clinical resolution of diarrhea in patients with recurrent Clostridium difficile infection: a randomized clinical trial. JAMA 2016;315:142–9.

83. Youngster I, Sauk J, Pindar C, et al. Fecal microbiota transplant for relapsing Clostridium difficile infection using a frozen inoculum from unrelated donors: a randomized, open-label, controlled pilot study. Clin Infect Dis 2014;58:1515–22.

84. Bajaj J, Hylemon P, Ridlon J, et al. Colonic mucosal microbiome differs from stool microbiome in cirrhosis and hepatic encephalopathy and is linked to cognition and inflammation. Am J Physiol 2012;303:G675–85.

85. Liu J, Wu D, Ahmed A, et al. Comparison of the gut microbe profiles and numbers between patients with liver cirrhosis and healthy individuals. Curr Microbiol 2012;65:7–13.

86. Garcia-Tsao G, Albillos A, Barden GE, et al. Bacterial translocation in acute and chronic portal hypertension. Hepatology 1993;17:1081–5.

87. Chang CS, Chen GH, Lien HC, et al. Small intestine dysmotility and bacterial overgrowth in cirrhotic patients with spontaneous bacterial peritonitis. Hepatology 1998;28:1187–90.

88. Shukla S, Shukla A, Mehboob S, et al. Meta-analysis: the effects of gut flora modulation using prebiotics, probiotics and synbiotics on minimal hepatic encephalopathy. Aliment Pharmacol Ther 2011;33:662–71.

89. Bajaj J, Saeian K, Christensen L, et al. Probiotic yogurt for the treatment of minimal hepatic encephalopathy. Am J Gastroenterol 2008;103:1707–15.

90. Sharma P, Sharma B, Puri V, et al. An open-label randomized controlled trial of lactulose and probiotics in the treatment of minimal hepatic encephalopathy. Eur J Gastroenterol Hepatol 2007;20:506–11.

91. Agrawal A, Sharma BC, Sharma P, et al. Secondary prophylaxis of hepatic en-cephalopathy in cirrhosis: an open-label, randomized controlled trial of lactu-lose, probiotics, and no therapy. Am J Gastroenterol 2012;107:1043–50.
92. Malaguarnera M, Gargante M, Malaguarner G, et al. Bifidobacterium combined with fructo-oligosaccharide versus lactulose in the treatment of patients with he-patic encephalopathy. Eur J Gastroenterol Hepatol 2009;22:199–206.
93. Lunia MK, Sharma BC, Sharma P, et al. Probiotics prevent hepatic encephalop-athy in patients with cirrhosis: a randomized controlled trial. Clin Gastroenterol Hepatol 2014;12:1003–8.
94. Eguchi S, Takatsuki M, Hidaka M, et al. Perioperative synbiotic treatment to pre-vent infectious complications in patients after elective living donor liver trans-plantation: a prospective randomized study. Am J Surg 2011;4:498–502.
95. Sawas T, Al Halabi S, Hernaez R, et al. Patients receiving prebiotics and probi-otics before liver transplantation develop fewer infections than controls: a sys-temic review and meta-analysis. Clin Gastroenterol Hepatol 2015;13:1567–74.
96. Spencer M, Hamp T, Reid R, et al. Association between composition of the hu-man gastroenterology microbiome and development of fatty liver with choline deficiency. Gastroenterology 2011;140:976–86.
97. Miloh T. Probiotics in pediatric liver disease. J Clin Gastroenterol 2015;49:S33–6.
98. Aller R, De Luis D, Izaola O, et al. Effect of a probiotic on liver aminotransferases in nonalcoholic fatty liver disease patient, a double blind randomized clinical trial. Eur Rev Med Pharmacol Sci 2011;15:1090–5.
99. Malaguarnera M, Vacante M, Antic T, et al. Bifidobacterium longum with fructo-oligosaccharides in patients with non-alcoholic steatohepatitis. Dig Dis Sci 2012;57:545–53.
100. Wong VW, Won GL, Chim AM, et al. Treatment of nonalcoholic steatohepatitis with probiotics. A proof-of-concept study. Ann Hepatol 2013;12:256–62.
101. Vajro P, Mandato C, Licenziati MR, et al. Effects of Lactobacillus rhamnosus strain GG in pediatric obesity-related liver disease. J Pediatr Gastroenterol Nutr 2011;52:740–3.
102. Horvath A, Leber B, Schmerboeck B, et al. Randomised clinical trial: the effects of a multispecies probiotic vs. placebo on innate immune function, bacterial translocation and gut permeability in patients with cirrhosis. Aliment Pharmacol Ther 2016;44:926–35.
103. Ptaszyńska AA, Borsuk G, Zdybicka-Barabas A, et al. Are commercial probiot-ics and prebiotics effective in the treatment and prevention of honeybee nose-mosis C? Parasitol Res 2016;115:397–406.
104. Lecerf JM, Depeint F, Clerc E, et al. Xylo-oligosaccharide (XOS) in combination with inulin modulates both the intestinal environment and immune status in healthy subjects, while XOS alone only shows prebiotic properties. Br J Nutr 2012;108:1847–58.
105. Lin SH, Chou LM, Chien YW, et al. Prebiotic effects of xylooligosaccharides on the improvement of microbiota balance in human subjects. Gastroenterol Res Pract 2016;2016:5789232.

Small Intestinal Bacterial Overgrowth

Nutritional Implications, Diagnosis, and Management

Abimbola Adike, MD, John K. DiBaise, MD*

KEYWORDS

- Small intestinal bacterial overgrowth • Malabsorption • Breath test
- Small bowel aspirate • Antibiotic • Diagnosis • Treatment

KEY POINTS

- Small intestinal bacterial overgrowth (SIBO) is characterized by the presence of excessive bacteria in the small intestine.
- Small bowel motility is the most important protective mechanism preventing SIBO.
- Macronutrient and micronutrient deficiencies may occur as a consequence of SIBO.
- There is no true gold standard for the diagnosis of SIBO.
- It is important to identify and treat the underlying disorder causing SIBO.

INTRODUCTION

Over the last decade, small intestinal bacterial overgrowth (SIBO) has been suggested to be underrecognized and to have important clinical implications,[1] yet there remains no consensus on the definition of SIBO. This relates, in part, to a lack of a diagnostic gold standard and the nonspecific clinical manifestations attributed to SIBO. As a consequence, its true prevalence and relationship with other clinical disorders (ie, cause, consequence, or epiphenomenon) are unclear.[2] For similar reasons, the treatment of SIBO also presents a challenge, particularly in patients with relapsing symptoms and without classic risk factors for the development of SIBO.

Although traditionally considered a malabsorptive disorder associated with severe gut stasis, SIBO has more recently been suggested to be a less specific disorder associated with diverse clinical conditions (eg, irritable bowel syndrome [IBS], nonalcoholic

Disclosure: The authors having nothing to disclose.
Division of Gastroenterology and Hepatology, Mayo Clinic, 13400 East Shea Boulevard, Scottsdale, AZ 85259, USA
* Corresponding author.
E-mail address: dibaise.john@mayo.edu

Gastroenterol Clin N Am 47 (2018) 193–208
https://doi.org/10.1016/j.gtc.2017.09.008
0889-8553/18/© 2017 Elsevier Inc. All rights reserved.

gastro.theclinics.com

fatty liver disease, and celiac disease) characterized by a variety of gastrointestinal and even nongastrointestinal symptoms thought to be related to the presence of excessive bacteria in the small intestine. Importantly, SIBO implies not only a quantitative assessment of bacteria but also the presence of particular species of bacteria in an atypical location in the small bowel. It is generally considered that only overgrowth of microbes that colonize the colon is clearly linked to clinically significant SIBO. As a corollary, if these microbes are reduced or eliminated from the small bowel, most commonly with antibiotics, then the clinical manifestations should resolve.

Reduced gastric acid production, deranged small bowel motility, altered bowel anatomy, and impaired systemic and/or local immunity are among the major intrinsic risk factors implicated in the development of SIBO. Although typically seen as a consequence of postsurgical stasis syndromes and profound intestinal dysmotility, SIBO is now considered by many investigators to result from less severe derangements in gut physiology. The objective of this article is to provide an up-to-date review of the nutritional implications, diagnosis, and management of SIBO. In the process, its risk factors and clinical manifestations are also discussed.

GUT MICROBES IN HEALTH

The gut microbiota of an infant is acquired from the mother during birth and, in the early stages of life, tends to be similar to that of the mother.[3,4] The diet and environment profoundly influence the composition of the gut microbiota during subsequent growth and development.[5] The commensal gut microbiota has multiple beneficial effects on the host, including the prevention of colonization by pathogenic bacteria, and maintenance of the integrity of intestinal epithelium and gut lymphoid tissue. In addition, certain gut microbes synthesize micronutrients such as vitamin K and folic acid, whereas others participate in drug metabolism.[6] Finally, colonic microbes are able to ferment undigested carbohydrates into short-chain fatty acids, which are used by colonocytes as an energy source and, in certain clinical scenarios (eg, short bowel syndrome), may be absorbed systemically and used as energy by the host.[6]

INTERNAL MECHANISMS REGULATING THE GUT MICROBIAL ECOSYSTEM

In the proximal small bowel of healthy individuals, gram-positive aerobic bacteria predominate with rare facultative anaerobes; together, these typically do not exceed more than 10^4 colony forming units (CFUs) per milliliter. In contrast, the distal small bowel acts as a transition zone with the microbiota in the small bowel consisting mostly of facultative anaerobes and sparse populations of aerobic bacteria, and the colon microbes consisting of a dense population of strict anaerobes; typically, greater than 10^{12} CFU/mL.[5]

SIBO may occur not only in the presence of excessive small bowel bacteria but also when there is an alteration in the distribution of the gut microbiota such that the microbes in the proximal small bowel reflect the usual microbes in the more distal gut. This typically is caused by a disturbance in factors normally preventing such alteration. The ileocecal valve has traditionally been considered important in regulating the composition of small intestine microbiota by preventing the reflux of colonic microbes into the small bowel. In support, a recent pilot study measured ileocecal valve pressures and found that individuals with a positive lactulose breath test for SIBO had defective ileocecal valve cecal distention reflex, which correlated with symptoms.[7] Additionally, Roland and colleagues[8] found that SIBO was more common in individuals with ileocecal valve dysfunction, as determined by impaired ileocecal junction pressures using a wireless motility capsule. In contrast, other studies suggest that the ileocecal valve may be less important in contributing to the development of SIBO and, instead, propose that it is the presence of normal distal small bowel motility that plays a primary role in preventing excessive colonization by colonic microbes.[9,10]

Additional physiologic mechanisms protecting against SIBO include small bowel motility, gastric acid, pancreaticobiliary secretions, and systemic and local immunity (**Table 1**). Small bowel motility is the most important mechanism preventing SIBO. The coordinated small intestinal motor patterns, both in the fasting and fed states, prevent colonization by inhibiting bacteria from attaching to the luminal wall. Both primary and secondary causes of intestinal dysmotility disrupt the enteric nervous system, visceral musculature, or both, and can result in SIBO.[3] Secondary causes of dysmotility can occur as a result of systemic diseases such as primary systemic sclerosis, Parkinson disease, hypothyroidism, and diabetes mellitus, or can be a result of treatments such as radiation or medications (eg, opioids, anticholinergics).[11] Additionally, surgical alteration of the small bowel can result in bacterial stasis. In patients with extensive surgical resection resulting in short bowel syndrome, SIBO seems to occur frequently.[12] Creation of blind intestinal loops, for example, after Roux-en-Y bypass surgery and the Billroth II procedure, also predisposes to SIBO because of ineffective bacteria clearance, decreased exposure to gastric acid, and/or retained food and

Table 1
Risk factors for small intestinal bacterial overgrowth

Mechanism	Examples
Failure of gastric acid barrier	Atrophic gastritis Hypochlorhydria Gastric bypass Gastrectomy Proton pump inhibitors
Failure of small bowel clearance	Primary visceral neuropathy or myopathy Connective tissue diseases (scleroderma, polymyositis) Amyloidosis Gastroparesis Radiation enteropathy Paraneoplastic syndrome Medications (opioids, anticholinergics)
Small bowel anatomic alteration	Short bowel syndrome Small bowel diverticulosis Small bowel strictures or fistulas Small bowel obstruction Blind loops (Roux-en Y) Ileocecal valve resection
Immunodeficiency	IgA deficiency Combined variable immune deficiency T cell deficiency
Multifactorial	Irritable bowel syndrome Cirrhosis Chronic pancreatitis Obesity Cystic fibrosis Chronic renal failure Celiac disease Diabetes mellitus Hypothyroidism

secretions. Anatomic risk factors intrinsic to the small bowel, such as from jejunal diverticulosis and strictures from Crohn disease or surgical anastomoses from small bowel resections, also predispose to stasis and increase the risk for SIBO.[11]

Gastric acid plays an important role in regulating the microbial population in the foregut and, perhaps, in more distal segments of the gut.[13] Fasting hypochlorhydria in asymptomatic patients may cause overgrowth of predominantly gram-positive organisms.[14] The clinical significance of excessive gram-positive bacteria in the proximal small bowel, however, remains controversial. Proton pump inhibitors (PPIs) have been implicated in the development of SIBO because of their marked effect on reducing gastric acid secretion. A meta-analysis of 11 studies comparing the risk of SIBO among adult users versus nonusers of PPIs found an odds ratio of SIBO in PPI users of 2.3 (95% CI 1.2–4.2).[15] This was, however, only statistically significant when using culture of small bowel aspirates for SIBO diagnosis and not when breath testing was used. Thus, the role of PPIs in causing clinically significant SIBO remains uncertain.

Immunodeficiency syndromes seem to increase the risk of SIBO because secretory immunoglobulin (Ig)-A-mediated system, non-IgA antibodies, and T lymphocytes are important in maintaining homeostasis of the internal gut environment.[16] The antimicrobial activity of pancreaticobiliary secretions also plays a role in limiting pathogenic gut microbes in the gut[17]; however, their role in causing SIBO is uncertain.[18]

NUTRITIONAL IMPLICATIONS OF SMALL INTESTINAL BACTERIAL OVERGROWTH

The adverse nutritional consequences of SIBO may involve multiple factors, including injury to the host epithelium, impact of bacterial metabolism, and diminished food intake due to the presence of gastrointestinal symptoms. These adverse consequences can contribute to malabsorption, weight loss, and altered micronutrient levels.

Malabsorption

Pathogenic bacteria can have direct toxic effect on the gut epithelium. Villous atrophy and varying degrees of epithelial inflammation have been described in association with SIBO.[19] These changes contribute to the reduction in intestinal absorptive surface area and play a role in the symptoms attributed to SIBO. Steatorrhea secondary to fat maldigestion and malabsorption may occur primarily as a result of deconjugation of bile acids by intraluminal bacteria and a subsequent deficiency of intraluminal bile acids necessary for adequate micelle formation.[20] These bacteria-derived deconjugated bile acids, such as lithocholic acid, may also exert a toxic injury on enterocytes that affects not only the absorption of fat but also carbohydrate and protein. Carbohydrate malabsorption may result from intraluminal degradation of sugars by the bacteria and by impaired activity of disaccharidase and other brush-border hydrolase activity responsible for absorption of sugars.[21] The production of toxins by bacteria may also directly impair carbohydrate and protein absorption. Bacterial products, however, do not contribute significantly to host protein catabolism. Although overt protein malnutrition is rarely seen in SIBO,[22] protein-losing enteropathy has been described.[23,24]

Altered Micronutrients

When fat malabsorption is present, deficiencies in the fat-soluble vitamins A, D, and E may occur,[25–27] although they are uncommon and usually remain clinically silent. As such, a high index of clinical suspicion and monitoring of micronutrient levels is suggested, particularly in those SIBO patients with more severe clinical manifestations. In contrast, levels of vitamin K, another fat-soluble vitamin, are usually normal or may be increased because of bacterial synthesis of menaquinones. Vitamin B12 deficiency may result from inhibition of normal B12 absorption by anaerobic organisms and by the consumption of vitamin B12 within the intestinal lumen by enteric microbes before it can be absorbed. Facultative gram-negative aerobes and anaerobes are capable of competitively using cobalamin.[28] In contrast, folate levels may be elevated in SIBO secondary to bacterial synthesis. Iron, thiamine, and nicotinamide deficiencies have also been described in the setting of SIBO although the mechanisms are not known.[29] A summary of nutritional consequences of SIBO is shown in **Table 2**.

CLINICAL MANIFESTATIONS OF SMALL INTESTINAL BACTERIAL OVERGROWTH

It is the negative effects on nutrient digestion just described that account for many of the clinical features seen in SIBO. Carbohydrate malabsorption is thought to lead to most of the symptoms ascribed to SIBO and the reduced dietary intake that may result in weight loss. For example, carbohydrate malabsorption may cause diarrhea and several gas symptoms, including abdominal discomfort and bloating. The malabsorption of fat may cause steatorrhea, foul-smelling flatus, weight loss, fat-soluble vitamin deficiencies with their clinical consequences and oxalate nephrolithiasis. Steatorrhea and other manifestations of fat malabsorption are generally seen only in association with the more classic postoperative stasis syndromes. Deconjugated bile acids may have secretomotor effects on the colon, also leading to diarrhea. Vitamin B12 deficiency may result in a megaloblastic anemia and, in severe cases, a rare neurologic syndrome. Alterations in gut peptide secretion due to differences in nutrient presentation to the more distal gut as a consequence of SIBO may lead to altered postprandial motility (eg, altered jejunal and ileal brakes) and its associated symptoms (eg, discomfort, fullness, bloating, nausea).[30]

Although SIBO, as currently considered, generally causes mild, nonspecific symptoms, it can also result in more severe manifestations. It is important to recognize that the more severe manifestations most commonly result from the underlying disease process rather than SIBO itself. SIBO may also be clinically silent and considered in the setting of abnormal laboratory studies. In addition, although diarrhea is more

Table 2
Mechanisms contributing to nutritional deficiencies in small intestinal bacterial overgrowth

Nutrient	Mechanism
Fat	• Deconjugation of bile acids resulting in decreased bile acids available for micelle formation • Production of toxins such as lithocholic acid that may directly inhibit absorption
Carbohydrate	• Production of toxins such as lithocholic acid that may directly inhibit absorption • Degradation of sugars by bacteria • Impaired activity of brush border disaccharidase and hydrolase
Protein	• Production of toxins such as lithocholic acid that may directly inhibit absorption
Vitamin B12	• Consumption of B12 by bacteria • Inhibition of B12 absorption in the terminal ileum
Vitamin A, D, and E	• Deconjugation of bile acids resulting in decreased bile acids available for fat absorption

commonly present in the setting of SIBO, methane-predominant SIBO (see following section) seems to be associated with constipation.[31,32]

DIAGNOSIS OF SMALL INTESTINAL BACTERIAL OVERGROWTH

The signs and symptoms associated with SIBO are nonspecific and cannot be used in isolation to aid in the diagnosis. Indeed, they may lead to diagnostic confusion because these symptoms and SIBO may coexist but be unrelated. At present, the most commonly used tests to diagnose SIBO in clinical practice are hydrogen breath tests and the culture of small bowel aspirates. Both have significant limitations (**Table 3**), however, precluding a true diagnostic gold standard for SIBO.[33] As a consequence, there is currently no consensus on the optimal test for the diagnosis of SIBO and the symptomatic response to a trial of antibiotics is often substituted for objective testing in clinical practice.

Small Bowel Aspirate or Culture

The gold standard test for SIBO has traditionally been considered the quantitative culture of a jejunal aspirate. Small bowel aspiration and culture, however, is invasive and costly because it generally requires endoscopy for sample collection and rapid delivery to the microbiology laboratory for aerobic and anaerobic processing. Nevertheless, because endoscopy is commonly performed in patients with symptoms that may be caused by SIBO, sampling of small bowel fluid can be readily performed with use of a commercially available sterile catheter passed through the working channel of the endoscope, thereby limiting potential contamination, while minimizing air insufflation.[34] Another limitation of small bowel aspirates is the possibility that SIBO may be patchy or preferentially located in the mid or distal small bowel, which may be missed by an aspirate obtained in the more proximal small bowel.[35] Yet, the reliability of the aspirate at different locations in the proximal jejunum has been demonstrated by some investigators and the clinical significance of distal SIBO remains to be validated.[36] It seems likely that the discrepancies identified in the reliability of the culture of jejunal aspirates may have arisen from differences in sampling the microbiological analytical techniques.

A critical and unresolved issue with use of the small bowel aspirate remains the lack of clarity on the optimal microbiological cutoff that defines a positive aspirate. The traditional cutoff level diagnostic of SIBO is greater than or equal to 10^5 (or even $\geq 10^6$) CFU/mL of aerobic gram-negative or strict anaerobic bacteria obtained from a jejunal aspirate.[36,37] This was based on highly symptomatic patients with high-risk conditions. In contemporary clinical practice, the patients selected for testing often

---

Table 3
Potential limitations of diagnostic testing for small intestinal bacterial overgrowth

Small Bowel Aspirates or Culture	Breath Testing
• Invasive and costly • Bacterial colonization may be patchy or located in more distal aspects of the small bowel • Improper handling of samples • Contamination may occur from oropharyngeal flora • Controversy regarding diagnostic cutoff	• Requires proper preparation • False positive tests may be seen with chronic lung disease and in smokers • Glucose may not detect bacterial overgrowth in the more distal portions of the small bowel • Lactulose shortens orocecal transit time • Wide variation in interpretation and diagnostic criteria

have no apparent risk factors for SIBO and only present with nonspecific symptoms. Furthermore, it is more common at present to obtain the aspirate from the distal duodenum because of the limited reach of a standard upper endoscope, yet the same cutoff level for SIBO is generally used. There may be a difference in the threshold of normal bacteria count in the mid-distal duodenum versus the proximal jejunum with lower concentration expected in the duodenum given the closer proximity to gastric acid and pancreaticobiliary secretions.

Recently, there have been reports suggesting that a lower colony count (eg, $\geq 10^3$ or $\geq 10^4$) obtained from the distal duodenum should be used instead to diagnose SIBO. Indeed, a recent report from the North American consensus group recommended greater than or equal to 10^3 CFU/mL be used when the culturing of small bowel aspirate is being considered for diagnosis of SIBO.[38] This is based, in part, on a systematic review of diagnostic tests for SIBO which suggested that the validity of greater than or equal to 10^5 CFU/mL for conditions other than the stagnant loop syndrome could not be confirmed.[33] The lower cutoff threshold seems to be based on a study of subjects with IBS that found that there was no difference in jejunal aspirate colony counts between IBS subjects and controls when based on the standard greater than or equal to 10^5 colonic bacteria/mL; however, when using a lower threshold of greater than or equal to 5×10^3/mL (≥ 95 percentile in controls), mildly increased bacterial counts were more common in IBS subjects (43% vs 12%; $P = .002$).[39] Erdogan and colleagues[40] also used a duodenal threshold level of greater than or equal to 10^3 CFU/mL in 139 subjects with unexplained gas, bloating, and diarrhea, and normal endoscopy, radiology, or blood tests. Duodenal cultures were positive in 45% (18% using a $\geq 10^5$ CFU/mL threshold) although symptom scores correlated poorly with the results of the SIBO testing. In a study from Greece, 320 consecutive subjects presenting for upper endoscopy were evaluated.[41] Duodenal aspirates were obtained in all subjects and a range of colony count thresholds ($\geq 10^3$, $\geq 10^4$, and $\geq 10^5$ CFU/mL) were analyzed to compare subjects with IBS to those without IBS. At all thresholds, more IBS subjects (67%–69%) had SIBO compared with non-IBS subjects (27%–31%). Of course, use of a lower threshold level is prone to false positivity from oral contamination.

Hydrogen (and Methane)-Based Breath Testing

Breath testing is an inexpensive, noninvasive, and relatively simple way to test for SIBO. Despite limitations and generally inferior performance characteristics compared with the small bowel aspirate, at least in patients at high risk of SIBO, these qualities have caused breath testing to be the most common test used in the diagnosis of SIBO. Healthy humans produce about 100 mL of intestinal gas composed of hydrogen, carbon dioxide, methane, and hydrogen sulfide. Of these, hydrogen and methane are produced exclusively by fermentation of carbohydrate by gut microbes. A sugar, most commonly glucose or lactulose, is used as a substrate for breath testing. Glucose is a monosaccharide that is absorbed primarily in the proximal small bowel, whereas lactulose is a synthetic nonabsorbable disaccharide that undergoes fermentation in the colon.

In normal physiologic conditions, glucose is almost entirely absorbed in the proximal small bowel. In the presence of excessive small bowel bacteria, however, glucose is fermented, releasing its gases, which are then absorbed into the bloodstream and expired via the lungs, which can then be measured in exhaled air using a breath analyzer. Similarly, with lactulose, in the presence of excessive bacteria in the small bowel, lactulose undergoes fermentation earlier than expected. The glucose breath test has been reported to have better test characteristics than the lactulose breath test with a sensitivity of 63% versus 52%, a specificity of 82% versus 86%, and a diagnostic accuracy of 72% versus 55%.[1] In comparison with the small bowel aspirate, a systematic review of 11 studies found the sensitivity of the lactulose breath test to range from 31% to 68% and specificity from 44% to 100%.[33]

In the conduct of SIBO breath testing, the Rome consensus group recommends 50 g of glucose in 250 mL of water with breath samples collected every 15 to 20 minutes for a total of 120 to 180 minutes,[42] whereas the recent recommendation from the North American consensus group is to use 75 g of glucose in 1 cup of water for a total testing period of 120 minutes.[38] It seems that the higher dose was preferred mainly because of ease of access because it is the dose available for use in the more commonly performed glucose tolerance testing. An increase in breath hydrogen after oral administration of glucose is diagnostic of SIBO although the absolute level of increase diagnostic of SIBO remains somewhat controversial. An increase greater than or equal to 20 parts per million (ppm) over baseline and sustained over at least 2 time points within 90 minutes is recommended by the North American consensus group, although an increase greater than 10 to 12 ppm from baseline has also been suggested.[42]

A potential limitation of glucose as the sugar substrate in breath testing is that, because glucose is absorbed primarily in the proximal small bowel, it may not detect SIBO occurring in more distal sections of the small bowel. The clinical significance of distal SIBO, however, remains ill-defined.[43] Furthermore, glucose malabsorption has been has been associated with rapid intestinal transit.[44] Lin and Massey[45] found that, when concurrent orocecal technetium (^{99m}Tc) scintigraphy findings were considered, almost half of their subjects with abnormal breath tests using glucose breath testing were falsely positive for SIBO because of colonic fermentation; most had prior upper gastrointestinal surgery, which likely influenced transit time. This counters the view that glucose is only absorbed in the proximal small bowel, cannot reflect more distal SIBO, and has greater specificity in the diagnosis of SIBO. Nevertheless, because of this perceived limitation of glucose as a substrate, some suggest that lactulose is a preferred sugar substrate for breath testing for SIBO.[46]

The test protocol for the lactulose breath test involves the ingestion of 10 g of lactulose in 200 mL of water, with breath samples collected every 15 minutes for 120 to 240 minutes.[38] An increase in hydrogen of greater than or equal to 20 ppm within 90 minutes is usually considered consistent with SIBO, although several other criteria are also used (eg, $\geq$20 ppm within 180 minutes, presence of a double peak).[38,42] Lactulose is an osmotic laxative that can accelerate orocecal transit, potentially resulting in false-positive results of SIBO breath testing because it may be prematurely metabolized in the colon. Yu and colleagues[47] found that when combining lactulose breath testing with orocecal ^{99m}Tc scintigraphy, the time of increase in breath hydrogen levels corresponded with an increase in accumulation of ^{99m}Tc in the cecum in 88% of cases, suggesting that positive breath test results from colonic bacteria metabolizing lactulose and not as a result of SIBO. Similar results have been found by other investigators.[48,49] Nevertheless, it remains a subject of debate whether the arrival of a small portion of the overall radiolabeled material in the colon proves that the fermentation is from colonic rather than small bowel bacteria.[50,51] Because of this limitation of both lactulose and glucose breath testing, it has been suggested that the combined use of breath test with orocecal scintigraphy is preferred to more accurately diagnose SIBO by identifying when the head of the meal has reached the colon. Using this technique, a recent report found that antibiotic treatment improved symptoms in subjects with IBS and healthy controls who were diagnosed with SIBO using the diagnostic criteria of an increase in breath hydrogen of 5 ppm before the head of the bolus reached the colon.[52] Despite the many limitations of the lactulose breath test in the diagnosis of SIBO, this test may serve as a useful biomarker predicting symptom response to antibiotic therapy.[53]

Because lactulose is not absorbed and undergoes fermentation by colonic bacteria, this is generally identified by a late peak in hydrogen (after 90 minutes) and has been used as a measure of orocecal transit. It should be recognized, however, that the average orocecal transit time as assessed by the lactulose breath test is only slightly longer.[54] Therefore, healthy individuals may seem to have SIBO and conditions with rapid transit will confound interpretation. Indeed, the measurement of orocecal transit time by lactulose breath testing has a wide variation in interpretation, poor reproducibility, and is not recommended for clinical use.[42] In the presence of SIBO, lactulose undergoes fermentation sooner than expected, which is detected as an early peak in hydrogen breath content. Typically, the presence of a double peak, with the first peak representing SIBO and the later peak representing colonic fermentation, was thought to be representative of the presence of SIBO using the lactulose breath test. The sensitivity and specificity of the double peak criteria to diagnose SIBO, however, are poor. As such, the North American consensus guidelines recommend against use of the double peak to diagnose SIBO.[38]

Up to 30% of the general population does not produce hydrogen on breath testing,[34] a phenomenon resulting predominantly from the presence of hydrogen-utilizing, methane-producing methanogenic microbes in the gut. Consequently, the measurement of breath methane in addition to hydrogen improves the sensitivity of the test. Therefore, both hydrogen and methane should be measured simultaneously during breath testing. The North American consensus group recommends that an increase in breath methane of greater than or equal to 10 ppm be used as an additional criterion diagnostic of SIBO.[38] It remains unclear how to interpret breath tests with no hydrogen or methane production (ie, flat lines), a not infrequent occurrence. This may occur because of the presence of bacteria in the gut, producing predominantly hydrogen sulfide, which cannot be measured by currently available techniques.

Proper preparation for breath tests (**Box 1**) is necessary because low fasting levels of breath hydrogen are important in the interpretation of results. Controversy exists

---

Box 1
Recommended preparation instructions for patients before breath testing

1. No antibiotics for 4 weeks before the test

2. Avoid laxatives and promotility agents for at least 1 week before the test

3. Avoid colon cleansing for 4 weeks before test

4. Can continue proton pump inhibitors and H_2-receptor antagonists

5. Insufficient evidence to recommend continuing or discontinuing prebiotics or probiotics before the test

6. Avoid complex carbohydrates and dairy products on the day before the test. Instead, consume plain baked or broiled chicken, turkey, or fish (salt and pepper only); plain or steamed white rice; eggs or egg substitute; and beef or vegetable broth for 24 hours before the test.

7. Fast 8 to 12 hours before the test

8. Avoid smoking, sleeping, or exercising 30 minutes before and during the test

9. Consider using a mouth wash with chlorhexidine before substrate administration

regarding the significance of an increased baseline or fasting hydrogen or methane level.[38] It has been suggested that an elevated hydrogen baseline of greater than 20 ppm is suggestive of SIBO; however, an elevated baseline level more often represents poor preparation for the test rather than a variant of SIBO. The clinical context should be taken into consideration before making a diagnosis of SIBO based on an elevated baseline hydrogen level.

MANAGEMENT OF SMALL INTESTINAL BACTERIAL OVERGROWTH

Because of the described limitations of the tests used to diagnose SIBO, a therapeutic trial of antibiotics is often used in clinical practice, although how best to define a response to such therapy remains unclear. In addition, the nonspecific clinical presentation and broad differential diagnosis make the pretest confidence of an accurate clinical diagnosis of SIBO difficult.[11] Furthermore, the use of antibiotics is not without risk (eg, serious adverse reactions, antibiotic resistance, and potential of *Clostridium difficile* infection) and when a patient does not respond or seems to respond but symptoms rapidly recur following discontinuation of a therapeutic trial, this often leads to repeated antibiotic use, misuse, and increased expense. Ultimately, reserving this approach to those patients with classic risk factors and symptoms of SIBO is advised.

The most important aspect of SIBO treatment is, whenever possible, to identify and correct its underlying cause. For example, the use of gut prokinetic agents (eg, metoclopramide or erythromycin) may be used to enhance motility. Such an approach has been shown to be superior to placebo in cirrhotic patients in normalizing breath tests[55] and in delaying symptom recurrence following antibiotic treatment in patients with suspected SIBO-associated IBS.[56] Nocturnal use of low-dose octreotide for 3 weeks was found to stimulate fasting intestinal motility; improve symptoms of nausea, bloating, and abdominal pain; and normalize glucose breath hydrogen testing in scleroderma patients with SIBO.[57] For similar reasons, opioids and other antimotility drugs should, whenever possible, be avoided in this patient population.

Unfortunately, the ability to correct most underlying causes of SIBO is uncommon. As such, the treatment generally involves identification and correction of nutritional deficiencies and modification of the altered microbial population. In those with identified micronutrient deficiencies, periodic monitoring of levels is recommended. In the individual with weight loss and malnutrition, oral nutritional supplements should be provided. Rarely, enteral or parenteral nutrition support may be needed for the severely malnourished patient with SIBO.

The role of dietary changes in the management of SIBO is poorly understood. Carbohydrate intolerance is common in SIBO,[32] and carbohydrate may act as a primary substrate for bacteria and provide a rich environment for bacterial growth. Thus, carbohydrate restriction (eg, lactose restriction) may theoretically be of benefit in SIBO in some individuals; however, this has not been subjected to rigorous study. Similarly, the much more involved low fermentable oligosaccharides, disaccharides, monosaccharides, and polyols (FODMAP) diet may have merit in the treatment of SIBO, particularly in patients with irritable bowel symptoms. FODMAPs are short-chained carbohydrates that are readily metabolized by small bowel bacteria. Although the role of a low FODMAP diet in SIBO deserves further study, it is generally agreed that the clinical symptoms of SIBO, which are not specific to SIBO, may improve with avoidance of fermentable foods. Fat restriction would seem to be of benefit only to those SIBO patients with evidence of fat malabsorption (eg, short bowel syndrome, chronic pancreatitis).

It was speculated that an elemental diet may be helpful in SIBO because the macronutrients from the elemental diet are absorbed primarily in the first few feet of the small bowel and potentially can limit delivery of nutrients to bacteria in the more distal small bowel. Based on this rationale, a retrospective study of 124 subjects with hydrogen-predominant or methane-predominant SIBO who were treated with an elemental diet, Vivonex Plus (Novartis Nutrition Corp, Minneapolis, MN, USA), for at least 2 weeks showed that 80% had normalization of the lactulose breath test at week 3; breath test normalization correlated with symptom improvement in 66% of these subjects.[58] These results have yet to be confirmed by other investigators and several factors limit the widespread use of such a dietary strategy, including the cost and palatability of elemental formulas. Such an approach, however, might be considered in SIBO patients in whom treatment options are limited, such as those with multiple antibiotic allergies, those who prefer to avoid antibiotics, or those with a relapsing course. For similar reasons, there has been an interest in the use of probiotic and prebiotic agents in the management of SIBO. Although suggested to be of benefit in small studies, their use in the management of SIBO remains unproven and requires further study.[59,60]

While nutritional repletion is ongoing, efforts should also be focused on addressing the microbial imbalance. At present, oral antibiotics are the mainstay of therapy in SIBO. In a metaanalysis of 10 randomized, placebo-controlled studies using different antibiotics to treat SIBO, the overall breath test normalization rate, the primary outcome measured, was 51.1% for antibiotics compared with 9.8% for placebo.[1] Despite the heterogeneity of the measures of clinical response used, symptom response tended to correlate with breath test normalization. Importantly, the studies were limited by fair quality, small sample size, and heterogeneous design. Because SIBO typically involves both aerobic and anaerobic microbes,[61] broad spectrum antibiotics are often recommended. **Table 4** lists a variety of commonly used antibiotics, generally used for 7 to 14 days. Rifaximin is the most studied antibiotic for SIBO and has been suggested to be preferred because of its limited absorption and systemic effects.[62] Rifaximin is, however, not currently FDA-approved for use in this indication and its cost can be prohibitive.

Clinical response is generally used as a guide to successful therapy; however, the duration of improvement is variable depending on the underlying cause of SIBO. SIBO is considered a relapsing disease with up to 44% of patients at 9 months having a recurrence of symptoms after initial successful antibiotic treatment.[63] This is particularly problematic in those with the classic stasis syndromes associated with SIBO.

Table 4
Oral antibiotics commonly used to treat small intestinal bacterial overgrowth

Antibiotics	Dosage
Amoxicillin-Clavulanate	500/125 mg tid
Ciprofloxacin	250–500 mg bid
Doxycycline	100 mg bid
Metronidazole	250 mg bid or tid
Neomycin	500 mg bid
Norfloxacin	400 mg bid
Rifaximin	550 mg bid or tid
Tetracycline	250–500 mg qid
Trimethoprim-sulfamethoxazole	160/800 mg bid

Depending on the rapidity of return of symptoms and their severity, a cyclical regimen consisting of a rotation of a variety of different antibiotics for 1 to 2 weeks each month has been recommended.[3] The efficacy and safety of such a cyclical regimen, however, has not been subjected to rigorous study. Furthermore, given the risks and expense associated with repeated courses of antibiotics, consideration should be given to retesting before repeating antibiotic treatment in patients with recurring symptoms after treatment with antibiotics.[1]

The predominant methane-producing bacteria in the gut, *Methanobrevibacter smithii*, are resistant to many antibiotics. Accordingly, antibiotic monotherapy seems to be insufficient in methane producers. A combination of rifaximin and neomycin was recently shown to be more effective than either antibiotic alone in methane-producers.[64] Individuals in this retrospective study who received either rifaximin or neomycin had a response rate of 28% and 33%, respectively (determined by normalization of breath tests after treatment), compared with 87% of patients treated with both rifaximin and neomycin. These results were confirmed in a subsequent randomized controlled trial in patients with methane-positive constipation-predominant IBS; the symptom reduction was predicted by a reduction in breath methane posttreatment.[65]

Recently, there has been interest in use of 3-hydroxy-3-methylglutaryl-coenzyme A reductase inhibitors (ie, statin drugs) in the treatment of methane-positive SIBO.[66] Statins have been shown to inhibit methane production by an effect on cell biosynthesis and by directly interfering with methanogenesis.[67] However, whether this translates into a meaningful clinical benefit requires further study.

SUMMARY

SIBO is characterized by the presence of an excessive concentration of either overall bacteria or specific types of bacteria in the small bowel. The most important physiologic mechanisms protecting against SIBO are small bowel motility and gastric acid. Potential nutritional consequences of SIBO include malabsorption of fat and carbohydrate, micronutrient deficiencies, and weight loss. There are significant limitations in the tests clinically available to diagnose SIBO, small bowel aspirates, and breath tests. As a result, there is currently no true gold standard for its diagnosis. Rapid advances in DNA-sequencing have enabled better understanding the diversity of the human gut microbiota. In the future, molecular sequencing of the microbiome in the small bowel may help characterize the enteric microbial population and elucidate pathologic bacterial colonies.[68] It is important to identify and treat the underlying cause of SIBO. Nutritional deficiencies should be identified and corrected when present. Antibiotics remain the cornerstone of treatment of SIBO. Clinical trials involving larger patient samples using standardized and objective measures of clinical response and longer follow-up to assess durability and relapse risk are needed to better understand the optimal treatments of SIBO.

REFERENCES

1. Shah SC, Day LW, Somsouk M, et al. Meta-analysis: antibiotic therapy for small intestinal bacterial overgrowth. Aliment Pharmacol Ther 2013;38(8):925–34.

2. Abu-Shanab A, Quigley EM. Diagnosis of small intestinal bacterial overgrowth: the challenges persist! Expert Rev Gastroenterol Hepatol 2009;3(1):77–87.

3. Bohm M, Siwiec RM, Wo JM. Diagnosis and management of small intestinal bacterial overgrowth. Nutr Clin Pract 2013;28(3):289–99.

4. Rautava S. Early microbial contact, the breast milk microbiome and child health. J Dev Orig Health Dis 2016;7(1):5–14.

5. Simrén M, Barbara G, Flint HJ, et al, and the Rome Foundation Committee. Intestinal microbiota in functional bowel disorders: a Rome foundation report. Gut 2013;62(1):159–76.

6. Lane ER, Zisman TL, Suskind DL. The microbiota in inflammatory bowel disease: current and therapeutic insights. J Inflamm Res 2017;10:63–73.

7. Miller LS, Vegesna AK, Sampath AM, et al. Ileocecal valve dysfunction in small intestinal bacterial overgrowth: a pilot study. World J Gastroenterol 2012;18: 6801–8.

8. Roland BC, Ciarleglio MM, Clarke JO, et al. Low ileocecal valve pressure is significantly associated with small intestinal bacterial overgrowth (SIBO). Dig Dis Sci 2014;59(6):1269–77.

9. Singleton AO, Redmond DC, McMurray JE. Ileocecal resection and small bowel transit and absorption. Ann Surg 1964;159:690–4.

10. Fich A, Steadman CJ, Phillips SF, et al. Ileocolonic transit does not change after right hemicolectomy. Gastroenterology 1992;103:794–9.

11. Krajicek EJ, Hansel SL. Small intestinal bacterial overgrowth: a primary care review. Mayo Clin Proc 2016;91(12):1828–33.

12. DiBaise JK, Young RJ, Vanderhoof JA. Enteric microbial flora, bacterial overgrowth, and short-bowel syndrome. Clin Gastroenterol Hepatol 2006;4(1):11–20.

13. Seto C, Jeraldo P, Orenstein R, et al. Prolonged use of proton pump inhibitors in healthy individuals reduces microbial diversity: implications for clostridium difficile susceptibility. Microbiome 2014;2:42, eCollection 2014.

14. Husebye E, Skar V, Hoverstad T, et al. Fasting hypochlorhydria with gram positive gastric flora is highly prevalent in healthy old people. Gut 1992;33:1331–7.

15. Lo WK, Chan WW. Proton pump inhibitor use and the risk of small intestinal bacterial overgrowth: a meta-analysis. Clin Gastroenterol Hepatol 2013;11(5):483–90.

16. Pignata C, Budillon G, Monaco G, et al. Jejunal bacterial overgrowth and intestinal permeability in children with immunodeficiency syndromes. Gut 1990;31: 879–82.

17. Kruszewska D, Ljungh A, Hynes SO, et al. Effect of the antibacterial activity of pig pancreatic juice on human multiresistant bacteria. Pancreas 2004;28(2):191–9.

18. Van Felius ID, Akkermans LM, Bosscha K, et al. Interdigestive small bowel motility and duodenal bacterial overgrowth in experimental acute pancreatitis. Neurogastroenterol Motil 2003;15(3):267–76.

19. Kaufman SS, Loseke CA, Lupo JV, et al. Influence of bacterial overgrowth and intestinal inflammation on duration of parenteral nutrition in children with short bowel syndrome. J Pediatr 1997;131:356–61.

20. Kim YS, Spritz N, Blum M, et al. The role of altered bile acid metabolism in the steatorrhea of experimental blind loop. J Clin Invest 1966;45(6):956–62.

21. Sherman P, Wesley A, Forstner G. Sequential disaccharidase loss in rat intestinal blind loops: impact of malnutrition. Am J Physiol 1985;248(6 Pt 1):G626–32.

22. Jones EA, Craigie A, Tavill AS, et al. Protein metabolism in the intestinal stagnant loop syndrome. Gut 1968;9(4):466–9.

23. Jain A, Reif S, O'Neil K, et al. Small intestinal bacterial overgrowth and protein-losing enteropathy in an infant with AIDS. J Pediatr Gastroenterol Nutr 1992; 15(4):452–4.

24. Su J, Smith MB, Rerknimitr R, et al. Small intestine bacterial overgrowth presenting as protein-losing enteropathy. Dig Dis Sci 1998;43(3):679–81.

25. Hasan M, Finucane P. Intestinal malabsorption presenting with night blindness. Br J Clin Pract 1993;47(5):275–6.
26. Stotzer PO, Johansson C, Mellström D, et al. Bone mineral density in patients with small intestinal bacterial overgrowth. Hepatogastroenterology 2003;50(53): 1415–8.
27. Brin MF, Fetell MR, Green PH, et al. Blind loop syndrome, vitamin E malabsorption, and spinocerebellar degeneration. Neurology 1985;35(3):338–42.
28. Welkos SL, Toskes PP, Baer H. Importance of anaerobic bacteria in the cobalamin malabsorption of the experimental rat blind loop syndrome. Gastroenterology 1981;80(2):313–20.
29. Sachdev AH, Pimentel M. Gastrointestinal bacterial overgrowth: pathogenesis and clinical significance. Ther Adv Chronic Dis 2013;4(5):223–31.
30. Stotzer PO, Björnsson ES, Abrahamsson H. Interdigestive and postprandial motility in small-intestinal bacterial overgrowth. Scand J Gastroenterol 1996; 31(9):875–80.
31. Kunkel D, Basseri RJ, Makhani MD, et al. Methane on breath testing is associated with constipation: a systematic review and meta-analysis. Dig Dis Sci 2011;56: 1612–8.
32. Rezaie A, Pimentel M, Rao SS. How to test and treat small intestinal bacterial overgrowth: an evidence-based approach. Curr Gastroenterol Rep 2016;18(2):8.
33. Khoshini R, Dai SC, Lezcano S, et al. A systematic review of diagnostic tests for small intestinal bacterial overgrowth. Dig Dis Sci 2008;53:1443–54.
34. Saad RJ, Chey WD. Breath testing for small intestinal bacterial overgrowth: maximizing test accuracy. Clin Gastroenterol Hepato 2014;12(12):1964–72.
35. Tillman R, King C, Toskes P. Continued experience with the xylose breath test: evidence that the small bowel culture as the gold standard for bacterial overgrowth may be tarnished. Gastroenterology 1981;80:1304.
36. Corazza GR, Menozzi MG, Strocchi A, et al. The diagnosis of small bowel bacterial overgrowth. Reliability of jejunal culture and inadequacy of breath hydrogen testing. Gastroenterology 1990;98(2):302–9.
37. Donaldson RM Jr. Normal bacterial populations of the intestine and their relation to intestinal function. N Engl J Med 1964;270:938–45.
38. Rezaie A, Buresi M, Lembo A, et al. Hydrogen and methane-based breath testing in gastrointestinal disorders: the North American Consensus. Am J Gastroenterol 2017;112(5):775–84.
39. Poserud I, Stotzer PO, Björnsson ES, et al. Small intestinal bacterial overgrowth in patients with irritable bowel syndrome. Gut 2007;56(6):802–8.
40. Erdogan A, Rao SS, Gulley D, et al. Small intestinal bacterial overgrowth: duodenal aspiration vs glucose breath test. Neurogastroenterol Motil 2015;27: 481–9.
41. Pyleris E, Giamarellos-Bourboulis EJ, Tzivras D, et al. The prevalence of overgrowth by aerobic bacteria in the small intestine by small bowel culture: relationship with irritable bowel syndrome. Dig Dis Sci 2012;57(5):1321–9.
42. Gasbarrini A, Corazza GR, Gasbarrini G, et al. Methodology and indications of H2-breath testing in gastrointestinal diseases: the Rome Consensus Conference. Aliment Pharmacol Ther 2009;29(Suppl 1):1–49.
43. Quigley EM. Small intestinal bacterial overgrowth: what it is and what it is not. Curr Opin Gastroenterol 2014;30(2):141–6.
44. Sellin JH, Hart R. Glucose malabsorption associated with rapid intestinal transit. Am J Gastroenterol 1992;87(5):584–9.

45. Lin EC, Massey BT. Scintigraphy demonstrates high rate of false-positive results from glucose breath tests for small bowel bacterial overgrowth. Clin Gastroenterol Hepatol 2016;14(2):203–8.
46. Pimentel M. Breath testing for small intestinal bacterial overgrowth: should we bother? Am J Gastroenterol 2016;111(3):307–8.
47. Yu D, Cheeseman F, Vanner S. Combined oro-caecal scintigraphy and lactulose hydrogen breath testing demonstrate that breath testing detects oro-caecal transit, not small intestinal bacterial overgrowth in patients with IBS. Gut 2011; 60:334–40.
48. Walters B, Vanner SJ. Detection of bacterial overgrowth in IBS using the lactulose H2 breath test: comparison with 14C-D-xylose and healthy controls. Am J Gastroenterol 2005;100(7):1566–70.
49. Riordan SM, McIver CJ, Walker BM, et al. The lactulose breath hydrogen test and small intestinal bacterial overgrowth. Am J Gastroenterol 1996;91(9):1795–803.
50. Triantafyllou K, Pimentel M. Understanding breath tests for small intestinal bacterial overgrowth. Clin Gastroenterol Hepatol 2016;14(9):1362–3.
51. Massey BT, Lin EC. Reply. Clin Gastroenterol Hepatol 2016;14(9):1363–4.
52. Zhao J, Zheng X, Chu H, et al. A study of the methodological and clinical validity of the combined lactulose hydrogen breath test with scintigraphic oro-cecal transit test for diagnosing small intestinal bacterial overgrowth in IBS patients. Neurogastroenterol Motil 2014;26(6):794–802.
53. Pimentel M, Chow EJ, Lin HC. Eradication of small intestinal bacterial overgrowth reduces symptoms of irritable bowel syndrome. Am J Gastroenterol 2000;95(12): 3503–6.
54. Hirakawa M, Iida M, Kohrogi N, et al. Hydrogen breath test assessment of orocecal transit time: comparison with barium meal study. Am J Gastroenterol 1988; 83(12):1361–3.
55. Madrid AM, Hurtado C, Venegas M, et al. Long-Term treatment with cisapride and antibiotics in liver cirrhosis: effect on small intestinal motility, bacterial overgrowth, and liver function. Am J Gastroenterol 2001;96:1251–5.
56. Pimentel M, Morales W, Lezcano S, et al. Low-dose nocturnal tegaserod or erythromycin delays symptom recurrence after treatment of irritable bowel syndrome based on presumed bacterial overgrowth. Gastroenterol Hepatol (N Y) 2009;5: 435–42.
57. Soudah HC, Hasler WL, Owyang C. Effect of octreotide on intestinal motility and bacterial overgrowth in scleroderma. N Engl J Med 1991;325(21):1461–7.
58. Pimentel M, Constantino T, Kong Y, et al. A 14-day elemental diet is highly effective in normalizing the lactulose breath test. Dig Dis Sci 2004;49:73–7.
59. Rosania R, Giorgio F, Principi M, et al. Effect of probiotic or prebiotic supplementation on antibiotic therapy in the small intestinal bacterial overgrowth: a comparative evaluation. Curr Clin Pharmacol 2013;8:169–72.
60. Khalighi AR, Khalighi MR, Behdani R, et al. Evaluating the efficacy of probiotic on treatment in patients with small intestinal bacterial overgrowth (SIBO)–a pilot study. Indian J Med Res 2014;140(5):604–8.
61. Bouhnik Y, Alain S, Attar A, et al. Bacterial populations contaminating the upper gut in patients with small intestinal bacterial overgrowth syndrome. Am J Gastroenterol 1999;94(5):1327–31.
62. Gatta L, Scarpignato C. Systematic review with meta-analysis: rifaximin is effective and safe for the treatment of small intestine bacterial overgrowth. Aliment Pharmacol Ther 2017;5(5):604–16.

63. Lauritano EC, Gabrielli M, Scarpellini E, et al. Small intestinal bacterial overgrowth recurrence after antibiotic therapy. Am J Gastroenterol 2008;103:2031–5.

64. Low K, Hwang L, Hua J, et al. A combination of rifaximin and neomycin is most effective in treating irritable bowel syndrome patients with methane on lactulose breath test. J Clin Gastroenterol 2010;44:547–50.

65. Pimentel M, Chang C, Chua KS, et al. Antibiotic treatment of constipation-predominant irritable bowel syndrome. Dig Dis Sci 2014;59(6):1278–85.

66. Gottlieb K, Wacher V, Sliman J, et al. Review article: inhibition of methanogenic archaea by statins as a targeted management strategy for constipation and related disorders. Aliment Pharmacol Ther 2016;43(2):197–212.

67. Muskal SM, Sliman J, Kokai-Kun J, et al. Lovastatin lactone may improve irritable bowel syndrome with constipation (IBS-C) by inhibiting enzymes in the archaeal methanogenesis pathway. Version 3. F1000Res 2016;5:606.

68. Giamarellos-Bourboulis E, Tang J, Pyleris E, et al. Molecular assessment of differences in the duodenal microbiome in subjects with irritable bowel syndrome. Scand J Gastroenterol 2015;50:1076–87.

Nutritional Interventions in Chronic Intestinal Pseudoobstruction

Donald F. Kirby, MD, AGAF, CNSC, CPNS[a],*,
Sulieman Abdal Raheem, MD[b],
Mandy L. Corrigan, MPH, RD, LD, CNSC, FAND[c]

KEYWORDS

- Chronic intestinal pseudo-obstruction • Gastrointestinal dysmotility
- Venting gastrostomy • Cecostomy • Parenteral nutrition • Intestinal transplant

KEY POINTS

- Chronic intestinal pseudo-obstruction is a rare disorder; its spectrum of disease ranges from abdominal bloating to severe gastrointestinal dysfunction.
- Goals should be to improve motility, when possible, and provide sufficient hydration and nutrition, orally, enterally, and/or parenterally.
- It is important to screen patients for nutrient deficiencies, especially if there is either chronic poor intake or evidence of malabsorption.
- Intestinal transplant is an option when all other conservative measures fail.

INTRODUCTION

Chronic intestinal pseudo-obstruction (CIPO) is a rare disorder that is characterized by the simulation of mechanical obstruction of either the small or large bowel when no anatomic explanation can be found. It is a motility disorder that is associated with dilation that differentiates itself from the small bowel disorder of chronic intestinal dysmotility or the colonic entities of slow transit constipation and colonic inertia.[1] Although etiologies can involve myopathic, neuropathic, or intestinal cells of Cajal, they can be primary or secondary to another disease or idiopathic. Further discussion of the etiology or the diagnostic work up are beyond the scope of this article. CIPO can also occur in both pediatric and adult patients; however, most of the comments will be concentrated on the adult population.

Disclosure Statement: The authors have nothing to disclose.
[a] Intestinal Transplant Program, Center for Human Nutrition, Cleveland Clinic, 9500 Euclid Avenue/A51, Cleveland, OH 44195, USA; [b] Center for Human Nutrition, Cleveland Clinic, 9500 Euclid Avenue/A51, Cleveland, OH 44195, USA; [c] Home Nutrition Support and Center for Gut Rehabilitation and Transplant, Center for Human Nutrition, Cleveland Clinic, 9500 Euclid Avenue/A100, Cleveland, OH 44195, USA
* Corresponding author.
E-mail address: kirbyd@ccf.org

Gastroenterol Clin N Am 47 (2018) 209–218
https://doi.org/10.1016/j.gtc.2017.09.005
0889-8553/18/© 2017 Elsevier Inc. All rights reserved.

CLINICAL MANIFESTATIONS

The most common symptoms include abdominal pain and distension with high associations of nausea, vomiting, and constipation.[2–4] Because of the nonspecific nature of these symptoms, delays in diagnosis with significant testing and/or unneeded surgery are common. Diarrhea may be seen in up to 20% of patients, but is usually seen with small intestinal bacterial overgrowth or in patients who have undergone surgical resections resulting in short bowel syndrome. Abdominal pain and distension are worse during exacerbations, which may wax and wane or in the most severely affected may be a more chronic feature.[4] The normal provision of nutrition may be difficult, because eating may be associated with worsening symptoms that then results in food avoidance. The most difficult issue is the unpredictable nature of acute and intermittent exacerbations that have no detectable causation and vary widely from patient to patient.[5] This wide spectrum of disease can result in delays in action on the physician's part and can contribute to the worsening of nutritional status, which clinicians should strive to prevent.

MEDICAL AND NUTRITIONAL THERAPIES

Joly and colleagues[6] have nicely summarized the 2 main goals in treating CIPO as follows: "(1) improvement of intestinal propulsion and (2) maintenance of adequate nutritional status including fluid and mineral balances." These 2 goals are very much interrelated, as improvement in motility may allow oral or a form of enteral therapy, whereas failure to improve the GI motility and symptoms may preclude the use of the gastrointestinal (GI) tract for feeding and necessitate the need for parenteral nutrition (PN) with the possibility of intestinal transplantation in some.

Medications and Other Therapies

Medications are often the first treatment attempted to try to ameliorate symptoms and improve nutritional intake. However, there are few true motility medications that are available for use in the United States. **Table 1** lists the medications that have been used, but many have either limited usefulness or are not available in the United States except under special US Food and Drug Administration (FDA) protocol for compassionate usage or off-label usage.[7–26] An in-depth discussion of these medications is beyond the scope of this article, but trials of some of these medications may be required to help ameliorate symptoms before resorting to either parenteral nutrition or an intestinal transplant.

The most common symptom is abdominal pain. Different classes of medication have been used including prokinetics like prucalopride and somatostatin, pain modulators such as tricyclic antidepressants, serotonin-norepinephrine reuptake inhibitors, and GABA analogues, in addition to narcotics.[16,19,20,23,24] Special attention should be used to look for potential side effects of these medications that can worsen some of the symptoms of CIPO, such as nausea and constipation.

Nausea is a common symptom, sometimes occurring on daily basis, and it can be associated with vomiting during episodes of exacerbations, interfere with oral intake, and impact quality of life. Antiemetics are used with variable efficacy and should be individualized based on the clinical presentation.

Antibiotics are often used to treat bacterial overgrowth syndrome.

Fecal transplant is an intriguing potential treatment. Gu and colleagues[26] prospectively studied 9 adult patients for 8 weeks after receiving fecal transplant from volunteer donors via nasojejunal tube (NJT) daily for 6 days after 3 days of daily NJT administration of 500 mg of liquid vancomycin. This reportedly resulted in significant

Table 1
Medications that have been used for chronic intestinal pseudo-obstruction

Medication	Comments
Erythromycin[7–10]	Off-label use, macrolide antibiotic with motilin agonist properties Has been useful in patients with acute attacks of CIPO, used as intravenous infusion at a dose of 3 mg/kg every 8 h for several days
Metoclopramide[11]	Available in United States Dopamine agonist with prokinetic effects Has been useful for acute exacerbations No convincing data of usefulness used long term Can have severe extrapyramidal side effects
Cisapride[12–14]	Taken off the US market in 1999 due to cardiac arrhythmia issues and drug interactions, available by FDA compassionate use many consider it the most effective
Domperidone[15,16]	Not available in the United States except by FDA compassionate use Dopamine agonist, but does not pass the blood-brain barrier May be useful for gastroparesis, good treatment for nausea
Tegaserod[16]	Taken off the US market in 2007 for concerns of increased cardiac issues, not available in the US except by FDA compassionate use
Neostigmine[17,18]	Off label, used for acute pseudo-obstruction (Ogilvie syndrome) Has also been used for acute on CIPO, given intramuscularly or intravenously, but usually done with cardiac monitoring
Octreotide[19,20]	Long-acting somatostatin analogue Reported beneficial in scleroderma patients with CIPO and has also been studied with erythromycin May improve enteral nutrition tolerance, better studied in children
Leuprolide[21,22]	Gonadotropin-releasing hormone analogue shown to decrease symptoms in patients with irritable bowel syndrome and CIPO – no large trials
Prucalopride[23,24]	5-HT4 receptor antagonist, not available in the United States It enhances motility through stomach, small bowel, and colon Could be promising treatment
Linaclotide[25]	Stimulates intestinal guanylate cyclase receptors Used to treat chronic constipation and irritable bowel syndrome with constipation Not systematically studied in CIPO
Fecal Transplant[26]	In the United States, an IND is required for use other than treatment of severe or recurrent C difficle infection Small open-label study from China showed some reduction in symptoms and increased tolerance of enteral nutrition via nasojejunal tube
Antibiotics	Aimed at treating small intestinal bacterial overgrowth – see **Box 1**

improvements in the bloating, abdominal pain, enteral feeding tolerance, and radiologic score of intestinal obstruction.[26] However, based on this 1 study, there are many more questions that need to be answered. In the United States, a special investigational new drug (IND) application must be filed with the FDA for use of fecal transplants other than those being used for the treatment of *Clostridia difficle* infections.

Bacterial Overgrowth

Bacterial overgrowth can be seen with any form of anatomic small bowel alteration,[27] after intraabdominal surgeries,[28] chronic small intestinal pseudo-obstruction, and intestinal dysmotility.[29] It is more commonly seen secondary to dysmotility present in many systemic diseases such as diabetes mellitus, hypothyroidism, systemic sclerosis, and Parkinson disease, and with the use of certain medications, especially narcotics and possibly proton pump inhibitors.[29,30] It is usually referred to as bacterial overgrowth, but other synonyms include small intestinal bacterial overgrowth (SIBO), blind loop, or stagnant loop syndrome.[31] This disorder is defined by excessive amount in the bacteria in the small bowel, 10^3-10^5 CFU/mL.[32] SIBO can be diagnosed in up to 15% of healthy individuals and can be higher in others with more medical comorbidities.[33]

The dysbiosis of the colonic type bacteria in the small bowel produces gas during carbohydrate metabolism. CIPO and SIBO symptoms overlap; like in CIPO, the symptoms of SIBO can include decreased appetite from bloating, abdominal pain, and increased flatulence.[34] Unlike CIPO, diarrhea, especially steatorrhea, is encountered more often than constipation in SIBO.[35] The nutritional implications of either disease or in case of overlap syndrome include weight loss; protein, fat, and carbohydrate malabsorption; altered hydration status; nutrition deficiencies of the fat-soluble vitamins A, E, D, the water soluble vitamin B_{12}, and iron; and development or worsening of osteoporosis.[36]

Some clinicians like to pursue an empiric diagnostic and therapeutic antibiotic trial for SIBO. Unfortunately, the diagnosis cannot be excluded in nonresponders. Breath testing is widely available, but the definitive test to confirm SIBO remains jejunal fluid aspiration and culture.[32]

Treatment of SIBO is often empiric, and antibacterial medications are the mainstay of SIBO management and are superior to placebo.[37] **Box 1** lists the most commonly used antibiotics to treat SIBO. Rifaximin has shown good success in alleviating symptoms.[37,38] However, it can be challenging to successfully obtain insurance authorization for rifaximin so it may not be the first antibiotic selected for SIBO treatment. In case of drug side effects, resistance, or if the patient elects to avoid antibiotic use, an elemental diet has been used in the short term with clinical improvement and normalization of the breath test.[39]

Diet

When devising an oral diet, it must be considered if gastroparesis is also present. This is usually associated with early satiety and possibly nausea and abdominal pain. Whereas a small bowel-predominant disorder might have nausea, abdominal pain, diarrhea, and varying degrees of bowel dilation. **Box 2** lists the suggestions for an oral diet, when possible. Thus, liquid, blenderized food, or soft food may be tolerated best with dietary features that will optimize motility. These would include low lactose and fructose, low fiber, and low fat, as well as eliminating foods that

---

Box 1
Antibiotics for small intestinal bacterial overgrowth treatment

Amoxicillin-clavulanate 500 mg three times daily by mouth for 7 to 10 days

Ciprofloxacin 500 mg twice daily by mouth for 7 to 10 days

Doxycycline 100 mg twice daily by mouth for 7 to 10 days

Metronidazole 250 mg three times daily by mouth for 7 to 10 days

Neomycin 500 mg twice daily by mouth for 7 to 10 days

Rifaximin 550 mg twice daily by mouth for 7 to 10 days

Tetracycline 250 mg 4 times a day by mouth for 7 to 10 days

generate gas such as carbonated beverages and legumes.[6,10,40–42] Dividing feedings into 5 or 6 meals per day is also important. It is key to attempt oral or enteral nutrition prior to initiating parenteral nutrition (PN) with the exception of the most severely malnourished, where nutritional rehabilitation might help to improve bowel function.

If patients are too intolerant of oral nutrition, then a trial of nasoenteric feeding should be done where the tube is placed in the distal duodenum or jejunum. If patients cannot tolerate continuous tube feeding at a rate that will keep them both hydrated and adequately nourished, then a trial of octreotide and erythromycin may be beneficial, as previously noted.[16] Otherwise, PN will be required. If patients tolerate the nasoenteric tube feeding, then a more permanent form of access in the jejunum, placed endoscopically or surgically, may be appropriate. However, initial success of enteral feeding does not guarantee long-term tolerance of enteral nutrition, and PN may still be required in the future (**Fig. 1**).

When weight loss leads to severe malnutrition that is unable to be ameliorated with delivery of adequate volumes through the enteral route, PN is utilized. PN formulation, initiation, and monitoring are beyond the scope of this article.[43] Use of PN is not without risk, including infectious complications, metabolic complications, and mechanical catheter complications (**Table 2**). Coverage for home PN through government payers can be challenging for patients with dysmotility.[44,45] Every effort should be made to regain nutritional autonomy through the enteral route.

Nutrient Deficiencies

In addition to obtaining a detailed diet history, a full nutrition assessment with a registered dietitian will also include screening for potential micronutrient deficiencies. A daily multivitamin with mineral supplement is commonly recommended if patients are not receiving adequate nutrition via the enteral route. Calcium supplements may be warranted for the prevention of osteoporosis if dietary intake of calcium is inadequate due to restrictions of lactose contacting foods and raw vegetables that are good sources of calcium. Often patients with pseudo-obstruction suffer from SIBO, and assessment for both macrocytic (vitamin B_{12}, folate) and microcytic (iron) anemia

---

Box 2
Oral diet alterations to maximize tolerance in chronic intestinal pseudo-obstruction

Small, frequent meals (5–6 per day)

No/low lactose and fructose

Low fiber

Low fat foods - under 30% fat

No carbonated drinks

No chewing gum

Soft foods and liquid foods preferred (including oral nutritional supplements)

Juicing is good - takes much of the fiber out

Cooked vegetables only - no raw

No legumes = beans - causes gas and have fiber

Data from Refs.[6,10,40–42]

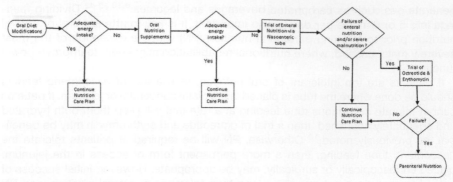

Fig. 1. Escalation algorithm for nutrition support interventions.

is needed. Serum electrolytes should also be monitored and corrected if abnormal values are noted.

SURGICAL INTERVENTIONS AND THE USE OF VENTING GASTROSTOMIES/FEEDING JEJUNOSTOMIES/CECOSTOMIES

If dietary manipulations and medications fail to improve the patient's symptoms, venting gastrostomies, feeding jejunostomies, and/or cecostomies have been used. In general, surgery should play a limited role in the CIPO patient. However, many patients undergo operation before a diagnosis of CIPO is made and then may have additional surgeries later.[46] Once surgery has been performed, the odds of reoperation are significant (44% at 1 year, 66% at 5 years).

Frequently performed surgeries include the creation of a venting ostomy, which can include a venting gastrostomy, jejunostomy, ileostomy, cecostomy, or colostomy.[46–52] The venting and draining of air and fluids can decrease the patient's nausea and vomiting. However, if the use of venting procedures does not provide adequate

Table 2	
Complications of parenteral nutrition	
Complication Classification	**Examples**
Metabolic	Metabolic bone disease
	Electrolyte abnormalities
	Dehydration
	Intestinal failure-associated liver disease
Infectious	Catheter-related blood stream infections
	Exit site or port pocket infections
Mechanical/non-infectious catheter	Catheter breaks
	Catheter occlusions
	Thrombosis
	Deep vein thrombosis
	Superior vena cava syndrome
	Air embolism

Modified from Ukleja A, Romano MM. Complications of parenteral nutrition. Gastroenterol Clin North Am 2007;36:23–46; with permission.

relief, then subtotal enterectomy has been performed for palliation.[53] This may be in addition to long-term PN and/or in preparation to an intestinal transplant.

PARENTERAL FEEDING

Parenteral Nutrition, when done well, can be lifesaving, and medically refractory CIPO is a definite indication.[43,54] Despite bowel rehabilitation and advances in nutrition support interventions, patients can be at risk for life-threatening complications. These complications include liver failure, catheter-related blood stream infections, central venous thrombosis, and impaired health-related quality of life.[55] PN will not be considered further in this article.

INTESTINAL TRANSPLANT

CIPO is a main cause of gut failure in both pediatric and adult populations, and between 60% to 80% of patients require PN at some point.[56–58] Intestinal transplantation has been increasingly used for the management of intestinal failure secondary to CIPO, accounting for about 9% of the transplants performed.[59]

The severity of bowel disease and liver status dictate the type of the transplant, isolated small bowel or multivisceral transplantation. The survival rate at 5 years after bowel transplantation is close to 60%.[60,61] Early referral to specialized tertiary centers is key, allowing for timely intervention and ultimately a better outcome. Transplantation can be a life-saving procedure with good long-term survival for selected patients with end-stage CIPO and intestinal failure who have failed more conservative management.

SUMMARY

Chronic intestinal pseudo-obstruction is a GI motility disorder with a broad spectrum of symptoms. Disease progression can be insidious with a late diagnosis because of the lack of specificity of the clinical presentation. This can lead to unnecessary interventions. Management can be challenging and requires a comprehensive approach to include nutritional evaluation, dietary modifications, and nutrition support. Symptom control with medications and occasionally endoscopic or surgical procedures is commonly used, and if everything fails, then visceral transplantation can be lifesaving.

REFERENCES

1. De Giorgio R, Sarnelli G, Corinaldesi R, et al. Advances in our understanding of the pathology of chronic intestinal pseudo-obstruction. Gut 2004;53:1549–52.
2. Stanghellini V, Cogliandro RF, De Giorgio R, et al. Chronic intestinal pseudoobstruction: manifestations, natural history and management. Neurogastroenterol Motil 2007;19:440–52.
3. De Giorgio R, Cogliandro RF, Barbara G, et al. Chronic intestinal pseudo-obstruction: clinical features, diagnosis and therapy. Gastroenterol Clin North Am 2011;40:787–807.
4. Gabbard SL, Lacy BE. Chronic intestinal pseudo-obstruction. Nutr Clin Pract 2013;28:307–16.
5. Stanghellini V, Cogliandro R, De Giorgio R, et al. Natural history of chronic intestinal pseudo-obstruction in adults: a single center study. Clin Gastroenterol Hepatol 2005;3:449–58.
6. Joly F, Amiot A, Messing B. Nutritional support in the severely compromised motility patient: when and how? Gastroenterol Clin North Am 2011;40:845–51.

7. Catnach SM. Fairclough. Erythromycin and the gut. Gut 1992;33:397–401.
8. Emmanuel AV, Shand SG, Kamm MA. Erythromycin for the treatment of chronic intestinal pseudo-obstruction: description of six cases with a positive response. Aliment Pharmacol Ther 2004;19:687–94.
9. Lacy BE, Loew BJ. Diagnosis, treatment and nutritional management of chronic intestinal pseudo-obstruction. Pract Gastroenterol 2009;8:9–24.
10. Minami T, Nishibayashi H, Shinomura Y, et al. Effects of erythromycin in chronic idiopathic pseudo-obstruction. J Gastroenterol 1996;31:855–9.
11. Lipton AB, Knauer CM. Pseudo-obstruction of the bowel. Therapeutic trial of metoclopramide. Am J Dig Dis 1977;22:263–5.
12. Camilleri M, Brown ML, Malagelada JR. Impaired transit of chyme in chronic intestinal pseudoobsruction. Correction by cisapride. Gastroenterology 1986;91: 619–26.
13. Camilleri M, Malagelada JR, Abell TL, et al. Effects of six weeks of treatment with cisapride in Gastroparesis and intestinal pseudoobstruction. Gastroenterology 1989;96:704–12.
14. Camilleri M, Balm RK, Zinsmeister AR. Determinants of response to a prokinetic agent in neuropathic chronic intestinal motility disorder. Gastroenterology 1994; 106:916–23.
15. Turgeon DK. Domperidone in chronic intestinal pseudoobstruction. Gastroenterology 1990;99:1194 (letter to the editor).
16. Panganamamula KV, Parkman HP. Chronic intestinal pseudo-obstruction. Curr Treat Options Gastroenterol 2005;8:3–11.
17. Ponec RJ, Saunders MD, Kimmey MB. Neostigmine for the treatment of acute colonic pseudo-obstruction. N Engl J Med 1999;341:137–41.
18. Borgaonkar MR, Lumb B. Acute on chronic intestinal pseudoobstruction responds to neostigmine. Dig Dis Sci 2000;45:1644–7.
19. Soudah HC, Hasler WL, Owyang C. Effect of octreotide on intestinal motility and bacterial overgrowth in scleroderma. N Engl J Med 1991;325:1461–7.
20. Verne GN, Eaker EY, Hardy E, et al. Effect of octreotide and erythromycin on idiopathic and scleroderma-associated intestinal pseudoobstruction. Dig Dis Sci 1995;40:1892–901.
21. Hammar O, Veress D, Montgomery A, et al. Expression of luteinizing hormone receptorin the gastrointestinal tract. Drug Target Insights 2012;6:13–8.
22. Mathias JR, Baskin GS, Reeves-Darby VG, et al. Chronic intestinal pseudoobstruction in a patient with heart-lung transplant. Therapeutic effect of leuprolide acetate. Dig Dis Sci 1992;37:1761–8.
23. Broad J, Kung VW, Boundouli G, et al. Cholinergic interactions between donepezil and prucalopride in the human colon: potential to treat severe intestinal dysmotility. Br J Pharmacol 2013;170:1253–61.
24. Emmanuel AV, Kamm MA, Roy AJ, et al. Randomised clinical trial: the efficacy of prucalopride in patients with chronic intestinal pseudo-obstruction – a double-blind, placebo-controlled, cross-over, multiple n=1 study. Aliment Phamacol Ther 2012;35:48–55.
25. Lacy BE, Levenick JM, Crowell MD. Linaclotide in the management of gastrointestinal tract disorders. Drugs Today 2012;48:197–206.
26. Gu L, Ding C, Tian H, et al. Serial frozen fecal microbiota transplantation in the treatment of chronic intestinal pseudo-obstruction: a preliminary study. J Neurogastroenterol Motil 2017;23:289–97.
27. Bures J, Cyrany J, Kohoutova D, et al. Small intestinal bacterial overgrowth syndrome. World J Gastroenterol 2010;16:2978–90.

28. Petrone P, Sarkisyan G, Fernández M, et al. Small intestinal bacterial overgrowth in patients with lower gastrointestinal symptoms and a history of previous abdominal surgery. Arch Surg 2011;146:444–7.

29. Jacobs C, Coss Adame E, Attaluri A, et al. Dysmotility and proton pump inhibitor use are independent risk factors for small intestinal bacterial and/or fungal overgrowth. Aliment Pharmacol Ther 2013;37:1103–11.

30. Lo W-K, Chan WW. Proton pump inhibitor use and the risk of small intestinal bacterial overgrowth: a meta-analysis. Clin Gastroenterol Hepatol 2013;11:483–90.

31. Miazga A, Osiński M, Cichy W, et al. Current views on the etiopathogenesis, clinical manifestation, diagnostics, treatment and correlation with other nosological entities of SIBO. Adv Med Sci 2015;60:118–24.

32. Khoshini R, Dai S-C, Lezcano S, et al. A systematic review of diagnostic tests for small intestinal bacterial overgrowth. Dig Dis Sci 2008;53:1443–54.

33. Dukowicz AC, Lacy BE, Levine GM. Small intestinal bacterial overgrowth: a comprehensive review. Gastroenterol Hepatol 2007;3:112–22.

34. Sachdev AH, Pimentel M. Antibiotics for irritable bowel syndrome: rationale and current evidence. Curr Gastroenterol Rep 2012;14:439–45.

35. Hwang L, Low K, Khoshini R, et al. Evaluating breath methane as a diagnostic test for constipation-predominant IBS. Dig Dis Sci 2010;55:398–403.

36. DiBaise J. Nutritional consequences of small intestinal bacterial overgrowth. Pract Gastroenterol 2008;12:15–28.

37. Shah SC, Day LW, Somsouk M, et al. Meta-analysis: antibiotic therapy for small intestinal bacterial overgrowth. Aliment Pharmacol Ther 2013;38:925–34.

38. Gratta L, Scarpignato C. Systematic review with meta-analysis: rifaximin is effective and safe for the treatment of small intestine bacterial overgrowth. Aliment Pharmacol Ther 2017;45:604–16.

39. Pimentel M, Constantino T, Kong Y, et al. A 14-day elemental diet is highly effective in normalizing the lactulose breath test. Dig Dis Sci 2004;49:73–7.

40. Billiauws L, Corcos O, Joly F. Dysmotility disorders; a nutritional approach. Curr Opin Clin Nutr Metab Care 2014;17:483–8.

41. Dutton DH, Harrell SP, Wo JM. Diagnosis and management of adult patients with chronic intestinal pseudoobstruction. Nutr Clin Pract 2006;21:16–22.

42. Camilleri M, Phillips SF. Acute and chronic intestinal pseudo-obstruction. Adv Intern Med 1991;36:287–306.

43. Worthington P, Balint J, Bechtold M, et al. When is parenteral nutrition appropriate? JPEN J Parenter Enteral Nutr 2017;41:324–77.

44. Allen P. Medicare coverage for home parenteral nutrition- an oxymoron? Part I. Pract Gastroenterol 2016;158:34–50.

45. Allen P. Medicare coverage for home parenteral nutrition- an oxymoron? Part II. Pract Gastroenterol 2017;159:24–38.

46. Sabbaugh C, Amiot A, Maggiori L, et al. Non transplantation surgical approach for chronic intestinal pseudoobstruction: analysis of 63 adult consecutive cases. Neurogastroenterol Motil 2013;25:e680–6.

47. Thompson AR, Pearson T, Ellul J, et al. Percutaneous endoscopic colostomy in patients with chronic intestinal pseudo-obstruction. Gastrointest Endosc 2004;59:113–5.

48. Han EC, Oh HK, Ha HK, et al. Favorable surgical treatment outcomes for chronic constipation with features of colonic pseudo-obstruction. World J Gastroenterol 2012;18:4441–6.

49. Chitnis M, Lazarus C, Simango I, et al. Laparoscopically inserted button colostomy as a venting stoma and access port for the administration of antegrade enemas in African degenerative leiomyopathy. S Afr J Surg 2011;49:44–6.
50. Pakarinen MP, Kurvinen A, Koivusalo AI, et al. Surgical treatment and outcomes of severe pediatric intestinal motility disorders requiring parenteral nutrition. J Pediatr Surg 2013;48:333–8.
51. Tun G, Bullas D, Bannaga A, et al. Percutaneous endoscopic colostomy: a useful technique when surgery is not an option. Ann Gastroenterol 2016;29:477–80.
52. Molina-Infante J, Mateos-Rodriguez JM, Vinagre-Rodriguez G, et al. Endoscopic-assisted colopexy and push percutaneous colostomy in the transverse colon for refractory chronic intestinal pseudo-obstruction. Surg Laparosc Endosc Percutan Tech 2011;21:e322–325.
53. Lapointe R. Chronic idiopathic intestinal pseudo-obstruction treated by near total small bowel resection: a 20-year experience. J Gastrointest Surg 2010;14:1937–42.
54. Pironi L, Goulet O, Buchman A, et al. Outcome on home parenteral nutrition for benign intestinal failure: a review of the literature and benchmarking with the European prospective survey of ESPEN. Clin Nutr 2012;31:831–4.
55. Ukleja A, Romano MM. Complications of parenteral nutrition. Gastroenterol Clin North Am 2007;36:23–46.
56. Mousa H, Hyman PE, Cocjin J, et al. Long-term outcome of congenital intestinal pseudoobstruction. Dig Dis Sci 2002;47:2298–305.
57. Lauro A, Zanfi C, Pellegrini S, et al. Isolated intestinal transplant for chronic intestinal pseudo-obstruction in adults: long-term outcome. Transplant Proc 2013;45:3351–5.
58. Lauro A, Zanfi C, Dazzi A, et al. Disease-relate transplant in adults: results from a single center. Transplant Proc 2014;46:245–8.
59. Bond GJ, Reyes JD. Intestinal transplantation for total/near-total aganglionosis and intestinal pseudo-obstruction. Semin Pediatr Surg 2004;13:286–92.
60. Lao OB, Healey PJ, Perkins JD, et al. Outcomes in children after intestinal transplant. Pediatrics 2010;125:e550–558.
61. Abu-Elmagd KM, Kosmach-Park B, Costa G, et al. Long-term survival, nutritional autonomy, and quality of life after intestinal and multivisceral transplantation. Ann Surg 2012;256:494–508.

The Need to Reassess Dietary Fiber Requirements in Healthy and Critically Ill Patients

Stephen J.D. O'Keefe, MBBS, MSc, MD, FRCP*

KEYWORDS

- Dietary fiber • Clinical studies • Fiber supplementation • Colon cancer
- *Clostridium difficile*

KEY POINTS

- Human dietary fiber requirements are based on the quantity known to be associated with cardiovascular health. It is more appropriate that they should be based on the nutritional needs of the colonic microbiota, which maintain colonic health and homeostasis.
- Diets containing more than 50 g of fiber per day are associated with low colon cancer risk.
- Current nutritional support of hospitalized patients overlooks the nutritional needs of the colonic microbiota, leading to colonic starvation and increased risk of dysbiosis, *Clostridium difficile* overgrowth, and acute colitis.

NORMAL HUMAN DIETARY FIBER REQUIREMENTS

The definition of dietary requirements is extremely difficult.[1] Traditionally requirements have been based on the quantity of food needed to maintain a normal body weight, or in the case of micronutrients to maintain normal blood levels. This presupposes that the definition of normal levels is known. People can be slim and fit or fat and fit. Blood levels of vitamins have to drop precipitously before tissue deficiency occurs and a pathologic phenotype is displayed.

The explanation for this problem is that nutrients are stored in good times that allow people to survive feasts and famines. Thus, overweight has been associated with improved outcome from the ICU.[2] On the other hand, slimness is associated with prolonged lifespan.[3]

Disclosure: The author has nothing to disclose.
Division of Gastroenterology and Nutrition, Department of Medicine, University of Pittsburgh, 853 Scaife Hall, 3550 Terrace Street, Pittsburgh, PA 15213, USA
* 479 Scaife Road, Sewickley, PA 15143.
E-mail address: sjokeefe@pitt.edu

Gastroenterol Clin N Am 47 (2018) 219–229
https://doi.org/10.1016/j.gtc.2017.10.005
0889-5553/18/© 2017 Elsevier Inc. All rights reserved.

gastro.theclinics.com

With dietary fiber, the definition of normal requirements becomes even more complex and difficult. Populations can survive on low fiber intakes for years, and patients with a colectomy do not need any fiber, as its chief role is to provide food for the colonic microbiota. However, the industrial and agricultural revolutions led to a massive increase in food production that supported the population explosion. Unfortunately, it also led to the progressive reduction in consumption of whole foods, which in turn led to dramatic reductions in food fiber content through food processing to promote storage and transportation. The development of fast foods through advanced food technology has culminated in the increased consumption of simple sugars, together with increased intake of processed meat and saturated fat, which characterize the western diet. This diet is responsible for the emergence of a group of chronic ailments, termed westernized diseases, which present the greatest challenge to health care in the United States today. Obesity, colon cancer, and cardiovascular diseases are perhaps the best examples. The lack of dietary fiber due to low intakes of coarse grains, fruits and vegetables is common to all, as their content of complex carbohydrate reduces satiety and glycemic responses to feeding, thereby reducing the risk of obesity. Obesity is associated with an increase in the incidence of at least 9 cancers, as documented by a recent review by the American Institute of Cancer Research, illustrated on **Fig. 1**.

The lack of fiber is particularly pertinent to the remarkably high incidence rates of colon cancer in westernized societies. For example, rates are uniformly high in all segments of the US population with levels of approximately 65 cases per 100,000 population in African Americans, 55 cases per 100,000 population in Caucasian Americans,[4,5] and as high as 100 cases or more per 100,000 population in Alaska Native People.[6] In stark contrast, colon cancer is rarely seen in rural African communities consuming their traditional high-fiber ($\sim$50 g/d), low-meat, and low-fat diets, at less than 5 cases per 100,000 population.

The explanation for this is the effect fiber has on the colonic microbiota. People have evolved over hundreds of million years on a high-fiber diet. Although people have characteristically been omnivores and hunter-gatherers, meat and fat intakes have been low and occasional, while foraging has been continual. Recent advances in dental microwear and stable isotope technology have provided evidence that grain consumption has always been part of the human diet.[7] Thus, human digestive tracts evolved in tandem with dietary exposure, but the few hundred years since the agricultural revolution have been insufficient to enable people to do without fiber. Basically, the small intestine is extremely efficient in digestion, absorbing 95% of what we eat. These absorbed nutrients maintain general body composition and health. However, some starches and proteins contain carbohydrate structures that are resistant to human enzymatic digestion and enter the colon. The anatomy of the colon evolved to produce a reservoir to hold up the digestive stream to allow infrequent defecation, just as the stomach evolved to become a reservoir to enable people to eat periodic meals, rather than having to nibble all day like a rat. The colonic reservoir increased the ability of the gastrointestinal (GI) tract to reabsorb all the fluid and electrolytes secreted by the upper GI tract to enhance the digestive efficiency of human enzymes. Perhaps more importantly, it created a home for environmental microbes that have the missing enzymes needed to complete the digestion of dietary residues, such as complex carbohydrates and dietary fibers. A perfect symbiotic, or mutualistic, relationship was set up where the fiber provided food for the microbes, while the microbes only partially broke the carbohydrate skeletons down to short chain fatty acids, notably acetate, butyrate, and propionate. These metabolites were released into the lumen and became the preferred nutritional sources for the colonic epithelium. The colonocytes differ from all other body cells in their preferred utilization of butyrate for energy production. Thus, naturally occurring foods provided sufficient fiber residues to maintain the health of the microbiota and the colon.

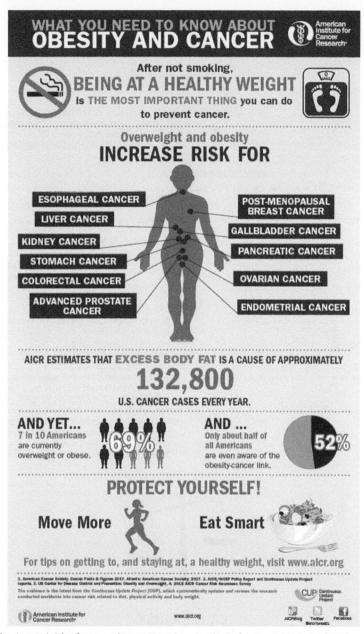

Fig. 1. Obesity and risk of cancer. (*From* American Institute for Cancer Research. What You Need to Know About Obesity and Cancer. AICR Infographics 2017. Available at: http://www.aicr.org/learn-more-about-cancer/infographics/infographic-obesity-and-cancer.html; © American Institute for Cancer Research, www.aicr.org; with permission.)

The author recently reviewed the overwhelming human study and experimental evidence for the overarching importance of butyrate in maintaining colonic health, resistance to disease, and prevention of colon cancer, summarized on **Fig. 2**.

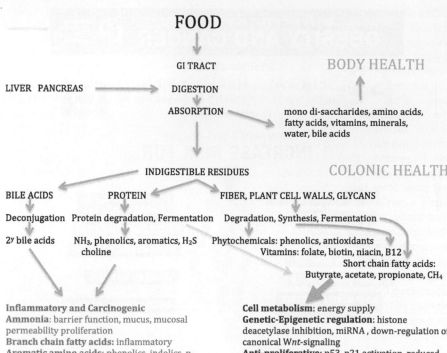

FOOD

GI TRACT

LIVER PANCREAS ⟶ DIGESTION

BODY HEALTH

ABSORPTION ⟶ mono di-saccharides, amino acids, fatty acids, vitamins, minerals, water, bile acids

INDIGESTIBLE RESIDUES

COLONIC HEALTH

BILE ACIDS   PROTEIN   FIBER, PLANT CELL WALLS, GLYCANS

Deconjugation Protein degradation, Fermentation Degradation, Synthesis, Fermentation

2^y bile acids NH_3, phenolics, aromatics, H_2S Phytochemicals: phenolics, antioxidants
choline   Vitamins: folate, biotin, niacin, B12
                                              Short chain fatty acids:
                                              Butyrate, acetate, propionate, CH_4

Inflammatory and Carcinogenic
Ammonia: barrier function, mucus, mucosal permeability proliferation
Branch chain fatty acids: inflammatory
Aromatic amino acids: phenolics, indolics, p-cresol, N-nitrosoamines
Hydrogen sulfide: inflammatory, DNA damage, genotoxic

Cell metabolism: energy supply
Genetic-Epigenetic regulation: histone deacetylase inhibition, miRNA , down-regulation of canonical Wnt-signaling
Anti-proliferative: p53, p21 activation, reduced cell cycling, apoptosis
Immunomodulatory and anti-inflammatory: GPR43, GPR109α activation, T_c reg activation of Foxp3 and IL-10 expression, NF-κB suppression
Mucosal health and defence: mucin synthesis, tight junctions, trefoil factors, antimicrobial peptides, heat shock proteins, transglutamase, β-glucoronidase acitivty
Microbiota homeostasis: phenolics, antioxidants

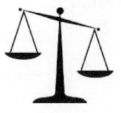

CANCER RISK

Fig. 2. Illustration of the influence of dietary composition on colonic microbial metabolism to enhance saccharolytic fermentation, colonic mucosal health, and cancer prevention, in the case of high fiber foods, or promote the production of inflammatory mediators or carcinogenesis in the case of fiber deficient, high-meat and high-fat diets. (*From* O'Keefe S. Diet, microbes and their metabolites, and colorectal cancer. Nat Rev Gastro & Hep 2016;13:691–706; with permission.)

This figure helps explain the mechanisms whereby diet affects colonic inflammation and colonic carcinogenesis. First, food is digested by the small intestine, releasing simple sugars, fats, amino acids, fluids and electrolytes and micronutrients into the bloodstream, supporting vital organ function and life. The content of fat, meat, and fiber determines what residues then enter the colon to provide substrate for the microbiota. The microbiota forms a complex system whose structure and activity depend upon what it is fed. Thus, a high-fiber diet stimulates the growth and function of microbes that contribute to saccharolytic fermentation, notably starch degraders such as *Ruminococcus. bromii* and *Bifidobacterium adolescentis* that cross-feed to produce acetate, which is the major energy source for the final major butyrate producers *Eubacterium rectale*, *Roseburia* subspecies, and *Faecalibacterium prausnitzii*.[8] Bifidobacteria are also induced by starch and soluble fiber to produce lactate, which is released into the lumen and fuels other butyrate-producers such as *E hallii*. Increased lactate production reduces luminal pH, which further stimulates the growth of butyrate producers and, importantly, suppresses overgrowth by pathogens. The figure outlines the remarkable pleotropic beneficial effects of butyrate on maintaining mucosal health and defense, immunologic modulation via stimulation of regulatory T cells, the promotion of microbial metabolism and homeostasis, and the epigenetic modulation (ie, butyrate acts as a histone deacetlyase inhibitor) of inflammation and epithelial proliferation, which suppresses long-term risk of carcinogenesis. Further reading on the evidence supporting each of these pathways is available elsewhere.[4] Microbes also digest the remaining plant cell walls, releasing phytochemicals at a mucosal level, where their powerful antioxidant, anti-inflammatory, and antineoplastic properties fortify the effects of short chain fatty acids in promoting mucosal health, microbial balance, and cancer resistance. Finally, increased colonic metabolism enables microbes to synthesize a remarkably wide spectrum of water-soluble vitamins, such as folate, B12, biotin, and nicotinamide, which are available in high local concentrations.[9,10] Recent studies have demonstrated that the view that such vitamins only become of benefit if copraphagia is practiced, as in rabbits, is incorrect, as specific transporters have been demonstrated in human colonic tissue.[11,12] Thus, the efficacy of these vitamins in regulating DNA synthesis and repair will likely further reduce the risk of neoplastic change and progression.

On the other hand, an unbalanced diet, rich in meat and fat, generates several mechanisms that increase mucosal inflammation, proliferation, and risk of colitis and cancer. A high-fat diet stimulates the liver to synthesize more bile acids, which are primarily needed for the small intestinal digestion and absorption of long chain fatty acids. Although most bile acids are reabsorbed in the proximal small intestine, a proportion enters the colon, where they are conjugated by specific microbes to secondary bile acids, which are recognized human carcinogens.[13] Furthermore, a recent study showed that high saturated fat consumption stimulated the production of taurine, one of the bile acids that has a high sulfur content.[14] On entering the colon, taurine stimulated a blossom of *Bilophila wadsworthiae*, which utilizes the sulfur to produce hydrogen sulfide, which caused acute colitis in experimental animals and has been shown to be genotoxic.[15]

High meat and protein diets are also not totally digested and stimulate colonic microbes to engage in proteolytic fermentation. Although this process also generates short chain fatty acids, it releases nitrogenous metabolites, such as nitrosamines, phenolics, and p-cresol, which are inflammatory and proneoplastic.[16] Furthermore, overcooked or burned meat produces heterocyclic amines, which are powerful carcinogens in their own right. Thus, the overall balance is shifted from colonic health to inflammation and neoplasia. It is critical to understand, however, that a high-fiber diet counteracts many of these inflammatory and neoplastic pathways,[17] and so a moderate quantity of meat and fat is well tolerated in a fiber-rich balanced diet.

Based on the fiber composition of the traditional African diet of greater than 50 g/d, which is associated with remarkably low rates of colon cancer, and the results of experimental studies that show there is a threshold quantity of fiber that needs to be met before the anti-inflammatory and antineoplastic effects of butyrate become active,[18] the author and colleagues believe the current US Department of Agriculture (USDA) recommendations that a normal diet should provide at least 22 g of fiber per day for women and 38 g/d for men, are insufficient. The author and colleagues believe that the ideal intake should be more like 50 g/d to prevent colitis and colon cancer. This proposal is further supported by the results of the Polyp Prevention Study, which recommended an increase on fiber to 35 g/d, and failed to achieve its primary endpoint, which was a reduction in adenomatous polyp recurrence.[19] Critically, it was demonstrated that in the segment of the population who increased their consumption of fiber rich foods and dry beans most, there was a significant reduction in the development of premalignant advanced polyps.[20] It is noteworthy that the current USDA dietary recommendations were based on the amount of fiber shown to reduce risk of cardiovascular diseases, not colonic health.

CLINICAL STUDIES

Following the previously cited evidence, the author and colleagues are concerned that the current nutritional recommendations for tube feeding of hospitalized patients are also inadequate. Most tube feed formulae have sufficient nutrients for maintain small intestinal health, but are grossly deficient for the support of colonic nutrition. Critically ill patients are commonly fed for prolonged periods on elemental diets that are either devoid of fiber, or only contain 4 g/L. A further concern is that most patients are treated with a variety of broad-spectrum antibiotics, which all but wipe out the microbes that are essential for using what little fiber there is to maintain colonic mucosal nutrition and defense. Thus, the colon is starved, increasing the risk of overgrowth of pathobionts such as *Clostridium difficile* and acute colitis.

In evidence, a recent study by Alverdy's group in a group of long-stay intensive care unit (ICU) patients[21] showed a dramatic contraction in the numbers of fecal microbial communities to between one1 to 4 taxa, mostly *Enterococcus* and *Staphylococcus* and the family *Enterobacteriaceae*. Furthermore, there was a rise in antimicrobial resistance, and overgrowth with fungal communities was common, including *Candida albicans* and *C glabrata*. **Fig. 3** illustrates one such patient who had received 14 courses of antibiotics and was left with a skeleton fecal microbiome consisting of 1 *Enterococcus* and 1 *Enterobacteraciae*.

FIBER SUPPLEMENTATION STUDIES

In an attempt to help the recovery of the colonic microbiota in a group of 13 critically ill ICU patients predominantly suffering from the consequences severe acute pancreatitis, the author and colleagues tested the utility of progressive soluble fiber supplementation of their enteral feeds for up to 36 days.[22] **Table 1** shows that all patients had been, or were receiving broad-spectrum intravenous antibiotics, and most were also treated with gastric acid suppression by proton pump inhibitors (PPIs). Previous studies had shown that PPIs were associated with disturbed gut function and small bowel bacterial overgrowth,[23] and had raised the concern that the combination of elemental diets, antibiotics, and PPIs were a prescription for *C difficile* infection and colitis.[24] The tube feed given was semielemental and contained 4 g soluble fiber per liter. Following fecal microbial analysis for microbes and short chain fatty acids, progressive supplementation was

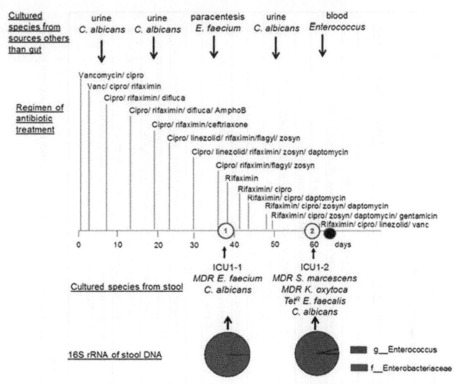

Fig. 3. Time course of 1 long-stay ICU patient who received multiple courses of antibiotics, illustrating the decimation of the fecal microbiota. (*From* Zaborin A, Smith D, Garfield K, et al. Membership and behavior of ultra-low-diversity pathogen communities present in the gut of humans during prolonged critical illness. MBio 2014;5:e01361–14; with permission.)

commenced at 4 g 3 times daily, and increased progressively every 3 days, with tolerance, to a goal of 24 g/d. The supplementation was well tolerated from a GI point of view, with no significant increase in stool output or diarrhea. In fact, bowel function was unchanged in those without diarrhea, and in the 4 with diarrhea, it improved in 2 patients, remained the same in 1 patient, and worsened in the fourth patient, whose progress was hindered by recurrent sepsis and the need for continued antibiotics.

Fecal studies revealed that microbial counts before fiber supplementation were dramatically suppressed in the group as a whole (**Fig. 4**), with a 97% reduction in the predominant potential butyrate producers at the genus level, namely *Clostridia* cluster XIVa (which include *Eubacterium rectale*, *Roseburia intestinalis*) and cluster IV (including *Faecalibacterium prausnitzii*), and in starch degraders (*Ruminococcus bromii* and *R obeum*). Similarly, fecal short chain fatty acid concentrations were several-fold lower. Following maximal fiber supplementation, there was partial, but not complete, restoration of microbial numbers and their metabolites, including butyrate (**Fig. 5**). The partial response could be explained by the continued use of antibiotics in some and to the well-recognized long-term disturbance of the microbiota following a course of antibiotics.[25]

Table 1
Results of testing the utility of progressive soluble fiber supplementation of patients enteral feeds for up to 36 days

Patient	Diagnosis	Age (y)	Sex	Body Mass Index (kg/m²)	Duration of Fiber Suppl (d)	Maximum Fiber (g/d)	Medications, Gastrointestinal Symptoms Before Feeding, Outcome
Group 1: bolus injections: short term							
1	Trauma	59	M	34.7	3	15	Metronidazole, lanzoprazole, diarrhea, d/c to snf
2	SAP	65	M	38.0	8	29	Cefepime, lanzoprazole, diarrhea, discharge home
3	SAP	85	F	31.0	3	24	Omeprazole, diarrhea, discharge home
4	SAP	89	F	29.4	6	32	Fluconazole, lanzoprazole, transfer rehab
5	SAP	43	M	34.7	9	12	Fluconazole, vancomycin, pantoprazole, discharge home
6	SAP	34	M	44.8	3	18	Ertapenem, omeprazole, diarrhea, d/c to snf
7	SAP	81	F	35.5	3	15	Omeprazole, discharge home
8	SAP	62	M	27.0	7	22	Famotidine, metronidazolel discharge home
9	SAP	56	M	28.7	6	24	Trimethoprim-sulfamethoxazole, voriconazole, pantoprazole, discharge home
Group 2: continuous infusions: long term							
10	SAP	88	F	30.3	19	35	Metronidazole, aztreonam, famotidine, diarrhea transfer to snf
11	SAP	65	F	27.6	36	36	Piperacillin-tazobactam, doripenem, metronidazole, pantoprazole, cefuroxime, diarrhea, distension, pain, d/c to snf
12	SAP	47	F	31.0	33	18	Piperacillin-tazobactam, pantoprazole, fluconazole, metronidazole, vancomycin, diarrhea, distention, d/c to snf
13	Chronic sepsis C diff	79	F	34.9	23	24	Metronidazole, vancomycin, lanzoprazole, diarrhea, distension, pain. C difficile, d/c to snf

Abbreviations: d/c, discharge; SAP, severe acute pancreatitis; snf, skilled nursing facility.
From O'Keefe SJ, Ou J, Delany JP, et al. Effect of fiber supplementation on the microbiota in critically ill patients. World J Gastrointest Pathophysiol 2011;2:138–45; with permission.

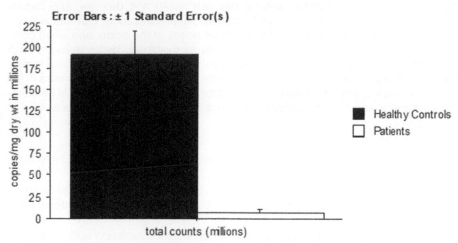

Fig. 4. Illustration of the gross suppression of fecal microbial counts in ICU patients recovering from severe acute pancreatitis. (*From* O'Keefe SJ, Ou J, Delany JP, et al. Effect of fiber supplementation on the microbiota in critically ill patients. World J Gastrointest Pathophysiol 2011;2:138–45; with permission.)

Indices of Fermentation before and after Fiber Supplementation

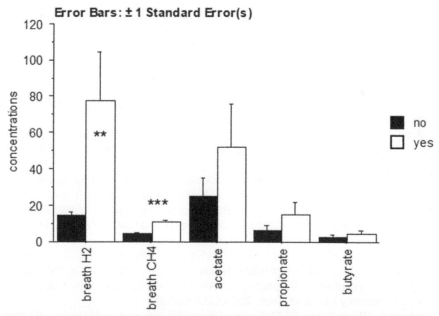

Fig. 5. Evidence of recovery of saccharolytic fermentation in ICU patients given progressive fiber supplementation of their tube feeds. (*From* O'Keefe SJ, Ou J, Delany JP, et al. Effect of fiber supplementation on the microbiota in critically ill patients. World J Gastrointest Pathophysiol 2011;2:138–45; with permission.)

SUMMARY

In conclusion, this article has provided evidence that current dietary fiber intake levels may be insufficient to maintain colonic mucosal health and defense, and reduce inflammation and cancer risk in otherwise healthy people. Secondly, current commercial tube feeds generally overlook the metabolic needs of the colon, and when combined with antibiotics may predispose patients to dysbiosis, bacterial overgrowth with pathogens such as C difficile, and acute colitis, thus perpetuating critical illness. These results raise concern about the wide-scale use of prophylactic antibiotics in the ICU and the use of elemental, fiber-depleted tube feeds. Nutrition support is not complete without the addition of sufficient fiber to meet colonic nutritional needs.

REFERENCES

1. O'Keefe SJD. The principles and practice of nutritional support. New York: Springer; 2015. p. 1–241.
2. Choban P, Dickerson R, Malone A, et al. A.S.P.E.N. Clinical guidelines: nutrition support of hospitalized adult patients with obesity. JPEN J Parenter Enteral Nutr 2013;37:714–44.
3. Yamada Y, Kemnitz JW, Weindruch R, et al. Caloric restriction and healthy life span: frail phenotype of nonhuman primates in the Wisconsin National Primate Research Center Caloric Restriction Study. J Gerontol A Biol Sci Med Sci 2017. [Epub ahead of print].
4. O'Keefe SJ. Diet, microorganisms and their metabolites, and colon cancer. Nat Rev Gastroenterol Hepatol 2016;13(12):691–706.
5. O'Keefe SJ, Li JV, Lahti L, et al. Fat, fibre and cancer risk in African Americans and rural Africans. Nat Commun 2015;6:6342.
6. Perdue DG, Haverkamp D, Perkins C, et al. Geographic variation in colorectal cancer incidence and mortality, age of onset, and stage at diagnosis among American Indian and Alaska Native people, 1990-2009. Am J Public Health 2014;104(Suppl 3):S404–14.
7. Balter V, Braga J, Telouk P, et al. Evidence for dietary change but not landscape use in South African early hominins. Nature 2012;489:558–60.
8. Flint HJ, Duncan SH, Scott KP, et al. Links between diet, gut microbiota composition and gut metabolism. Proc Nutr Soc 2015;74:13–22.
9. O'Keefe S, Sharma S, Aufreiter S, et al. Colonic microbiota folate production: Another piece of the folate-colon cancer puzzle? Am J Gastroenterol 2008;103: 1400.
10. O'Keefe SJD, Ou J, Aufreiter S, et al. Products of the colonic microbiota mediate the effects of diet on colon cancer risk. J Nutr 2009;139:2044–8.
11. Said HM, Ortiz A, McCloud E, et al. Biotin uptake by human colonic epithelial NCM460 cells: a carrier-mediated process shared with pantothenic acid. Am J Physiol 1998;275:C1365–71.
12. Subramanian VS, Chatterjee N, Said HM. Folate uptake in the human intestine: Promoter activity and effect of folate deficiency. J Cell Physiol 2003;196:403–8.
13. Bernstein C, Holubec H, Bhattacharyya AK, et al. Carcinogenicity of deoxycholate, a secondary bile acid. Arch Toxicol 2011;85:863–71.
14. Devkota S, Wang Y, Musch MW, et al. Dietary-fat-induced taurocholic acid promotes pathobiont expansion and colitis in Il10-/- mice. Nature 2012;487:104–8.
15. Attene-Ramos MS, Wagner ED, Plewa MJ, et al. Evidence that hydrogen sulfide is a genotoxic agent. Mol Cancer Res 2006;4:9–14.

16. Windey K, De Preter V, Verbeke K. Relevance of protein fermentation to gut health. Mol Nutr Food Res 2012;56:184–96.
17. Humphreys KJ, Conlon MA, Young GP, et al. Dietary manipulation of oncogenic microRNA expression in human rectal mucosa: a randomized trial. Cancer Prev Res (Phila) 2014;7:786–95.
18. Donohoe DR, Collins LB, Wali A, et al. The Warburg effect dictates the mechanism of butyrate-mediated histone acetylation and cell proliferation. Mol Cell 2012;48:612–26.
19. Schatzkin A, Lanza E, Corle D, et al. Lack of effect of a low-fat, high-fiber diet on the recurrence of colorectal adenomas. N Engl J Med 2000;342:1149–55.
20. Lanza E, Hartman TJ, Albert PS, et al. High dry bean intake and reduced risk of advanced colorectal adenoma recurrence among participants in the polyp prevention trial. J Nutr 2006;136:1896–903.
21. Zaborin A, Smith D, Garfield K, et al. Membership and behavior of ultra-low-diversity pathogen communities present in the gut of humans during prolonged critical illness. MBio 2014;5. e01361-14.
22. O'Keefe SJ, Ou J, Delany JP, et al. Effect of fiber supplementation on the microbiota in critically ill patients. World J Gastrointest Pathophysiol 2011;2:138–45.
23. Lewis SJ, Franco S, Young G, et al. Altered bowel function and duodenal bacterial overgrowth in patients treated with omeprazole. Aliment Pharmacol Ther 1996;10:557–61.
24. O'Keefe SJ. Tube feeding, the microbiota, and clostridium difficile infection. World J Gastroenterol 2010;16:139–42.
25. Dethlefsen L, Relman DA. Incomplete recovery and individualized responses of the human distal gut microbiota to repeated antibiotic perturbation. Proc Natl Acad Sci U S A 2011;108(Suppl 1):4554–61.

Nutritional Therapy in Gastrointestinal Cancers

Priscila Garla, MSc, RD[a], Dan Linetzky Waitzberg, PhD, MD[a,b,*],
Alweyd Tesser, RD[a]

KEYWORDS

- Cancer • Malnutrition • Nutrition screening • Cachexia • Early enteral nutrition
- Immunonutrition

KEY POINTS

- Malnutrition is highly prevalent in gastrointestinal cancer and negatively affects patient prognosis.
- Nutritional risk screening and assessment of nutritional status should be performed within the first 24 to 48 hours of hospital admission.
- Nutrition therapy in patients with cancer aims to provide optimal energy and protein to maintain nutritional status and avoid clinical and surgical complications.
- The perioperative nutritional intervention can favorably modify postoperative clinical outcome in patients undergoing elective gastrointestinal surgery.
- Preoperative immunonutrition has been associated with an improvement in immune and anti-inflammatory response, nutritional status, and reduction of postoperative complications in malnourished patients.

INTRODUCTION

Gastrointestinal cancer (GC), including the different organs of the digestive system: esophagus, stomach, liver, gallbladder, pancreas, small intestine, large intestine, rectum, and anus, is the most frequently diagnosed type of cancer worldwide. According to estimates from the World Health Organization, by 2030 the global incidence is expected to increase to 21.7 million cancer cases and 13 million cancer deaths due to the growth and aging of the population. In the United States, GC represents more than 20% of all newly diagnosed cancer cases, with gastric cancer considered the fourth most common type and the second leading cause of cancer death.[1] Most of the cases

Disclosure Statement: The authors have nothing to disclose.
[a] Department of Gastroenterology, School of Medicine, University of Sao Paulo, Av. Dr Arnaldo, 455, 2 andar, sala 2208–Cerqueira Cé sar, São Paulo, São Paulo CEP: 01246-903, Brazil;
[b] Grupo Apoio Nutrição Enteral Parenteral–Human Nutrition, Maestro Cardim, 1236 - Paraíso, São Paulo 01323-001, Brazil
* Corresponding author. Av. Dr Arnaldo, 455, 2° andar, sala 2208–Cerqueira César, São Paulo, São Paulo CEP: 01246-903, Brazil.
E-mail address: dan.waitzberg@gmail.com

Gastroenterol Clin N Am 47 (2018) 231–242
https://doi.org/10.1016/j.gtc.2017.09.009
0889-8553/18/© 2017 Elsevier Inc. All rights reserved.

occur in developed countries, and the highest incidence of stomach cancer is in East Asia, Eastern Europe, and Central and South America.[2]

Cancer is one of the diseases with the highest mortality in the world. Over the past decades, despite the considerable progress in reducing incidence and mortalities of cancers, GC remains the second leading cause of cancer-related mortality worldwide.[3]

It has been well reported that GC incidence increases progressively with increasing age, radiation exposure, genetic pattern, family history, central obesity, smoking, and alcohol addiction.[1–3] In epidemiologic studies, diet has been shown to directly affect GC risk. Most recently, the World Cancer Research Fund/American Institute for Cancer Research demonstrated that the excessive consumption of salt-preserved food and processed meats is strongly associated with an increased risk of developing GC. On the other hand, a healthy balanced diet rich in fiber, fruit, and vegetables seems to be associated with lower incidence and reduced overall mortality of all types of cancer.[4]

At cancer diagnosis, nutritional disorders become an emergent issue. Patients with cancer are frequently at risk of malnutrition, not only because of physical and metabolic effects of the disease but also because of adverse consequences of anticancer therapies, and intake changes related to inadequate food consumption or malabsorption.[5] It is now well known that malnutrition is an independent risk factor for increased morbidity, length of hospital stay, higher readmission rates, late recovery, poor quality of life, higher hospital costs, and mortality. For these reasons, the therapeutic approach should be initiated early through assessment and specific nutritional guidance. Individualized nutritional counseling, with or without artificial diets, might increase the food intake, which helps the prevention of important weight loss associated with antineoplastic therapy and improves clinical outcomes. Therefore, this present review has the aim of transmitting an updated and clear vision of the nutritional strategies on the impact of tumor and anticancer treatments on GC.[5–7]

NUTRITIONAL SCREENING AND ASSESSMENT

Early diagnosis of nutritional disorders in patients with cancer is essential to avoid further complications and to improve survival rate.[5–8] Nutritional risk screening and assessment of nutritional status should be performed within the first hours of admission, and factors such as tumor localization and gastrointestinal (GI) dysfunction caused by chemotherapy and radiotherapy treatments must be considered during the screening.

In recent research conducted in 12 countries of Latin America, the prevalence of malnutrition was identified in 40% to 60% of general patients at hospital admission. In addition, the investigators identified that the risk of disease-related malnutrition increased by 20% during the first 2 weeks of hospitalization and was directly associated with further infectious and noninfectious complications, longer hospitalization permanence, and higher treatment costs.[9] At GC diagnosis, the risk of malnutrition might reach up to 80% of patients according to the extension of surgical resection, anticancer treatment, and its related side effects.[10] In a recent systematic review[11] focused on older patients undergoing chemotherapy, the highest prevalence of malnutrition was found in patients with upper GC, mainly related to adverse effects of anticancer therapy. Symptoms such as dry mouth, nausea, stomach pain, and GI motility disorders were the most frequently reported chemotherapy-related symptoms causing impairment of nutritional status.

It is widely agreed the major challenge in patients with GI cancer is to avoid involuntary weight loss, which is frequently observed in clinical practice and must be considered as a warning sign for cachexia development.[12,13] The disorder is diagnosed in approximately 50% of patients with cancer, most commonly in advanced disease, malnourished individuals, age greater than 65 years, sarcopenia, upper GI tumor, and with acute systemic inflammation. Cancer cachexia is well established as a complex multifactorial syndrome characterized by severe and progressive muscle wasting with or without loss of fat mass.[14] The established diagnostic criteria include involuntary weight loss of more than 5%, or 2% in underweight individuals according to the body mass index (BMI; <20 kg/m^2) or presence of sarcopenia. The classification of the syndrome was recently proposed according to clinical severity, in precachexia, cachexia, and refractory cachexia. The first stage is defined by weight loss equal to or greater than 5%, anorexia, and metabolic changes; for inclusion in the second stage, weight loss equal to or greater than 5%, or 2% and BMI less than 20 kg/m^2, or sarcopenia accompanied by a loss of body weight equivalent or greater than 2%, is considered. The frequent presence of reduced intake and systemic inflammation is also mentioned in this stage. Finally, the third stage (refractory cachexia) includes patients with intense catabolism who do not respond to anticancer treatment and patients with low-performance score and survival expectancy of less than 3 months.[15] Future perspectives embrace the determination of plasma biomarkers such as proinflammatory cytokines and the early determination of cachexia by detection of genetic polymorphisms.[15,16] Together with nutritional support, cancer cachexia should be a multimodal treatment associated with muscle support consisting of routine physical activity, training exercises, and techniques to increase muscle mass or strength.

It has been consistently proven that progressive muscle loss is associated with severe complications that worsen prognosis through depletion of the body's energy and protein reserve, thereby contributing to the severity of treatment-related toxic effects, reduced response to anticancer drugs, and survival rate.[3,6,10–18] Findings from a cohort study,[16] including patients with solid cancer, showed that involuntary weight loss higher than 8% associated with muscle depletion resulted in lower survival rates, regardless of the initial BMI classification. These observational data are consistent with previous investigations that showed the loss of fat free mass might directly contribute to functional and immunity impairment and become a fatal complication when up to 30% of involuntary muscle depletion occurs.[16]

Considering the strong influence of nutritional status on better clinical outcomes in cancer, early nutritional screening has been recommended in all patients to identify any specific risk of malnutrition. Current recommendations of nutritional bodies[12–15] suggest that nutritional screening should be performed using validated tools in all individuals at cancer diagnosis, during the first 24 to 48 hours of hospital admission as well as regular assessments during treatment. The validated screening and assessment nutritional tools in patients with cancer[17] are shown in **Table 1**. The periodic rescreening might be assessed weekly in severe patients and those with advanced cancer.[12] More recently, the percentage of weight loss and BMI have both been clinically recognized as an important nutritional tool to predict overall survival in malnourished patients with advanced cancer.[12–14]

NUTRITION THERAPY FOR ANTICANCER TREATMENT

Radiation therapy uses high-energy radiation to cause destabilization and damage in the double-helices of nuclear DNA, leading to irreversible loss of the reproductive integrity of the cancer cell and resulting in death by apoptosis.[3] It is well Known the

Table 1
Nutrition therapy in patients with cancer

Screening Instrument	Main Measures
Malnutrition Screening Tool	Unintentional weight loss, appetite
Nutritional Risk Screening 2002	Weight loss, BMI, food intake
Malnutrition Universal Screening Tool	BMI, weight changes
Nutritional assessment	
Subjective Global Assessment (SGA)	Weight loss, food intake, GI symptoms, functional capacity
Patient-generated SGA	Weight loss, food intake, GI symptoms, functional capacity
Revised Mini Nutritional Assessment Short Form	BMI or calf circumference, weight loss, appetite
Nutritional requirements	
Energy	Resting energy expenditure by indirect calorimetry. If not possible, may be calculated by simplistic weight-based equation (25–30 kcal/kg/d)
Protein	1.2–1.5 g/kg/d. Up to 2 g in elderly (>65 y), inactivity and systemic inflammation In acute or chronic renal failure, do not exceed 1.2 g/kg/d
Fat intake	35%–50% of total energy requirement in patients at risk of malnutrition and advanced cancer
Oral nutritional supplements	If oral food intake is inadequate to reach nutrition requirements
Artificial nutrition: enteral and parenteral nutrition	Prefer enteral tube feeding; parenteral nutrition if enteral nutrition is contraindicated
Vitamins and minerals	Equal to the RDA; supplementation of high-dose micronutrients only in specific deficiencies
Omega-3 fatty acids or fish oil supplements	Most frequent dose (2–4 g/d) in malnourished patients with advanced cancer undergoing anticancer drug therapy

intensity and frequency of side effects depend on the tumor, site of irradiation, duration of treatment, dose, and fractionation.[3] Irradiation of the GI tract and the head and neck area is most often associated with side effects with the greatest nutritional impact.[11] The oropharyngeal mucous membranes are especially sensitive to radiation; therefore, stomatitis, esophagitis, mucositis, xerostomia, odynophagia, dysphagia, and dyspepsia are very frequent.[11,14] In these situations, there may be weight loss in about 90% of patients and an increased risk of malnutrition (**Fig. 1**).

Recent guidelines recommend nutritional counseling to increase food intake, prevent additional important weight loss, and to diminish the negative effect of anticancer treatment on nutritional status.[5,14] The initial goal of nutritional therapy is to correct or prevent nutritional deficiencies, improve the immune system to prevent further infections, and maintain/improve quality of life. The ultimate goals are to improve response and tolerance to treatment, increase survival, reduce complications of malnutrition, and promote early hospital discharge.[5,12–14,18]

Once the risk has been identified, individual nutritional therapy planning should be established.[5,12–14,18] In patients who are able to eat, the most effective form of nutritional therapy is hyperproteic and hypercaloric oral nutritional supplements together

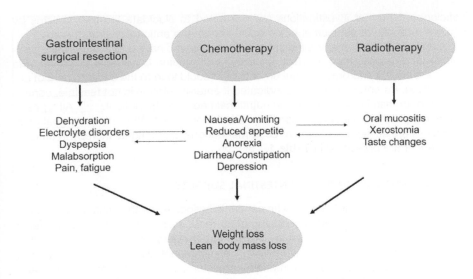

Fig. 1. Anticancer treatment side effects with negative impact on nutritional status.

with standard oral diet to reach nutritional requirements. Administering oral nutritional supplements to malnourished patients has demonstrated improvement of immunologic and anti-inflammatory biomarkers, nutritional status, and increased fat free mass.[18] Formula enriched with long-chain omega-3 fatty acids, eicosapentaenoic (EPA), and docosahexaenoic (DHA) acids has been shown to be an important nutrient in the nutritional treatment of cancer, proposed to increase appetite and lean body mass in patients with poor appetite undergoing radiotherapy and chemotherapy.[14] Many clinical findings point out the positive effects on the attenuation of anorexia/cachexia syndrome, especially in patients undergoing chemotherapy and radiotherapy, and in the treatment of patients with upper GC undergoing major elective surgery.[19–26]

In addition, experimental studies have speculated that omega-3 could improve the efficacy of antitumor therapies.[27,28] Although the proposed pathways by omega-3 EPA and DHA action on carcinogenesis remain unclear, studies in vitro and in vivo suggest the lower production of proinflammatory eicosanoids, upregulation of resolvins, protectins, and maresins, immune boosting, reduction in oncogenic protein signaling, and cell tumor growth inhibition might be possible explanations.[27,28] In a recent meta-analysis, dietary supplement for GI malignancy was effective in improving immune response by reducing the level of inflammatory markers, including C-reactive protein and interleukin-6, and for improvement of nutritional status with higher levels of albumin, and immune markers $CD3^+$ T cells, $CD4^+$ T cells, and $CD4^+/CD8^+$ ratio compared with the isocaloric nutrition regimen.[29]

The oral high-dose supplementation of other nutrients as vitamins and minerals in anticancer treatment is strongly debatable and still controversial by nutritional bodies.[14,30,31] Some experts think that the use of vitamin supplements may increase the response of the tumor to treatment; others think that some of those micronutrients could protect cells from damaging the antineoplastic treatment.[30,31] Presently, oral vitamins and minerals are suggested to be supplied in amounts approximately equal to the Recommended Daily Allowance (RDA), and the supplementation of high-dose micronutrients is not recommended in the absence of laboratory confirmed deficiency.[14] Further investigations are warranted to elucidate the mechanisms by which micronutrient supplementation could impact the anticancer drug therapy.

Enteral nutritional therapy is indicated for patients who have a total or partially functioning GI digestive tract, of which exclusive oral feeding is not able to provide the adequate energy and protein requirements, and could lead to the development of undernutrition. Parenteral nutrition is indicated if enteral nutrition is not feasible, contraindicated, or insufficient to meet the nutritional needs of the patient.[5,7,14] All types of nutritional planning should be monitored continuously until the proposed goals and objectives are achieved. The main recommendations of nutritional therapy in patients with cancer are presented in **Table 1**.

PERIOPERATIVE CARE IN GASTROINTESTINAL SURGERY

Major surgical trauma in patients with cancer is associated with simultaneous activation of proinflammatory and anti-inflammatory responses defined as SIRS (systemic inflammatory immune response) and CARS (compensatory anti-inflammatory immune response). The impaired balance between these immunologic responses in trauma is accompanied by postoperative immunosuppression and might contribute to elevated risk of infectious complications, longer length of stay, and mortality.[32] Many factors might contribute to elevating the risks of immune imbalance in elective surgical patients, such as the diagnosis of advanced cancer, age greater than 60 years, the type and extent of surgical trauma, predisposing genotype, and undernutrition.[7,13,16] Considering that all of these criteria are unmodifiable, except nutritional status, the need to favorably change the nutritional profile before elective surgery providing optimal support a few weeks before the event has been consistently linked to decreasing of postoperative complications and to better clinical outcomes.[7,14,32–36]

The major indications of perioperative specialized nutrition support in the patients with cancer are to prevent or reverse malnutrition before the surgical procedure and to minimize the effects of prolonged period of fasting in the perioperative period that results in severe catabolism and intense inflammatory activity.[5,14,32–36] Perioperative nutrition therapy is currently indicated in all malnourished patients or at risk of malnutrition, previously identified by screening.[5,14,36] The European Society for Clinical Nutrition and Metabolism[14] reinforces attention to nutritional risk situations in elective surgical patients: body weight loss of 10% to 15% within 6 months, BMI less than 18.5 kg/m^2, subjective global assessment grade C or Nutritional Risk Screening >5, and serum albumin less than 30 mg/dL (without evidence of hepatic and renal dysfunction). Severe nutritional risk is considered when there are at least one of the mentioned criteria. For these patients, 10 to 14 days of preoperative nutritional therapy to increase immunologic defense are recommended without expecting changes in body composition parameters and serum albumin.[6,14]

It is also important to highlight that the knowledge of metabolic changes in fasting is crucial for successful nutritional care. It has been well documented that, after a few hours of fasting, there is a progressive increase in the consumption of energy and protein reserves, which generates intense catabolism and the release of inflammatory mediators.[32–35,37] Multimodal protocol seeks to abbreviate the perioperative fasting to optimize the recovery of surgical trauma. Enhanced recovery of patients after surgery as "ERAS" has become an important focus of multimodal perioperative management in cancer treatment, designed to achieve early recovery after surgical procedures by reducing the stress response following surgery and improving the patient physical well-being in patients with GI cancer (**Fig. 2**).[5,14,33–35] Randomized clinical trials and meta-analysis in elective colorectal surgery have shown that this practice is safe,

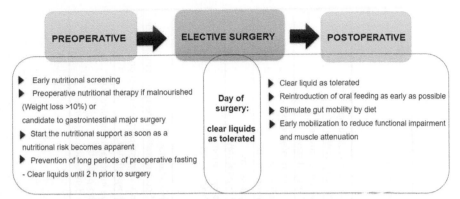

Fig. 2. Primary goals of nutritional care to early recovery after selective surgery.

but also useful for the faster recovery of surgical trauma, lower complications, and shorter length of hospital stay. It is thought that the ERAS protocol can also ameliorate the immunologic and nutritional status and improve GI permeability and bacterial translocation.[33–35]

After a digestive system surgical procedure, it is essential to consider cancer prognosis as well as the estimated period for postoperative refeeding. In those patients, postoperative undernutrition may be directly related to changes in food intake, digestion, and absorption processes.[6–8] The concept of early enteral nutrition (EEN) plays a major role in postoperative care and consists of the offering of nutritional therapy in the first 24 to 48 hours after the occurrence of a traumatic or infectious event.[33–35] This intervention is justified insofar as the absence of nutrients in the GI tract, especially in the intestine, is associated with intestinal hypotrophy, favoring the breakdown of the immunologic barrier, greater permeability, and possible microbial translocation, eventually resulting in the appearance of infectious complications and increased mortality. From the metabolic point of view, EEN can prevent excessive secretion of catabolic hormones by reducing the release of serum cortisol and glucagon. In addition, it maintains nutritional status and might prevent cachexia by reducing the loss of body weight, muscle attenuation, and negative nitrogen balance.[5,14] In a large meta-analysis including 835 patients with gastric cancer, EEN postoperatively resulted in increased levels of albumin and prealbumin, larger body weight gain, better immunologic parameters, as well as reducing hospital stay compared with patients who received parenteral nutrition therapy.[36]

Despite many clinical advantages, management of EEN is not free of metabolic, GI, or mechanical complications. Management of EEN should include attention to the advancement of feeding, glycemic control, and GI tolerance, especially in malnourished patients and advanced cancer.[5,24,37–40] In this regard, the use of protocols in enteral care is becoming a promising treatment option in nutrition support teams to improve decision making and to determine appropriate treatments. Periodic evaluation of quality indicators for enteral nutritional therapy is of great interest and allows identification of existing complications and the development of action plans to reduce morbidities.[37–40]

IMMUNONUTRITION

Strengthening the patient's immune defenses is a useful approach to help to reduce complications. In recent years, alongside standard artificial nutrition, solutions have

Table 2
Meta-analysis evaluating perioperative use of enteral immunonutrition in patients submitted to gastrointestinal tract surgery

Author, y	RCT	Number of Patients	Diet	Duration of Intervention	Clinical Outcomes
Waitzberg et al,[7] 2006	17	2305	EIN vs SEN	5–7 d before and/or after surgery	• Reduced postoperative infectious complications • Decreased length of hospital stay
Zheng et al,[42] 2007	13	1269	EIN vs SEN	Preoperative = 5–7 d Postoperative = 5–10 d	• Reduced postoperative infectious rate • Decreased length of hospital stay
Marik et al,[43] 2010	21	1918	EIN vs SEN	Preoperative = 2–5 d Postoperative = 7 d	• Reduced the risk of acquired infections • Reduced wound complications • Decreased length of hospital stay
Cerantola et al,[44] 2011	35	2730	EIN vs SEN	Preoperative = 5–7 d Postoperative = 10 d	• Reduced overall complications • Decreased length of hospital stay
Drover et al,[45] 2011	35	3445	EIN vs SEN	Preoperative = 2–7 d Perioperative = 5–10 d (pre + post) Postoperative = 10 d	• Reduced infectious complication • Decreased length of hospital stay
Zhang et al,[46] 2012	19	2331	EIN vs SEN	Preoperative = 5 d Postoperative = 5–8 d	• Decreased length of hospital stay • Reduced morbidity of postoperative infectious complication
Marimuthu et al,[47] 2012	26	2496	EIN vs SEN	5 d before and/or after surgery	• Decreased the incidence of postoperative infections • Decreased length of hospital stay
Osland et al,[48] 2014	20	2005	EIN vs SEN	Preoperative = 5 d Postoperative = 14 d	• Reduced postoperative infectious complications • Decreased length of hospital stay • Reduced anastomotic dehiscence incidence

Abbreviation: SEN, standard enteral nutrition.

been developed that are enriched in nutrients, with the aim of stimulating the host immune response, improving control of the inflammatory response, and increasing nitrogen balance after major surgery. These nutrients are arginine, glutamine, omega-3 polyunsaturated fatty acids, nucleotides, trace elements, and antioxidants. Their combination in the nutritional formula is called immunonutrition.[28,41] It is a strong and commonly held belief among nutrition clinicians that oral/enteral immunonutrition (EIN) is a preferable access route than a parenteral route.

For the past 35 years, many clinical trials have been performed to investigate the effect of immunomodulatory diet in elective surgery, particularly in patients at nutritional risk with upper GI cancer. Data from randomized clinical trials summarized in 9 meta-analyses provide convincing evidence that EIN in GC is safe and well tolerated in the perioperative period, effective for enhancing host immunity and relieving the inflammatory response, which contributed to healing of postoperative wounds, reduction of infectious complications, and lower length of stay in malnourished patients, but without affecting the mortality (**Table 2**).[7,42–48] Its use is recommended in the perioperative period for 5 to 7 days in major upper abdominal surgeries, head and neck cancer, and severe trauma. Nutrition guidelines recommend the oral administration of 500 to 1000 kcal/d of IEN, or an enteral offer to achieve the minimum of 60% of nutritional requirements. At present, there are no recommendations for the use of perioperative EIN in the presence of septic shock and in nourished patients.[5,14,28]

Despite immunonutrients showing a promising role as a pharmaconutritional therapy, their parenteral application remains unclear. Future research should attempt to improve understanding of the specific mechanisms of action and signaling pathways involved, to define the ideal patient characteristics, and to clarify the optimal parenteral doses to be used for each immunonutrient.

NUTRITIONAL CARE IN PALLIATIVE CARE

In advanced incurable cancer, the objectives of nutritional intervention are aimed at promoting the quality of life and relieving the patient's symptoms. The proposed nutritional care plan should involve discussion between the health professionals, patients, and their families. At this stage, it is important to know the preferences and eating habits of the patient to develop strategies to maximize comfort and quality of life. Changes in taste and smell, often present in those patients with cachexia and advanced cancer, are potential barriers to optimal oral intake. The reduction of this symptom burden and early satiety and intestinal functioning become crucial factors to favor food acceptance. Whenever possible, the goal is to maintain oral nutrition through the nutritional counseling of the patient and their family members. Artificial nutritional therapy has shown inconsistent effects on survival rate and quality of life. According to nutrition bodies, the palliative use of nutritional therapy in patients with end-stage cancer is rarely indicated, and there is no evidence that parenteral nutrition improves cachexia-anorexia syndrome in palliative care patients.[14,29,30,49,50]

SUMMARY

Reduced food intake associated with involuntary weight loss and body composition changes has a negative impact on clinical and surgical GI cancer treatment. Early nutrition screening, assessment, and intervention are recommended to prevent negative outcomes and increase life expectancy. The application of nutrition support protocols together with the health care team aims at a better understanding and greater assertiveness of the choices in clinical and nutritional management.

REFERENCES

1. Herszényi L, Tulassay Z. Epidemiology of gastrointestinal and liver tumors. Eur Rev Med Pharmacol Sci 2010;14:249–58.
2. Ferlay J, Soerjomataram I, Ervik M, et al. GLOBOCAN 2012 v1.1, cancer incidence and mortality worldwide: IARC Cancer Base No. 11. Lyon (France): International Agency for Research on Cancer; 2014. Available at: http://globocan.iarc.fr. Accessed January 16, 2015.
3. Karimi P, Islami F, Anandasabapathy S, et al. Gastric cancer: descriptive epidemiology, risk factors, screening, and prevention. Cancer Epidemiol Biomarkers Prev 2014;23(5):700–13.
4. Schwingshackl L, Hoffmann G. Adherence to Mediterranean diet and risk of cancer: an updated systematic review and meta-analysis of observational studies. Cancer Med 2015;4(12):1933–47.
5. Weimann A, Braga M, Harsanyi L, et al. ESPEN guidelines enteral nutrition: surgery including organ transplantation. Clin Nutr 2006;25:224–44.
6. Rosania R, Chiapponi C, Malfertheiner P, et al. Nutrition in patients with gastric cancer: an update. Gastrointest Tumors 2016;2:178–87.
7. Waitzberg DL, Saito H, Plank LD, et al. Postsurgical infections are reduced with specialized nutrition support. World J Surg 2006;30(8):1592–604.
8. Hiesmayr M, Schindler K, Pernicka E, et al. Decreased food intake is a risk factor for mortality in hospitalised patients: the NutritionDay survey 2006. Clin Nutr 2009; 28(5):484–91.
9. Correia MITD, Perman MI, Waitzberg DL. Hospital malnutrition in Latin America: a systematic review. Clin Nutr 2017;36(4):958–67.
10. Hébuterne X, Lemarié E, Michallet M, et al. Prevalence of malnutrition and current use of nutrition support in patients with cancer. JPEN J Parenter Enteral Nutr 2014;38(2):196–204.
11. Caillet P, Liuu E, Raynaud Simon A, et al. Association between cachexia, chemotherapy and outcomes in older cancer patients: a systematic review. Clin Nutr 2017;36(6):1473–82.
12. Caccialanza R, Pedrazzoli P, Cereda E, et al. Nutritional support in cancer patients: a position paper from the Italian Society of Medical Oncology (AIOM) and the Italian Society of Artificial Nutrition and Metabolism (SINPE). J Cancer 2016;7(2):131–5.
13. Mueller C, Compher C, Ellen DM, American Society for Parenteral and Enteral Nutrition (A.S.P.E.N.) Board of Directors. A.S.P.E.N. Clinical guidelines: nutrition screening, assessment, and intervention in adults. JPEN J Parenter Enteral Nutr 2011;35:16–24.
14. Arends J, Bachmann P, Baracos V, et al. ESPEN guidelines on nutrition in cancer patients. Clin Nutr 2017;36(1):11–48.
15. Fearon K, Arends J, Baracos V. Understanding the mechanisms and treatment options in cancer cachexia. Nat Rev Clin Oncol 2013;10:90–9.
16. Martin L, Birdsell L, MacDonald N, et al. Cancer cachexia in the age of obesity: skeletal muscle depletion is a powerful prognostic factor, independent of body mass index. J Clin Oncol 2013;31:1539–47.
17. Isenring E, Elia M. Which screening method is appropriate for older cancer patients at risk for malnutrition? Nutrition 2015;31(4):594–7.
18. Kim JM, Sung MK. The efficacy of oral nutritional intervention in malnourished cancer patients: a systemic review. Clin Nutr Res 2016;5(4):219–36.

19. Barber MD. Cancer cachexia and its treatment with fish-oil-enriched nutritional supplementation. Nutrition 2001;17:751–5.

20. de Luis DA, Izaola O, Aller R, et al. A randomized clinical trial with two omega 3 fatty acid enhanced oral supplements in head and neck cancer ambulatory patients. Eur Rev Med Pharmacol Sci 2008;12:177–81.

21. Mantovani G, Maccio A, Madeddu C, et al. A phase II study with antioxidants, both in the diet and supplemented, pharmaconutritional support, progestagen, and anti-cyclooxygenase-2 showing efficacy and safety in patients with cancer-related anorexia/cachexia and oxidative stress. Cancer Epidemiol Biomarkers Prev 2006;15:1030–4.

22. Murphy RA, Mourtzakis M, Chu QS, et al. Supplementation with fish oil increases first-line chemotherapy efficacy in patients with advanced nonsmall cell lung cancer. Cancer 2011;117:3774–80.

23. Weed HG, Ferguson ML, Gaff RL, et al. Lean body mass gain in patients with head and neck squamous cell cancer treated perioperatively with a protein- and energy-dense nutritional supplement containing eicosapentaenoic acid. Head Neck 2011;33:1027–33.

24. Fearon KC, Barber MD, Moses AG, et al. Double-blind, placebo-controlled, randomized study of eicosapentaenoic acid diester in patients with cancer cachexia. J Clin Oncol 2006;24:3401–7.

25. Moses AW, Slater C, Preston T, et al. Reduced total energy expenditure and physical activity in cachectic patients with pancreatic cancer can be modulated by an energy and protein dense oral supplement enriched with n-3 fatty acids. Br J Cancer 2004;90:996–1002.

26. Ryan AM, Reynolds JV, Healy L, et al. Enteral nutrition enriched with eicosapentaenoic acid (EPA) preserves lean body mass following esophageal cancer surgery: results of a double-blinded randomized controlled trial. Ann Surg 2009;249: 355–63.

27. Liu J, Xu M, Zhao Y, et al. n-3 polyunsaturated fatty acids abrogate mTORC1/2 signaling and inhibit adrenocortical carcinoma growth in vitro and in vivo. Oncol Rep 2016;35(6):3514–22.

28. Lim K, Han C, Dai Y, et al. Omega-3 polyunsaturated fatty acids inhibit hepatocellular carcinoma cell growth through blocking beta-catenin and cyclooxygenase-2. Mol Cancer Ther 2009;8(11):3046–55.

29. Yu J, Liu L, Zhang Y, et al. Effects of omega-3 fatty acids on patients undergoing surgery for gastrointestinal malignancy: a systematic review and meta-analysis. BMC Cancer 2017;17(1):271–80.

30. Macpherson H, Pipingas A, Pase MP. Multivitamin-multimineral supplementation and mortality: a meta-analysis of randomized controlled trials. Am J Clin Nutr 2013;97(2):437–44.

31. Velicer CM, Ulrich CM. Vitamin and mineral supplement use among US adults after cancer diagnosis: a systematic review. J Clin Oncol 2008;26(4):665–73.

32. Dąbrowska AM, Słotwiński R. The immune response to surgery and infection. Cent Eur J Immunol 2014;39(4):532–7.

33. McLeod RS, Aarts MA, Chung F, et al. Development of an enhanced recovery after surgery guideline and implementation strategy based on the knowledge-to-action cycle. Ann Surg 2015;262(6):1016–25.

34. Kehlet H, Wilmore DW. Evidence-based surgical care and the evolution of fast-track surgery. Ann Surg 2008;248(2):189–98.

35. Aguilar-Nascimento JE, Salomão AB, Caporossi C, et al. Clinical benefits after the implementation of a multimodal perioperative protocol in elderly patients. Arq Gastroenterol 2010;47(2):178–83.
36. Nikniaz Z, Somi MH, Nagashi S, et al. Impact of early enteral nutrition on nutritional and immunological outcomes of gastric cancer patients undergoing gastrostomy: a systematic review and meta-analysis. Nutr Cancer 2017;1:1–9.
37. Weimann A, Braga M, Carli F, et al. ESPEN guideline: clinical nutrition in surgery. Clin Nutr 2017;36:623–50.
38. Jensen GL, Mirtallo J, Compher C, et al, International Consensus Guideline Committee. Adult starvation and disease-related malnutrition: a proposal for etiology-based diagnosis in the clinical practice setting from the International Consensus Guideline Committee. Clin Nutr 2010;29(2):151–3.
39. McClave SA, Taylor BE, Martindale RG, et al, Society of Critical Care Medicine, American Society for Parenteral and Enteral Nutrition. Guidelines for the provision and assessment of nutrition support therapy in the adult critically ill patient: Society of Critical Care Medicine (SCCM) and American Society for Parenteral and Enteral Nutrition (A.S.P.E.N.). JPEN J Parenter Enteral Nutr 2016;40(2):159–211.
40. Verotti CC, Torrinhas RS, Cecconello I, et al. Selection of top 10 quality indicators for nutrition therapy. Nutr Clin Pract 2012;27(2):261–7.
41. Mariette C. Immunonutrition. J Visc Surg 2015;152:14–7.
42. Zheng Y, Li F, Qi B, et al. Application of perioperative immunonutrition for gastrointestinal surgery: a meta-analysis of randomized controlled trials. Asia Pac J Clin Nutr 2007;16(Suppl 1):253–7.
43. Marik PE, Zaloga GP. Immunonutrition in high-risk surgical patients: a systematic review and analysis of the literature. JPEN J Parenter Enteral Nutr 2010;34(4):378–86.
44. Cerantola Y, Hübner M, Grass F, et al. Immunonutrition in gastrointestinal surgery. Br J Surg 2011;98(1):37–48.
45. Drover JW, Dhaliwal R, Weitzel L, et al. Perioperative use of arginine-supplemented diets: a systematic review of the evidence. J Am Coll Surg 2011;212(3):385–99.
46. Zhang Y, Gu Y, Guo T, et al. Perioperative immunonutrition for gastrointestinal cancer: a systematic review of randomized controlled trials. Surg Oncol 2012; 21(2):e87–95.
47. Marimuthu K, Varadhan KK, Ljungqvist O, et al. A meta-analysis of the effect of combinations of immune modulating nutrients on outcome in patients undergoing major open gastrointestinal surgery. Ann Surg 2012;255(6):1060–8.
48. Osland E, Hossain MB, Khan S, et al. Effect of timing of pharmaconutrition (immunonutrition) administration on outcomes of elective surgery for gastrointestinal malignancies: a systematic review and meta-analysis. JPEN J Parenter Enteral Nutr 2014;38(1):53–69.
49. Haun MW, Estel S, Rücker G, et al. Early palliative care for adults with advanced cancer. Cochrane Database Syst Rev 2017;12(6):111–29.
50. August DA, Huhmann MB, American Society for Parenteral and Enteral Nutrition (A.S.P.E.N.) Board of Directors. A.S.P.E.N. clinical guidelines: nutrition support therapy during adult anticancer treatment and in hematopoietic cell transplantation. JPEN J Parenter Enteral Nutr 2009;33(5):472–500.

Nutritional Considerations in Liver Disease

Asim Shuja, MD*, Miguel Malespin, MD, James Scolapio, MD

KEYWORDS

- Malnutrition • Liver disease • Transplantation

KEY POINTS

- Nutrition is very important in liver disease.
- When it comes to the pathophysiology of malnutrition in liver diseases, malnutrition is multifactorial.
- Cirrhotic patients should avoid fasting for long periods of time.
- Liver transplantation is the only true "cure" of malnutrition in patients with end-stage liver disease.

Malnutrition occurs in up to 80% of patients with cirrhosis and is associated with higher rates of morbidity and mortality.[1] It is often underrecognized and undertreated despite improved outcomes with appropriate management. In this review, the authors discuss the pathophysiology of malnutrition and methods to optimize nutrition status in liver disease and include a brief section on perioperative and postoperative nutrition.

PATHOPHYSIOLOGY OF MALNUTRITION IN LIVER DISEASE

Malnutrition in chronic liver disease (CLD) is multifactorial (**Box 1**).

Decreased Intake of Nutrients

Anorexia and early satiety are well-known causes of decreased nutrient intake in patients with CLD. Anorexia could be explained by the fact that cirrhotic patients tend to have elevated circulating levels of certain proinflammatory cytokines, with known anorexic properties, for example, tumor necrosis factor-α, interleukin (IL)-1B, IL-6, and Leptin.[2–7] Similarly, alcohol-induced anorexia is another important reason for diminished nutrient intake in patients with alcoholic liver disease (ALD). Certain conditions, like esophagitis, gastritis, and pancreatitis, can further contribute to poor dietary

Disclosure: The authors have nothing to disclose.
Division of Gastroenterology and Hepatology, University of Florida College of Medicine, 4555 Emerson Street, Suite 300, Jacksonville, FL 32207, USA
* Corresponding author.
E-mail address: asim.shuja@jax.ufl.edu

Gastroenterol Clin N Am 47 (2018) 243–252
https://doi.org/10.1016/j.gtc.2017.09.010

Box 1
Factors associated with malnutrition in patients with chronic liver disease

Factors

Anorexia

Ascites

Altered taste perception

Metabolic and inflammatory derangements

Inadequate diet restrictions

Decreased social status

Polypharmacy

Multiple paracentesis

Variceal bleeding

Long fasting periods for laboratory tests and diagnostic procedures

---

intake.[8] Anorexia can also lead to zinc deficiency and hyperglycemia, whereas iatrogenic factors also contribute to poor oral intake. For example, most patients with CLD are advised to consume a low-salt diet in an effort to avoid fluid retention.[9] Consequently, this modified diet is generally unpalatable, leading to a decrease in caloric intake.[9] Many studies recommend against protein restriction given the higher degree of sarcopenia in these patients; however, many providers do not follow those recommendations, which further leads to malnutrition.[10] Furthermore, patients with decompensated liver disease suffer from complications that are generally associated with increased readmissions rates and are frequently kept nil per oral pending examinations and procedures.[8]

Early satiety can occur as a result of impaired gastric accommodation of the stomach likely because of the presence of ascites.[2,11,12] Studies have shown that these patients are also at high risk for the development of functional dyspepsia, secondary to autonomic neuropathy, further causing nausea and early satiety.[5,13]

Decreased Digestion and Absorption of Nutrients

Intestinal digestion and absorption can be impaired by portal hypertension because of congestion by intestinal mucosa.[13] Similarly, patients with cholestatic liver diseases (eg, primary biliary cirrhosis, primary sclerosing cholangitis) have decreased intraluminal bile salt concentration, which leads to fat malabsorption and deficiency of fat-soluble vitamins, such as vitamin A, D, E, and K.[14] Fat malabsorption is also common in patients with ALD, especially with concomitant pancreatic damage. Alcohol itself causes direct toxicity to small intestinal mucosa and brush border enzymes, leading to increased mucosal permeability, impaired salt and water absorption, and rapid intestinal transit.[14,15]

Altered Metabolism

Altered protein metabolism is the most significant metabolic disturbance in patients with CLD. These patients primarily are hypoalbuminemic as a result of decreased hepatic functional capacity and increased amino acid demands.[16] Cirrhotic patients also have diminished hepatic glycogen reserves due to impaired synthetic capacity of hepatocytes.[15] To compensate for this unavailable source of glucose, there is a higher rate of gluconeogenesis, causing mobilization of amino acids from skeletal muscles of the body, further precipitating amino acid shortage.[17] It addition to accelerated gluconeogenesis and protein catabolism, there is increased lipid peroxidation leading to loss of subcutaneous fat and muscle wasting. It is therefore recommended that these patients should avoid prolonged fasting periods and consume small frequent meals.[18–20] There are data suggesting the benefit of a nighttime carbohydrate snack.[9] The daily recommended protein intake for patients with cirrhosis is 1.2 g/kg/d to maintain nitrogen balance compared with 0.5 g/kg/d required for healthy individuals.[15,16] There is a popular misconception to place advanced liver disease patients on a protein-restricted diet given concerns for exacerbation of hepatic encephalopathy. This practice should be discouraged if any improvement in lean tissue mass is to be achieved.[21] Patton and Aranda-Michel[16] recommend that even when patients are hospitalized for management of hepatic encephalopathy, they should be managed with traditional medications (Lactulose, Rifaximin, Neomycin, and so forth) before placing them on protein restriction because the benefit is only minimal.

It has also been described that patients with CLD may have an impaired synthesis of polyunsaturated fatty acids, with increasing levels of n-6 and n-9 and decreases in n-3 fatty acids in adipose tissue.[22]

Nutrient Losses

Malnutrition in liver patients also occurs secondary to gastrointestinal bleeding and protein-losing enteropathy.[23] Similarly, iatrogenic interventions, such as the use of diuretics, lactulose, and frequent paracentesis, can lead to protein deficiency as well.[24] Renal losses of micronutrients, such as thiamine, also occur.[15]

Hypermetabolic State

Disturbances in metabolic rate are common in patients with CLD. Muller and his colleagues[25] performed the largest study to date, including 473 patients with cirrhosis, and found that 34% of them were hypermetabolic (based on elevated resting energy expenditure [REE]) on indirect calorimetry.[25,26] Hypermetabolism is also associated with poor survival in orthotopic liver transplant (OLT) patients.[27] The literature has demonstrated conflicting results regarding the exact cause of elevated REE in patients with cirrhosis. Logical causes of elevated REE include the presence of ascites, overt infections, or systemic inflammatory response syndrome.[28] The fact that hypermetabolism can persist even after liver transplantation suggests that extrahepatic factors may also contribute to this phenomenon.

METHODS TO MAXIMIZE NUTRITIONAL STATUS
Vitamins and Minerals

Most patients with liver disease have derangements in electrolytes balance and vitamin deficiencies. These micronutrients are important for metabolic utilization of macronutrients, such as protein, carbohydrate, and fat. Patients with cirrhosis of any origin, especially those with cholestatic liver disease, are at high risk of developing fat-soluble vitamin deficiencies. Almost 55% of patients undergoing OLT are found to have osteopenia/osteoporosis in the setting of vitamin D deficiency, putting them at higher risk for bone fractures. Patients with osteopenia and risk factors, such as smoking, obesity, older age, and history of prior fractures, are advised to take 1200 to 1500 mg of calcium and 400 to 800 IU of vitamin D. The addition of bisphosphonates is recommended in individuals with osteoporosis.[29] Despite the potential for its use, the role of RANKL antibody has not been studied well in patients with CLD. DEXA scan should be performed in patients considered for OLT to screen for osteoporosis.[16]

Similarly, vitamin A deficiency, which can cause night blindness, has been reported in 73% in patients evaluated for OLT (**Table 1**).[16]

Supplementation of vitamin K is recommended in patients at higher risk of bleeding, for example, those with elevated international normalized ratio, with esophageal varices, or before surgical intervention. In those cases, parenteral dose of 10 mg of vitamin K every 4 weeks is recommended.[29]

Patients with ALD are particularly prone to deficiency of zinc, vitamin C, thiamine, and folate. Therefore, all patients should receive balanced multivitamin and mineral preparation to avoid deficiency of the mentioned elements and vitamins. Patients with cirrhosis are generally in a state of hyperaldosteronism, which can lead to severe sodium and water retention. Therefore, a diet low in sodium, that is, less than 2 to 3 g/d, is advised in the presence of ascites and/or peripheral edema. Even though a low-sodium diet can make the food unpalatable, a fine balance should be maintained to avoid both inadequate nutrient intake and worsening fluid retention. Monitoring of electrolytes, such as magnesium and phosphorus, is very important, especially in patients with ALD and those at risk for refeeding syndrome.[8]

Energy and Protein Intakes

Protein energy malnutrition (PEM) is commonly seen in patients with CLD. There is ample evidence to suggest that PEM is an independent risk factor for both morbidity and mortality in patients with ESLD.[10] It is very vital to recognize malnutrition in these patients and manage it as early as possible.[16] Therefore, the primary goal for these patients should be to maintain their weight and sustain a balanced diet rich in macronutrients and micronutrients. Ideally, a diet with an energy intake of 35 to 40 kcal/kg and a protein intake of 1.2 to

Table 1	
Clinical examination for micronutrient deficiencies in alcoholic liver disease patients	
Vitamins	**Clinical Findings**
A (retinol)	Night blindness, increased fibrosis
E	Skin changes
D	Osteopenia and osteoporosis
B_1 (thiamine)	Wernicke encephalopathy, neuropathy, beriberi with high-output heart failure
B_3 (niacin)	Pellagra (dementia, diarrhea, and dermatitis)
B_6 (pyridoxine)	Neuropathy, sideroblastic anemia, elevated AST/ALT ratio
B_9 (folate)	Megaloblastic anemia
B12 (cyanocobalamin)	Megaloblastic anemia, subacute combined degeneration, neuropathy
C (ascorbic acid)	Scurvy
Minerals	**Clinical Findings**
Iron	Anemia
Calcium	Osteopenia and osteoporosis
Magnesium	Cardiomyopathy
Phosphorous	Cardiac arrhythmias, delirium tremens
Selenium	Cardiomyopathy
Zinc	Ageusia and skin changes

Adapted from Chao A, Waitzberg D, de Jesus RP, et al. Malnutrition and nutritional support in alcoholic liver disease: a review. Curr Gastroenterol Rep 2016;18(12):65; with permission.

1.5 g/kg is recommended.[2,9,24] This diet will not only maximize positive nitrogen balance but also preserve lean mass as well. In most patients with compensated cirrhosis, normal everyday diet is recommended without any special additions or restrictions. However, patients with decompensated cirrhosis may require supplementary meals like bedtime snacks and other caloric supplements.[30]

Early observations revealed that episodes of overt hepatic encephalopathy in patients with cirrhosis could be controlled by reducing the protein intake.[31] As previously noted, most recent studies actually suggest that low-protein diets have little or no effect on encephalopathy and may actually harm through worsening nutritional status.[10,32]

The American College of Gastroenterology Practice Guidelines on hepatic encephalopathy recommend that, for patients with cirrhosis and acute encephalopathy, protein intake should be started at 0.5 g/kg/d with subsequent progressive increase to 1.0 to 1.5 g/kg/d, depending on patient tolerance.[32]

In patients with advanced CLD, branched-chain amino acids (BCAA) supplement concentrations are low, whereas the concentrations of aromatic amino acids, such as phenylalanine and tyrosine, are high, conditions that may be closely associated with hepatic encephalopathy and the prognosis of these patients. Based on these basic observations, patients with advanced CLD have been treated clinically with BCAA-rich medicines, with positive effects. Randomized controlled trials have suggested that oral BCAA supplements can help achieve or maintain positive nitrogen balance in patients who are intolerant to dietary protein.[9,33,34] These supplements have been associated with decreased frequency and severity of hepatic encephalopathy when used as maintenance therapy. However, studies did not show any effects on mortality or quality of life.[35]

It is suggested that diets rich in vegetable and dairy protein may be beneficial, and they are recommended.[32] A recent consensus statement from the International Society for Hepatic Encephalopathy and Nitrogen Metabolism recommends that the patients with recurrent or persistent hepatic encephalopathy should consume a diet low in animal protein and rich in vegetable protein, because fewer aromatic amino acids are produced from vegetable sources.[31]

Carbohydrates and Fat

Patients with cirrhosis are at increased risk of hypoglycemia because of ineffective gluconeogenesis and diminished glycogen stores. Therefore, these patients should be advised to avoid fasting for longer than 3 to 6 hours and should be encouraged to take small, frequent meals distributed throughout the day.[9,16,32]

Similarly, fat intake should not be restricted unless there is evidence of malabsorption, in which case medium chain triglycerides (MCTs) are recommended.[36] MCTs should be taken with food to avoid common side effects, such as nausea and diarrhea, associated with it. A deficiency of essential fatty acids (EFA) has been described in CLD, which correlates with the degree of malnutrition and severity of liver disease, and thus EFA should be provided to these patients.[37,38]

Role of Parenteral Nutrition and Tube Feeds

Physicians should encourage oral intake as much as possible in patients with CLD; however, as discussed, anorexia is one of the major limitations to good oral intake.[39] In severely ill patients, supplemental enteral nutrition is advisable. Patients who cannot meet their caloric requirements through oral intake despite individual support are candidates for enteral nutrition. Tube feedings even in the presence of esophageal varices should not be delayed.[8,40–42]

BCAA-enriched formulas are used in patients with hepatic encephalopathy arising during enteral nutrition.[2] A soft small-bore feeding tube (8–10 French) is usually well tolerated for a short period of time, that is, less than 4 to 8 weeks. Use of a gastrostomy tube should be avoided given higher risk of leakage and peritonitis in cirrhotics with ascites.[43] One option that is more acceptable to the patient is to cycle tube feeds at night and allow a regular diet during the day.[16]

The use of parenteral nutrition (PN) should be limited because of the increased risk of catheter-related infection.[44] It should be reserved only for special circumstances, such as those who are unable to tolerate oral as well as enteral feeding, or in conditions such as bowel obstruction or ileus.[16] If PN is given to the patient with cholestatic liver disease (ie, elevated bilirubin), copper (hepatotoxic) and manganese (neurotoxic) should not be given because they are excreted via hepatic circulation.[45]

PERIOPERATIVE AND POSTOPERATIVE NUTRITION

Liver transplantation is the only true "cure" of malnutrition. Without a healthy liver, the body cannot process the raw material (protein) to restore muscle mass and health. Within 6 months of transplantation, malnutrition is corrected and muscle mass is restored despite intake of the same amount of calories and protein as pre-OLT.

Perioperative and postoperative nutrition recommendations are similar to those for other postoperative situations. It is very important to minimize interruptions of nutritional intake before and after the liver transplant surgery. The role of a professional dietitian is very vital in this regard. Post–liver transplant patients also have increased energy requirements after the surgery. Studies have shown that in the immediate postoperative phase, protein catabolism is markedly increased, and it is recommended that patients should receive about 1.5 to 2.0 g/kg of protein per day.[9] Similarly, because of the routine use of diuretics and surgical drains and the risk of refeeding syndrome, electrolytes such as serum potassium, magnesium, and phosphorus levels should be closely monitored.[46] Early postoperative diet or enteral nutrition (12 hour) after liver transplant is advisable as long as the patient can tolerate it.[47]

After liver transplant, patients need immunosuppressive medications lifelong. Most common immunosuppressive agents include tacrolimus, cyclosporine, and corticosteroids. These medications can have multiple side effects, the most common being glucose intolerance or new onset diabetes, and[48,49] can be managed with a diabetic diet; oral hypoglycemic agents and in some cases insulin regimen are required especially in the immediate postoperative period when patients are started on steroids. Similarly, the hyperglycemic potential of immunosuppressive medications such as tacrolimus may be lowered by reduction in dose.[9]

Hyperkalemia can be present in many patients because of the nephrotoxic effect of these medications. Hyperkalemia is more common in early posttransplant periods and resolves later on.[50] Hypomagnesemia is another electrolyte abnormality that can be seen. Thus, the intake of magnesium-rich foods, such as dark cocoa, whole grains, and green vegetables, should be encouraged.[9]

Although it is very important to recover the nutritional status (because the patients lose an average of 9kg during the course of liver disease) after transplant, unfortunately some patients have uncontrolled weight gain in subsequent years, leading to increased prevalence of obesity.[9] Studies have shown that there is a net gain of fat mass over muscle mass by the end of the first postoperative year, which leads to an increased risk of metabolic syndrome as well as morbidity and mortality.[51–53] Therefore, patients should be encouraged to avoid excessive weight gain and its consequences after liver transplantation.[52,54] These derangements may be prevented by adequate nutritional counseling and intervention, when necessary (Table 2).

Table 2
Guidelines for nutrition therapy in chronic liver disease

Chronic Liver Disease	Protein (g/kg/d)	Energy (kcal/kg/d)	Total Energy Intake		Goals
			% Carbohydrates	% Lipids	
Steatohepatitis alcoholic	1.2–1.5	25–30	50–65	25–30[a]	Prevent or treat malnutrition or obesity associated; promote regeneration
ALD[b]	1.2–1.5[b]	35–40[b]	55–65	30–35[a]	Prevent or treat ALD
Compensated cirrhosis	1.2–1.5	35–40	55–70	25–30[a]	Prevent malnutrition; promote regeneration
Compensated cirrhosis by					
PEM	1.5–1.8	35–50	72	28	Treat malnutrition
Cholestasis	1.0–1.5	30–40	73–80	20–27	Treat malabsorption
Hepatic encephalopathy (HE)					
Grade 1 or 2	1.2–1.6 80% of vegetable protein + dairy	25–40 —	60–75 —	25–30 —	Meet nutritional needs without precipitating HE
Grade 3 or 4	0.6 + 0.25 BCAA	25–40	60–75	25–30	
Specific conditions clinics:					
Liver transplantation					
Pretransplant	1.2–1.75	35–40	70–80	20–30	Restore or maintain Nutritional status
Posttransplant	1.2–1.5	30–35	>70	≤30	

Recommendations from American Association for the Study of Liver Diseases.
[a] Preference for polyunsaturated fatty acids.
[b] Recommendations from American Association for the Study of Liver Diseases.
Adapted from Chao A, Waitzberg D, de Jesus RP, et al. Malnutrition and nutritional support in alcoholic liver disease: a review. Curr Gastroenterol Rep 2016;18(12):65; with permission.

REFERENCES

1. Kalaitzakis E, Simren M, Olsson R, et al. Gastrointestinal symptoms in patients with liver cirrhosis: associations with nutritional status and health-related quality of life. Scand J Gastroenterol 2006;41(12):1464–72.
2. Plauth M, Schutz ET. Cachexia in liver cirrhosis. Int J Cardiol 2002;85(1):83–7.
3. Richardson RA, Davidson HI, Hinds A, et al. Influence of the metabolic sequelae of liver cirrhosis on nutritional intake. Am J Clin Nutr 1999;69(2):331–7.
4. McCullough AJ, Bugianesi E, Marchesini G, et al. Gender-dependent alterations in serum leptin in alcoholic cirrhosis. Gastroenterology 1998;115(4):947–53.
5. Hammad A, Kaido T, Uemoto S. Perioperative nutritional therapy in liver transplantation. Surg Today 2015;45(3):271–83.
6. Ferreira LG, Ferreira Martins AI, Cunha CE, et al. Negative energy balance secondary to inadequate dietary intake of patients on the waiting list for liver transplantation. Nutrition 2013;29(10):1252–8.
7. Madden AM, Bradbury W, Morgan MY. Taste perception in cirrhosis: its relationship to circulating micronutrients and food preferences. Hepatology 1997;26(1):40–8.
8. Tsiaousi ET, Hatzitolios AI, Trygonis SK, et al. Malnutrition in end stage liver disease: recommendations and nutritional support. J Gastroenterol Hepatol 2008;23(4):527–33.
9. Anastacio LR, Davisson Correia MI. Nutrition therapy: integral part of liver transplant care. World J Gastroenterol 2016;22(4):1513–22.
10. Ney M, Abraldes JG, Ma M, et al. Insufficient protein intake is associated with increased mortality in 630 patients with cirrhosis awaiting liver transplantation. Nutr Clin Pract 2015;30(4):530–6.
11. Izbeki F, Kiss I, Wittmann T, et al. Impaired accommodation of proximal stomach in patients with alcoholic liver cirrhosis. Scand J Gastroenterol 2002;37(12):1403–10.
12. Aqel BA, Scolapio JS, Dickson RC, et al. Contribution of ascites to impaired gastric function and nutritional intake in patients with cirrhosis and ascites. Clin Gastroenterol Hepatol 2005;3(11):1095–100.
13. Thuluvath PJ, Triger DR. Autonomic neuropathy and chronic liver disease. Q J Med 1989;72(268):737–47.
14. Taylor RM, Bjarnason I, Cheeseman P, et al. Intestinal permeability and absorptive capacity in children with portal hypertension. Scand J Gastroenterol 2002;37(7):807–11.
15. Saunders J, Brian A, Wright M, et al. Malnutrition and nutrition support in patients with liver disease. Frontline Gastroenterol 2010;1:105–11.
16. Patton KM, Aranda-Michel J. Nutritional aspects in liver disease and liver transplantation. Nutr Clin Pract 2002;17(6):332–40.
17. Reeds PJ, Fjeld CR, Jahoor F. Do the differences between the amino acid compositions of acute-phase and muscle proteins have a bearing on nitrogen loss in traumatic states? J Nutr 1994;124(6):906–10.
18. McCullough AJ, Tavill AS. Disordered energy and protein metabolism in liver disease. Semin Liver Dis 1991;11(4):265–77.
19. Owen OE, Reichle FA, Mozzoli MA, et al. Hepatic, gut, and renal substrate flux rates in patients with hepatic cirrhosis. J Clin Invest 1981;68(1):240–52.
20. Owen OE, Trapp VE, Reichard GA Jr, et al. Nature and quantity of fuels consumed in patients with alcoholic cirrhosis. J Clin Invest 1983;72(5):1821–32.

21. Swart GR, van den Berg JW, van Vuure JK, et al. Minimum protein requirements in liver cirrhosis determined by nitrogen balance measurements at three levels of protein intake. Clin Nutr 1989;8(6):329–36.
22. Thomas EL, Taylor-Robinson SD, Barnard ML, et al. Changes in adipose tissue composition in malnourished patients before and after liver transplantation: a carbon-13 magnetic resonance spectroscopy and gas-liquid chromatography study. Hepatology 1997;25(1):178–83.
23. Stanley AJ, Gilmour HM, Ghosh S, et al. Transjugular intrahepatic portosystemic shunt as a treatment for protein-losing enteropathy caused by portal hypertension. Gastroenterology 1996;111(6):1679–82.
24. Kondrup J. Nutrition in end stage liver disease. Best Pract Res Clin Gastroenterol 2006;20(3):547–60.
25. Muller MJ, Bottcher J, Selberg O, et al. Hypermetabolism in clinically stable patients with liver cirrhosis. Am J Clin Nutr 1999;69(6):1194–201.
26. Scolapio JS, Bowen J, Stoner G, et al. Substrate oxidation in patients with cirrhosis: comparison with other nutritional markers. JPEN J Parenter Enteral Nutr 2000;24(3):150–3.
27. Michel H, Bories P, Aubin JP, et al. Treatment of acute hepatic encephalopathy in cirrhotics with a branched-chain amino acids enriched versus a conventional amino acids mixture. A controlled study of 70 patients. Liver 1985;5(5):282–9.
28. Nutritional status in cirrhosis. Italian multicentre cooperative project on nutrition in liver cirrhosis. J Hepatol 1994;21(3):317–25.
29. Gundling F, Teich N, Strebel HM, et al. Nutrition in liver cirrhosis. Med Klin (Munich) 2007;102(6):435–44.
30. Nakaya Y, Okita K, Suzuki K, et al. BCAA-enriched snack improves nutritional state of cirrhosis. Nutrition 2007;23(2):113–20.
31. Nguyen DL, Morgan T. Protein restriction in hepatic encephalopathy is appropriate for selected patients: a point of view. Hepatol Int 2014;8(2):447–51.
32. Amodio P, Bemeur C, Butterworth R, et al. The nutritional management of hepatic encephalopathy in patients with cirrhosis: International Society for Hepatic Encephalopathy and nitrogen metabolism consensus. Hepatology 2013;58(1): 325–36.
33. Fialla AD, Israelsen M, Hamberg O, et al. Nutritional therapy in cirrhosis or alcoholic hepatitis: a systematic review and meta-analysis. Liver Int 2015;35(9): 2072–8.
34. Metcalfe EL, Avenell A, Fraser A. Branched-chain amino acid supplementation in adults with cirrhosis and porto-systemic encephalopathy: systematic review. Clin Nutr 2014;33(6):958–65.
35. Gluud LL, Dam G, Les I, et al. Branched-chain amino acids for people with hepatic encephalopathy. Cochrane Database Syst Rev 2017;(5):CD001939.
36. Sanchez AJ, Aranda-Michel J. Nutrition for the liver transplant patient. Liver Transpl 2006;12(9):1310–6.
37. Cabre E, Abad-Lacruz A, Nunez MC, et al. The relationship of plasma polyunsaturated fatty acid deficiency with survival in advanced liver cirrhosis: multivariate analysis. Am J Gastroenterol 1993;88(5):718–22.
38. Cabre E, Nunez M, Gonzalez-Huix F, et al. Clinical and nutritional factors predictive of plasma lipid unsaturation deficiency in advanced liver cirrhosis: a logistic regression analysis. Am J Gastroenterol 1993;88(10):1738–43.
39. Chao A, Waitzberg D, de Jesus RP, et al. Malnutrition and nutritional support in alcoholic liver disease: a review. Curr Gastroenterol Rep 2016;18(12):65.

40. Cabre E, Gonzalez-Huix F, Abad-Lacruz A, et al. Effect of total enteral nutrition on the short-term outcome of severely malnourished cirrhotics. A randomized controlled trial. Gastroenterology 1990;98(3):715–20.
41. Kearns PJ, Young H, Garcia G, et al. Accelerated improvement of alcoholic liver disease with enteral nutrition. Gastroenterology 1992;102(1):200–5.
42. De Ledinghen V, Beau P, Mannant PR, et al. Early feeding or enteral nutrition in patients with cirrhosis after bleeding from esophageal varices? A randomized controlled study. Dig Dis Sci 1997;42(3):536–41.
43. Scolapio JS. Nutrition therapy in liver disease. Nutr Clin Pract 2002;17(6):331.
44. O'Connor A, Hanly AM, Francis E, et al. Catheter associated blood stream infections in patients receiving parenteral nutrition: a prospective study of 850 patients. J Clin Med Res 2013;5(1):18–21.
45. Abunnaja S, Cuviello A, Sanchez JA. Enteral and parenteral nutrition in the perioperative period: state of the art. Nutrients 2013;5(2):608–23.
46. Sugihara K, Yamanaka-Okumura H, Teramoto A, et al. Recovery of nutritional metabolism after liver transplantation. Nutrition 2015;31(1):105–10.
47. Montejo Gonzalez JC, Mesejo A, Bonet Saris A, Metabolism and Nutrition Working Group of the Spanish Society of Intensive Care Medicine and Coronary units. Guidelines for specialized nutritional and metabolic support in the critically-ill patient: update. consensus SEMICYUC-SENPE: liver failure and liver transplantation. Nutr Hosp 2011;26(Suppl 2):27–31.
48. Bodziak KA, Hricik DE. New-onset diabetes mellitus after solid organ transplantation. Transpl Int 2009;22(5):519–30.
49. Pham PT, Pham PC, Lipshutz GS, et al. New onset diabetes mellitus after solid organ transplantation. Endocrinol Metab Clin North Am 2007;36(4):873–90, vii.
50. Bethke PC, Jansky SH. The effects of boiling and leaching on the content of potassium and other minerals in potatoes. J Food Sci 2008;73(5):H80–5.
51. Tsien C, Garber A, Narayanan A, et al. Post-liver transplantation sarcopenia in cirrhosis: a prospective evaluation. J Gastroenterol Hepatol 2014;29(6):1250–7.
52. Giusto M, Lattanzi B, Di Gregorio V, et al. Changes in nutritional status after liver transplantation. World J Gastroenterol 2014;20(31):10682–90.
53. Ukleja A, Scolapio JS, McConnell JP, et al. Nutritional assessment of serum and hepatic vitamin A levels in patients with cirrhosis. JPEN J Parenter Enteral Nutr 2002;26(3):1848.
54. Garcia AM, Veneroso CE, Soares DD, et al. Effect of a physical exercise program on the functional capacity of liver transplant patients. Transplant Proc 2014;46(6):1807–8.

Printed and bound by CPI Group (UK) Ltd, Croydon, CR0 4YY

07/10/2024

01040504-0010